Essentials of
HEALTH CARE MARKETING

Second Edition

ERIC N. BERKOWITZ, PhD
Professor of Marketing
Isenberg School of Management
The University of Massachusetts

JONES AND BARTLETT PUBLISHERS
Sudbury, Massachusetts
BOSTON   TORONTO   LONDON   SINGAPORE

World Headquarters
Jones and Bartlett Publishers
40 Tall Pine Drive
Sudbury, MA 01776
978-443-5000
info@jbpub.com
www.jbpub.com

Jones and Bartlett Publishers
Canada
6339 Ormindale Way
Mississauga, Ontario, L5V 1J2
CANADA

Jones and Bartlett Publishers
International
Barb House, Barb Mews
London W6 7PA
UK

Jones and Bartlett's books and products are available through most bookstores and online booksellers. To contact Jones and Bartlett Publishers directly, call 800-832-0034, fax 978-443-8000, or visit our website at www.jbpub.com.

Substantial discounts on bulk quantities of Jones and Bartlett's publications are available to corporations, professional associations, and other qualified organizations. For details and specific discount information, contact the special sales department at Jones and Bartlett via the above contact information or send an email to specialsales@jbpub.com.

Library of Congress Cataloging-in-Publication Data
Berkowitz, Eric N.
    Essentials of health care marketing / Eric N. Berkowitz. — 2nd ed.
        p. cm.
    Includes bibliographical references and index.
    ISBN: 10-0-7637-8350-1
    ISBN: 13-978-0-7637-8350-1
    1. Medical care—Marketing.   I. Title.
    [DNLM: 1. Marketing of Health Services.   W 74.1 B513e 2006]
    RA410.56.B46 2006
    362.1068'8--dc22

                                                2005027417

6048

Production Credits
Publisher: Michael Brown
Manufacturing and Inventory Coordinator:
    Amy Bacus
Associate Editor: Kylah Goodfellow McNeill
Production Director: Amy Rose
Production Editor: Tracey Chapman
Associate Marketing Manager:
    Marissa Hederson

Manufacturing and Inventory Coordinator:
    Amy Bacus
Text Design: Anne Spencer
Composition: Publishers' Design and
    Production Services, Inc.
Cover Design: Tim Dziewit
Printing and Binding: Malloy, Inc.
Cover printing: Malloy, Inc.

Printed in the United States of America
10 09 08 07   10 9 8 7 6 5 4 3

Contents

PART II ■ Understanding the Consumer

Preface

Health care marketing is now recognized as a functional discipline to be utilized in the management of a health care organization. While not always practiced effectively, the perspective that marketing is more than advertising has gained greater recognition. Over the past 30 years since the term "marketing" first appeared in the health care management literature, the industry has gone through dramatic changes as a function of reimbursement in a move from cost-based payment systems to a capitated payment system to today's discounted fee-for-service approach. Now, as we move deeper into the 21st century, the system is undergoing another radical transformation, whereby a greater responsibility of the cost of care is being shifted back to consumers in what some are almost defining as a return to the days of true fee-for-service. In the months prior to this book going to press, one of the largest corporations in America, General Motors, reworked their agreements with the United Auto Workers union in terms of health care coverage to also shift more of its health care cost to retirees and employees. Many health care experts believe this will be another bellwether change for the industry. The implications being that an ever greater number of employees across all corporations will pay more for the care they receive. This change will have the greatest impact on marketing since the concept was first introduced into health care 30 years ago.

Now, as we begin to see the ultimate user, the consumer, pay for care and be sensitive to the price, health care services move closer to other industries. And, in this way, the marketing concepts as practiced in other industries also have ever greater relevance to the practice of health care providers. Relevant questions for health care organizations now become; What is the value being provided to the consumer? What customer does the organization want to go after? Once that customer is gained with their dollars spent in a high deductible plan, how can a relationship be built so that if appropriate care is needed again they will return to that particular provider (relationship marketing)? These are basic marketing issues faced in a slightly different way by hotels, computer manufacturers, and now health care providers.

Few industries are as dramatic in the pace of change as health care. Driven by technology, which can impact business in a moment, such as drug-coated stents, or pills that might reduce the need for screening colonoscopies, or reimbursement shifts that reduced length of stays for inpatient surgeries, health care in the United States today is now facing global competition from Asia and the Mideast. Possibly, the greatest impact on all providers and health care organizations is in the home of every potential patient and at the fingertips of every potential buyer of health care service—the Internet through their computer. This technology portal provides access to data on competitors, quality, and prices and can alter shopping behaviors in ways that may make strategy more complicated for any organization. Marketing will be more complicated and more essential to succeed.

In this book, the essentials of health care marketing are presented. The purpose of the book is to provide a thorough understanding of the principles and concepts as they apply to health care organizations. This book examines the essential elements of marketing in the hopes that readers will recognize the application of marketing tools and strategies in today's fast changing and dynamic health care environment. Few industries are more challenging within which to work.

Introduction

This book is divided into three main parts. Part I, "The Marketing Process," looks first at what marketing is, the nature of marketing strategy, and the environment in which marketing operates. Chapter 1 provides a perspective on the meaning of marketing, how marketing has evolved in health care, and the marketing planning process. Additionally, this chapter outlines how marketing health care is changing in light of restructuring that is occurring in this industry. Chapter 2 provides an overview of marketing strategy and an understanding of the strategic options available to a health care organization. It also presents a discussion of the importance of having a differential advantage for a health care organization as a component of marketing strategy. Chapter 3 focuses on the environment in which health care is formulated, and the impact of changes in the environment on marketing strategy for organizations whether these changes are technological, sociological, competitive, or regulatory.

At the core of marketing is the focus on the consumer which is covered in Part II, "Understanding the Consumer." In today's health care world that consumer may be the individual patient, or another organization such as a company buying health care for its employees, or an insurance company deciding whom they should contract with for care. Chapter 4 provides an overview of the consumer decision making process as it pertains to both consumers and organizations. In order to assess the consumer, marketing research is an important tool. Chapter 5 describes the marketing research process and the alternative methodologies used within marketing research. It is important to recognize that not all consumers or organizations make decisions the same way. Marketing strategies must often be tailored to groups of consumers or particular types of companies. This refinement of marketing strategy often occurs as a result of market segmentation, which is the focus of Chapter 6. Finally, it is important to recognize that in dealing with consumers or companies the key is to develop their loyalty, the focus of Chapter 7. This is the focus of a new chapter in this edition in which creating customer value and developing relationship marketing strategy is presented.

The last section of this book, Part III, is "The Marketing Mix." The Four Ps of product, price, place, and promotion form the basis around which all organizations develop their marketing plans and strategies. Chapter 8 reviews concepts and marketing strategies involved in the product or service being delivered. Chapter 9 discusses pricing objectives and strategies and how the role of positioning price is more important with the advent of medical savings accounts. In today's health care marketplace, the Internet is a new way to deliver service and takes its place within the discussion of distribution as presented in Chapter 10. Chapters 11, 12, and 13 involve the promotional element of the marketing mix. Understanding the communication process and the range of promotional elements is discussed in Chapter 11. Chapter 12 discusses the advertising components of marketing, while personal selling is presented in Chapter 13. Chapter 14, the final chapter, provides an overview of monitoring and controlling the marketing process. Measuring the outcome of marketing decisions is necessary in order to continue to refine effective marketing strategies.

■ Chapter Organization

Readers of this book will find that six sections appear in each chapter. These are: Learning Objectives, Conclusions, Key Terms, Chapter Summary, Chapter Problems, and Notes. All Key Terms appear with their definitions in the glossary and at the end of the book is an index for the reader's convenience.

Acknowledgments

As any author of a textbook knows, often one name is listed on the cover yet the development and actual outcome of the project are the result of the valuable input of many individuals. Over the past 30 years in which I have been interested in health care marketing, several individuals and organizations have contributed to my understanding and education in this field. At the risk of leaving some people unmentioned, I would like to express my thanks to two early colleagues at the University of Minnesota. First, William Flexner, now Emeritus Partner of Options Technologies, Inc. Bill and I first collaborated while Assistant Professors at the University of Minnesota. At that time, Bill was a research professor in the Center for Health Services Research at the University of Minnesota where he had a particular interest in applying marketing to health care and I was an assistant professor in the School of Management. Together, Bill and I published some of the first articles on health care marketing. At this time, I acknowledge my appreciation for the early role Bill played in introducing me to an exciting industry. A second colleague who also became a co-author is Steve Hillestad. Together Steve and I have written *Health Care Market Strategy: From Planning to Action*, now in its third edition with Jones and Bartlett (2004). Steve, in his early career, practiced marketing as the Vice President of Marketing at Fairview Health Care System in Minneapolis St. Paul and now is an active consultant and speaker in health care marketing and strategy.

Over the past 30 years in health care marketing there are many individuals with whom I have worked and collaborated who have impacted my thinking on marketing and health care strategy. At the risk of not mentioning all, let me name a few; Carla Windhorst who led the Alliance for Health Care Marketing and Strategy, Bill Gombeski, Priscilla Clarke, the late Trevor Fisk, the late Frank Weaver, Steve Gelineau, and from another discipline of health care finance, J.B. Silvers and Hugh Long in Health Care Finance. Most importantly, my closest colleague, Robert Kauer was a gifted teacher and a critical thinker. He helped shape my own thinking around the role of marketing and its impact on strategy was most shaped these past 15 years, prematurely deceased was a gifted teacher and a critical thinker.

I express my great appreciation to the American College of Physician Executives and its Executive Vice President, Roger Schenke. My conversations with Roger continually push my own thinking as to the transformation of health care and its impact on marketing. The American College of Physician Executives is the largest organization of physicians in management. Since 1978, I have had the opportunity to be a regular faculty presenter in the College's education programs. And, in 1985, I was made an honorary member of the College. As a faculty member, I realize that I have learned far more from my association with this organization than any knowledge I will ever be able to transmit to its membership. It is through this organization that I have had the opportunity to meet thousands of physicians that who have given me great insight and appreciation into the most valuable service provided to society.

In developing and preparing this book, several other individuals have been of great help. Foremost I want to acknowledge the staff in the Graduate Programs Office of the Isenberg School of Management who has had to work around me for the time I have spent in preparing the revision of this text. Cari Carpenter, the Executive Director of the MBA Programs, is the person to whom all faculty and staff go and who is the consummate professional. Also, I want to express my appreciation to a dedicated staff of professionals who make our office the excellent place it is in terms of customer service and builds the relationships with our constituencies in a way similar to what I discuss in some of the concepts in this text. In order of seniority in the office, Mary Beth Kimball, Keri Jane Crist, Charles Mutigwe, Amy Bergin, Nicole Tominsky, and DeDe Beach, all deserve my greatest appreciation. Several people at Jones and Bartlett have been helpful throughout this project: Mike Brown, Kylah Goodfellow McNeill, and Tracey Chapman, who collectively in different phases have all contributed to this revision.

Finally, I express my appreciation to my family, who most often had to endure directly the pressures that I felt in bringing this project to completion. While my daughters Anne and Julia have little desire to enter marketing, it is for them that I undertook this project. My best friend and partner of more than 30 years, my wife, fortunately again has tolerated my anxieties as another text is completed.

The Marketing Process

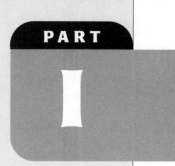

The Meaning of Marketing

Primary care satellites, integrated delivery systems, managed care plans, and physician–hospital organizations are but a few of the elements that dominate the structure of the health care industry today, as the government, employers, consumers, providers, and health care suppliers deal with a new health care market. This marketplace is typified by massive restructuring in the way health care organizations operate, health care is purchased, and care is delivered. Competing in this environment will require an effective marketing strategy to deal with these forces of change. This book will focus on the essentials for effective marketing and their implementation in this health care marketplace. This discussion begins with an examination of what marketing is and how it has evolved within health care since first being discussed as a relevant management function in 1976.

■ Marketing

For anyone involved in health care during the past 10 to 15 years, the term *marketing* generates little emotional reaction. Yet, health care marketing—a commonplace concept today—was considered novel and controversial when first introduced to the industry three decades ago. In 1975, Evanston Hospital, in Evanston, Illinois, was one of the first hospitals to establish a formal marketing staff position. Now, more than 30 years later, marketing has diffused throughout health care into hospitals, group practices, rehabilitation facilities, and other health care organizations. In this book, fundamental marketing concepts and marketing strategies are discussed. Although health care is undergoing significant structural change, the basic elements of marketing will be at the core of any organization's successful position in the marketplace.

The Meaning of Marketing

There are several views and definitions of marketing. The most widely accepted definition is that of the American Marketing Association, the professional organization for marketing practitioners and educators, which defines **marketing** as "the process of planning and executing the conception, pricing, promotion, and distribution of ideas, goods, and services to create exchanges that satisfy individual and organizational objectives."[1]

Central to this definition of marketing is the focus on the consumer, whether that is an individual patient, physician, or organization such as a company contracting for industrial medicine. This definition also contains the key ingredients of marketing that lead to consumer satisfaction. Increasingly in health care, customer satisfaction is the key issue.

The Joint Commission on Accreditation of Healthcare Organizations, the industry's major accrediting agency for operating standards of health care facilities, required—in its 1994 accreditation manual—that hospitals improve on nine measures of performance, one of which is patient satisfaction. This focus on patient satisfaction for hospital accreditation is an overt recognition of the need for health care facilities to be marketing oriented and, thus, customer responsive.

Prerequisites for Marketing

This book's definition of marketing includes several prerequisite conditions that must exist before marketing occurs. First, there must be two or more parties with unsatisfied needs. One party might be the consumer trying to fulfill certain needs; the second, a company seeking to exchange a service or product for economic gain. A second prerequisite for marketing is the desire or ability of one party to meet the needs of another. Third, parties must have something to exchange. For example, a physician has the clinical skills that will meet an individual patient's need to have a torn meniscus repaired. A consumer must have the health insurance or financial resources to exchange for the receipt of these medical services. Finally, there must be a means to communicate. In order to facilitate an exchange between two parties, each party must learn of the other's existence. It is this last aspect of health care that has formally evolved in recent years.

Until 1975, advertising and promotion really did not exist within health care. Communication to facilitate exchange occurred by word of mouth. One would consult with a physician, and that individual in turn recommended the physician to other consumers who would then seek out that particular physician. Prior to 1975, the American Medical Association (AMA) had within its codes of ethics a prohibition against advertising. That very year, the U.S. Supreme Court ruled that professional associations were subject to federal antitrust laws. The AMA revised its code of ethics to be less stringent regarding advertising. Further legal actions between the Federal Trade Commission (FTC) and the AMA had, by 1982, removed even those restrictions. The FTC believed the restriction on advertising deprived consumers of the free flow of information regarding health care alternatives and services. The FTC and the federal courts recognized the value of communication to consumers. Communication is a prerequisite for marketing. It is only in the last two decades that more formal means of communication have evolved within health care and that marketing strategies have become more visible.

Who Does Marketing?

Traditionally, only for-profit commercial businesses in consumer or industrial settings conducted marketing. In this text, they will be referred to as traditional businesses. Yet, the application of marketing broadened in the late 1960s.

In 1969, two marketing academics—Philip Kotler and Sidney Levy—at Northwestern University in Illinois published an article about broadening the concept of marketing. Their writing was the first attempt to recognize that for-profit and nonprofit businesses engaged in marketing activities. They recognized that marketing activities occurred in both service and product businesses. At the core of these organizations' activities was the notion of "exchange."[2]

Viewing the concept of exchange as the core of marketing allowed people to consider other areas where marketing might also be useful. Fine arts centers and museums, hospitals, and school districts began to see the relevance of marketing strategies and tactics to their settings. A consumer exchanges time and money for the pleasure of seeing a display of fine art. A patient pays for medical services provided by a free-standing diagnostic clinic, while a school district provides education in exchange for public support through tax levies.

The scope and nature of who markets has broadened considerably. Marketing is conducted by individuals and organizations. Marketing is relevant to for-profit and nonprofit entities. Throughout this book, examples of marketing programs at businesses such as General Motors (GM) or Johnson & Johnson will be discussed, along with the marketing programs of health care providers such as the Geisinger Health System in Danville,

Pennsylvania, or the Mayo Clinic in Rochester, Minnesota. While there are distinct aspects within any industry that require the modification of marketing principles to fit particular needs, the core of marketing and the marketing mix is relevant for almost every organization.

■ The Elements of Successful Marketing

Marketing Research

Within the definition of marketing is the discussion of a process of planning and executing to meet consumer needs. Marketing requires an understanding of consumer wants and needs. This understanding is derived through an assessment of these needs. Within this book, Chapter 5 focuses on marketing research. **Marketing research** is a process in which there is a systematic gathering of data from customers to identify their needs.

The Four Ps

The heart of marketing strategy is the development of a response to the marketplace. As noted in the definition, marketing is the "execution of the conception, pricing, promotion, and distribution of the goods, ideas, and services." To respond to customers, an organization must develop a product, determine the price customers are willing to pay, identify what place is most convenient for customers to purchase the product or access the service, and finally, promote the product to customers to let them know it is available.

Product, price, place, and promotion are referred to as the **four Ps** of marketing strategy.[3] It is these four controllable variables that a firm uses to define its marketing strategy. The mix of these four controllable variables that a business uses to pursue a desired level of sales is referred to as the **marketing mix**. The definitions of the four major elements of marketing as discussed below provide the focus of this book.

Product

Product represents goods, services, or ideas offered by a firm. In this text, the term "product" also will be used interchangeably with health care services and ideas. In health care, the nature of the product has changed dramatically. Thirty years ago, one could define the product simply as a medical procedure or as an orthotic device to correct a physical disability. In today's climate, the discussion of the health care product includes not only these traditional products, but also products and services such as health insurance plans offered by managed care organizations (MCOs), or a group purchasing contract such as that offered by Premier, Inc., an alliance of independent hospitals in 50 states.

Price

Price focuses on what customers are willing to pay for a service. What price represents is addressed in the definition of marketing in terms of exchanges. A company provides a service and customers exchange dollars for receipt of a service that satisfies their needs. An employee paying an annual premium to an MCO or an insurance company reimbursing a physician's fee are both exchanges involving some determined price.

As will be discussed in Chapter 9, the issue of pricing for health care services has become a major concern of marketing strategy as the health care environment changes. Several factors are contributing to the greater role that the pricing variable is playing in developing marketing strategy. Corporations are directly feeling the costs of health care. In 2005, GM, one of the largest corporations in America, indicated that a major source of its financial problems financially was the cost of health care and union contractual obligations. In 2003, GM's health care expenditures were $800 million dollars and were forecasted to rise to $5.6 billion in 2005.[4] More employers, like Chrysler, are requiring that employees pay a greater percentage of their health care insurance premiums. In 2005, Chrysler amended its United Auto Workers contract in negotiations with the union such that annual health care deductibles rose from $100 to $1000. Many insurance companies also now require consumers to make a co-payment for medical services, whereas in the past, insurance companies paid the full medical bill. As mentioned earlier, companies that historically have paid the full premium for health care costs have become concerned about the price of medical services. These employers are now looking for ways to become more efficient buyers of health care coverage.

Finally, within the health care system itself, new approaches are being considered to control costs and reduce prices in the long run. The most interesting experiment being undertaken currently is the pay-for-performance model being attempted by Medicare. Marshfield Clinic in Marshfield, Wisconsin, is one of the medical groups participating in this three-year pilot program in which the organization will receive a bonus based on achieving a higher health status for the patients.[5] For marketers, the issue of price involves understanding what level of dollars a customer is willing to exchange for the receipt of some want-satisfying services or products. In the current health care climate, determining the value of these services—represented by the price—is the major challenge facing health care organizations.

Place

Place represents the manner in which goods or services are distributed by a firm for use by consumers. Place might include decisions regarding the location or the hours a medical service can be accessed. Chapter 10 reviews the marketing considerations for place that have assumed greater importance in today's managed care environment.

Increasingly, as more health care organizations establish managed care plans to enroll consumers in an insurance option that provides for all their health care needs, the place variable assumes a more critical role. Companies offering prepaid health care plans must consider location and primary care access for potential enrollees. While 40, 20, or even 10 years ago, a physician would establish an office in a location convenient for the physician, today the consumer dictates this variable element of the marketing mix. However, in the digital and wireless age, the entire definition of *place* in terms of patient/provider interaction may also shift.

Promotion

The final P represents promotion. For many people this has historically meant advertising, and advertising has meant marketing. Yet, as can be seen in the definition, promotion is just one part of marketing; promotion alone is not marketing. **Promotion** represents any way of informing the marketplace that the organization has developed a response to meet its needs, and that the exchange should be consummated. Promotion itself involves a range of tactics involving publicity, advertising, and personal selling, which are described in Chapters 11, 12, and 13, respectively.

As discussed earlier, formal communication in the form of advertising was not allowed as recently as 1975. Yet while the past 30 years have seen a change in terms of the amount of advertising, other promotional tactics such as personal selling have become more relevant to compete effectively in today's marketplace. Health insurance companies and MCOs all employ sales forces. Even local acute-care hospitals now often have physician referral staff who call on physicians to ensure that their needs are being met at the facility where they admit patients.

■ The Dilemma of Needs and Wants

One of health care marketing's major concerns pertains to the issues of needs and wants. Health care professionals often speak of the fact that what consumers want may not be what they need. Clinical and professional responsibility demands treatment of the need. A **need** has been defined as a "condition in which there is a deficiency of something, or one requiring relief."[6] A **want** is defined as the "wish or desire for something."[7] A consumer *needs* to have medication for hypertension. A person may *want* medication to suppress the appetite and thus lose weight. To which need or want should the health care marketer respond?

Underlying any response in health care must be whatever constitutes providing quality care for the patient. Meeting medical needs must be the primary purpose of the system. Yet wants should not be ignored. For the health care professional, consider the just-cited dilemma of a pill for weight reduction. Should the system respond to this want? A marketer's response would most likely be yes, but the response must be medically appropriate. In fact, the marketer would try to understand more closely what it is the consumer wants (or is buying). In this instance, it is less likely to be a pill and more probably a more attractive appearance through weight reduction. The request for medication might be met more appropriately with creation of an eating disorders program or a wellness center that helps establish an exercise and fitness regimen. The ultimate want that the customer has can be satisfied, but the methodology must observe appropriate practice standards.

Identifying the Customer

In health care, this need/want dilemma often masks the major question, "Who is the customer?" Consider recent trends in the field of obstetrics. For many years, the consumer—the expectant mother—wanted to have her significant other with her in the delivery room. The medical community responded by claiming that this want was inappropriate. It would compromise good standards of care. In fact, the issue had less to do with standards of care and more with standards of convenience for the provider. Now, in most delivery rooms in the United States, a woman in labor will be accompanied by her significant other, a nurse midwife, and possibly, the obstetrician.[8]

The medical community argued that the need to restrict access to the labor suite was for "good standards in obstetrical care." In reality, medicine lost sight of who the customer was and how her needs and wants could be met. In the delivery process, the physician may be viewed as part of the production line, not as the customer. Medical needs are not compromised in modern labor rooms, but customer needs are being more closely addressed. A community hospital like Cooley Dickinson in Northampton, Massachusetts, offers a postpartum doula program linked with the childbirth center. The doula service representative visits the mother after birth and can help provide a range of services from helping the new mother bond with the child, to preparing snacks, running errands, or transmitting messages.

In our current health care marketplace, most health care organizations have multiple markets or customers to whom they must be attentive. FIGURE 1-1 shows an array (but probably not all-encompassing) of potential markets for a health care organization. An organization offering a mental health or substance abuse program for adolescents might have to accommodate the needs of judges, probation officers, or social workers. Schools might be the market for a sports medicine program. Long-term care facilities might be the market for a geriatric assessment program. Also included are the more traditional markets represented by physicians, nurses, patients, referring physicians, employee assistance personnel at companies, managed care plans, and regulators. One increasingly important market includes employers. For many years, this segment was considered of secondary importance, since companies paid the full insurance premiums for their labor force. Now, however, companies are

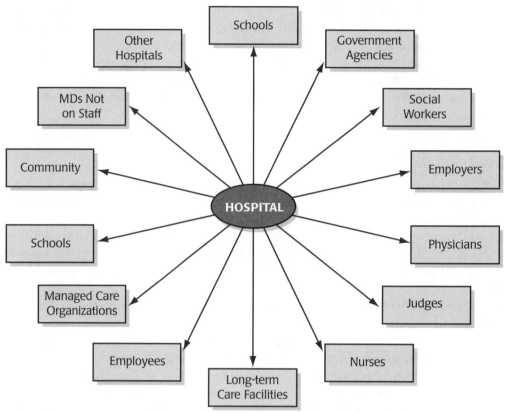

FIGURE 1-1 The Many Hospital Markets

controlling rising health care costs (a factor discussed further in Chapter 3) by dealing directly with providers to meet their employees' health care needs.

As the topic of markets is discussed in this book, it is important to be aware that health care organizations have multiple markets—the importance of each one is a function of the program or issue being addressed.

■ The Evolution of Marketing

In both traditional businesses and in health care, the marketing concept has taken several decades to evolve. In health care, this evolution has occurred in a relatively short time period. As previously noted, one of the first hospitals to hire a person with a marketing title was Evanston Hospital in Illinois in 1975. In traditional product businesses, the evolution of the marketing concept took longer.

Production Era

To understand how marketing has evolved, let's consider its development in a corporation such as Pillsbury Company of Minneapolis–St. Paul, long known as a manufacturer of flour, baking goods, and other food products. Let's also trace this same evolution in the typical hospital.

Pillsbury located itself in the Minneapolis–St. Paul, Minnesota, market in the 1800s. The location, along the Mississippi River, offered the company a source of water power. (In that era, the Mississippi River had waterfalls that far north.) This location was also close to the raw materials needed for the production of Pillsbury's product. Robert Keith, a former Pillsbury president, described the company at this stage of its development. "We are professional flour millers. Blessed with a supply of the finest North American wheat, plenty of water power, and excellent milling machinery, we produce flour of the highest quality. Our basic function is to mill high-quality flour, and of course we must hire salesmen to sell it, just as we hire accountants to keep the books."[9] At this stage of the company's evolution, the primary focus of the business was producing a high-quality product—flour. The sales and even the consumption or purchase of the product were incidental to the firm's focus—it was assumed that people would buy Pillsbury flour because it was high quality.

Many hospitals were and are at this stage in their own evolution. One might rewrite Keith's statements for a production-oriented hospital to say, "Our basic function is to provide high-quality medicine. Accompanied by the highest forms of technology, we have physicians, nurses, and allied health personnel to provide this service and we have administrators to keep the books." For a production-oriented hospital or health care organization, the focus is on providing high-quality medicine. As can be seen in Table 1-1, the health care organization's focus is on delivering clinical quality.

Sales Era

For many traditional businesses such as Pillsbury, the production orientation worked well until the early 1900s. By 1920, the automobile became part of our way of life and changed the world for consumers and companies. The federal government began to finance the construction of a roadway system in the United States. Consumers became more mobile in the everyday life of work, shopping, and recreation. For companies, the strategic change was in the hiring of traveling salespeople. Competition

Table 1-1	The Evolution of Marketing	
Orientation	Pillsbury	Hospital
Production	Product quality focus	Clinical quality focus
Sales	Generating volume	Filling beds
Marketing	Satisfying needs and wants	Identifying health care needs and meeting them

heightened as competing sales forces fought for customers who formerly were the domain of manufacturers in their particular region. Robert Keith so characterized Pillsbury's business focus at this stage: "We are a flour-milling company, manufacturing a number of products for the consumer market. We must have a first-rate sales organization which can dispose of all the products we make at a favorable price."[10]

For hospitals, the sales era occurred in the mid-1970s with the change in reimbursement. Under cost-based reimbursement, competition with other hospitals was not a major concern. Hospitals had patients, lengths of stay were not an issue, and occupancy rates were high. Hospitals treated patients and passed along the actual cost, along with an appropriate profit margin, for reimbursement by the third-party payers. The focus for a hospital administrator in the sales stage was twofold. The first and top priority was to get as many patients as possible. Traditionally, this goal was accomplished by attracting as many physicians as possible to admit patients to the hospital. Since this era preceded the days of utilization reviews, hospitals had no concerns about attracting efficient physicians who could care for patients in some limited time period. The hospital wanted to ensure that as many patients as possible wanted to be admitted into the facility who were so directed by their physicians.

Changing Mr. Keith's statement, one might characterize the focus of a sales-oriented hospital as: "We are a high-quality hospital providing numerous medical services to the market. We must attract physicians in the community to want to admit to our facility. And, we must encourage patients to want to come here." This stage of marketing evolution focused on sales. Hospitals tried to entice physicians to admit to a particular facility. Hospitals built medical office buildings attached to their facilities offering physicians the convenience of admitting patients at the hospital contiguous to their offices. Hospitals developed physician relations programs to bond with the providers. They sponsored seminars for physicians or provided valet parking and attractive lounges. All these were attempts to build the census, fill the beds.

At this time, hospitals also recognized that the patient might play a role in the hospital selection decision.[11] A second, concurrent strategy of selling to the public also occurred. In the mid-1970s, many hospitals adopted mass advertising strategies to promote their programs, including the use of billboard displays and television and radio commercials touting a particular service. The advertising goal was to encourage patients to use the hospital facilities when the physician presented a choice, or to self-refer if necessary. In health care, this was the evolution to sales.

Marketing Era

The evolution to marketing occurred after World War II. In the late 1940s, many companies found that their level of technological sophistication had increased dramatically as a result of their wartime efforts. Moreover, consumers were returning from the war and establishing households, escalating the demand for products and services. For many companies the major question became one of deciding which products or services to offer. Pillsbury's perspective changed to: "We are in the business of satisfying the wants and needs of consumers." With this focus, it is the customer who drives the production process and directs the organization's efforts.

So, too, in health care, a similar perspective can and is being achieved. Health care providers can offer any number of services by reallocating their financial resources. The underlying question, however, becomes which service to offer? This is where a marketing-oriented perspective is valuable. In health care, the focus of a marketing-oriented institution can be viewed as "We address the health care needs of the marketplace." Such a marketing-oriented focus might lead to a product or service line that includes home health care, geriatric medicine, after-hours care, or wellness centers. The trend toward integrated delivery systems (a concept discussed in greater detail later in this text) is a response to a marketplace that does not want to deal with a fractionated health care system of providers, free-standing medical centers, a hospital, and an insurance firm. The integrated system formation can deliver a seamless health care product to the buyer that involves not only delivering the clinical care, but also accepting the risk for the cost of that care through a managed care product. It is a focus that begins with the consumer; the organization responds to this demand.

■ The Marketing Culture

Some organizations achieve a final level of evolution, where marketing becomes part of the corporate culture, diffused throughout all levels of the organization. The focus of marketing no longer lies solely under the responsibility of the marketing department. Rather, in the health care setting, marketing is performed by the clinical nurse administrator for the neurology program. The admitting desk clerks and the house maintenance staff understand and appreciate the need to maintain a customer orientation.

The evolution to this stage may be seen in organizations that have adopted a patient-focused system. Sentara, an integrated delivery system in Hampton, Virginia, and Lakeland Regional Medical Center, a large tertiary hospital in Lakeland, Florida, are two such institutions. These organizations have made the customer the central focus of all their activities. Admitting is accomplished on the floor where the patient is assigned a bed, employees cross-train for skills that allow them to be the most patient-responsive possible without compromising the quality of care delivered. Whenever possible, certain diagnostic equipment is brought to the patient rather than having the patient move through the hospital. It is the primary responsibility of each employee to respond to customer needs first. The development of patient-focused care in such organizations is the transference of a marketing culture throughout the organization. Rather than having the patient (customer) go to the provider (such as when the patient moves through the delivery system for treatment or clinical testing), the provider goes to the patient whenever possible to administer the necessary clinical interventions.

For organizations at this stage, the concept of a marketing orientation has taken hold. A **marketing orientation** has five distinct elements:

1. Customer orientation—having a sufficient understanding of the target buyers to be able to create superior value for them continuously
2. Competitor orientation—recognizing competitors' (and potential competitors') strengths, weaknesses, and strategies
3. Interfunctional coordination—coordinating and deploying company resources in a manner that focuses on creating value for the customer
4. Long-term focus—adopting a perspective that includes a continuous search for ways to add value by making appropriate business investments
5. Profitability—earning revenues sufficient to cover long-term expenses and satisfy key constituencies[12]

■ The Nonmarketing-Driven Planning Process

While the patient-focused health care approach represents the diffusion of a marketing orientation throughout a health care institution, such an approach has not always been the perspective taken by health care providers. Most health care organizations have been characterized by a nonmarket-driven culture and planning process. In no place is the difference between being marketing-oriented and nonmarketing-oriented more apparent than when a health care organization goes about its long-range planning process.

To understand the difference between a marketing-driven and nonmarketing-driven process, it is important to recognize the implications of the difference between the two concepts on long-range planning.[13]

FIGURE 1-2 shows the sequence involved when a non-marketing-driven organization conducts long-range planning. In most health care organizations, long-range planning is assigned to a committee comprising administrators, key members of the hospital's

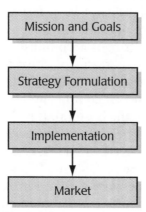

FIGURE 1-2 Nonmarket-Based Planning Sequence

board of directors, and a few influential physicians. Typically, the first step involves a review of the organization's mission and goals. A hospital might reaffirm its mission "to provide high-quality health care regardless of race, creed, religion, and [in small print] ability to pay."

The second step of the planning process—strategy formulation—is often difficult and time-consuming. At this point, members of the long-range planning committee debate what objectives should be included in the hospital's five-year plan. Now, the real implications of the nonmarketing-driven approach become evident. Often, a senior physician stands up at the strategy formulation stage and makes a speech such as the following: "I've been at this hospital since the day I entered the medical profession. This hospital is my life and I never even admitted a patient to another facility. Of course, I'm also being recognized as an expert in the future of medicine. I've been invited to conferences to speak on the future of medicine and I've just published an article in the *New England Journal of Medicine*. As I think about what services we need to provide in the new ambulatory care wing of the hospital, it's clear to me that we need a sports medicine program." Usually, the physician making this recommendation appears to be a self-serving orthopedic surgeon.

At this stage in the planning process, several committee members become dismayed. Some think the hospital should, instead, offer an expanded geriatric medicine program; other committee members want to get into rehabilitative medicine. Yet this physician is very influential and has lined up committee votes in favor of a sports medicine program before the committee met. The vote is taken and the final tally is seven to five in favor of a sports medicine program, which becomes part of the strategic plan.

The next stage of the long-range planning process—implementation—is more difficult. The hospital realizes it has no staff members trained in sports medicine. The hospital hires a physician recruiting firm to find a new medical director for sports medicine. The position is filled and it is at this stage of the process where conflict often occurs within the organization. Many committee members opposed opening a sports medicine program, yet now, the new director and new program require resources. Other services within the hospital find their budgets for the coming fiscal year are reduced in order to reallocate dollars to sports medicine. Other program directors are upset because they lose space in the new ambulatory care wing because of the needs of the sports medicine service. The new sports medicine director has an aggressive agenda. She has hired her staff, purchased the necessary equipment, and is setting up shop.

A state of anxiety soon takes hold of the hospital's administrators. As the date moves closer to the grand opening of the sports medicine program, they ask, "Who is really going to use the service?" Recognizing the need for patient volume, they attempt to market the program. But what happens is not marketing but sales. The hospital administrator typically places a frantic call to the public relations director requesting an open house for the new sports medicine program. Advertisements are placed in the local community paper. Invitations to tour the facility are distributed to influential people. The goal is to attract visitors to the new program. On the day of the open house, attendance is disappointing. Four months later the finance committee convenes to review the performance of the sports medicine program. It is a failure. Why?

The first response is to blame public relations; the public relations director didn't promote the service well. This may be a possible explanation. A second hypothesis suggests the failure is the fault of the new sports medicine director, whose interpersonal style is discouraging other physicians from referring patients to the program. Yet, there may be a third, more viable explanation—the sports medicine program wasn't needed. The program differed little from the competition's offering; hence, patients had no reason to switch facilities.

This scenario is a common result of a nonmarketing-driven planning process. The problem with a nonmarketing-driven process is that it requires a group of people (or one powerfully persuasive committee member) to have insight into what kinds of health care service the marketplace wants, how it wants that service configured, and what it is willing to pay for it. This approach to delivering a service or health care product to the market is an internal-to-external development process. The product is sold first. The challenge then is finding enough buyers willing to use the service or product at a level sufficient to make a profit. This approach is risky at best because it relies on the market forecasting ability of people within the organization.

The limitations of the internal-to-external perspective of the nonmarketing-driven approach, as well as overcoming the political power of some people within the organization, are addressed by taking a marketing-driven approach to planning.

■ A Marketing-Driven Planning Sequence

A marketing-driven planning sequence is dramatically different from a nonmarketing-driven process, as illustrated in FIGURE 1-3. The first step is the same; every organization has the right to determine its mission and goals. Yet the marketing-driven approach is substantially different at step two. It is at this stage of needs assessment where market research, as will be discussed in Chapter 5, begins to make its contribution. The hospital conducts a survey to determine which services are most needed. Should sports medicine, geriatric medicine, or women's health services be offered in the new ambulatory care wing of the hospital?

When determining the most needed service, it is essential to examine the competition. If there are existing competing services in the market, the necessary differential advantage for these new offerings must be identified. While the sources of a differential advantage are discussed later in this chapter, a **differential advantage** is the incremental benefits of a product relative to competing products that are important to the buyer and perceived by the buyer. In our example, the hospital's survey reveals that 20% of the market wants sports medicine, 25% would like to see a new geriatric program, and 50% wants women's health. Further research shows that the major differential advantages that would lead women to use this service over their existing providers are convenient location and hours.

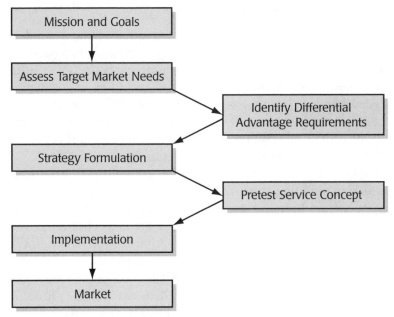

FIGURE 1-3 **Market-Driven Planning Sequence**

With the market research completed, the strategy is clear. A conveniently located, accessible women's health program is written into the hospital's long-range plan. Prior to full-scale implementation, however, market research is employed again in the form of a pretest. Pretesting involves returning to the market with a product sample to ensure that the specifications meet customer expectations. In a service business such as health care, the pretesting stage is particularly difficult. Unlike many product businesses that can manufacture a prototype without incurring major fixed costs, a new health program might require a redesign of physical space, the hiring of trained personnel, and acquisition of new technologies. Pretesting must still be done, however, without the addition of all these costs.

To pretest a service in health care effectively, the personnel involved with the program and with customer relations must develop a detailed concept description of the service. Then they assemble a sample of potential female patients similar to those in the target market and walk them through a concept test of the service. Consumers can be questioned about hours, service location, and appointment procedure. Reactions to the concept generate appropriate modifications. Full-scale implementation then begins. At this point, the hospital needs to market—not sell—the program. Market research has determined the product, the price customers are willing to pay, and how the service should be distributed (i.e., locations, hours). All that remains for the hospital is to inform the target market about the availability of the desired new service through the appropriate promotions.

Is Marketing Planning Approach Needed?

A comparison of Figures 1-2 and 1-3 shows that using market research can lead to a dramatically different result in long-range planning. Yet, is a marketing-driven planning process needed in health care? Twenty or 30 years ago, a nonmarketing-driven process was sufficient. Competition wasn't a prime factor. In most communities, including major metropolitan areas, demand exceeded supply. A hospital would offer a new service and the major issue was how to meet demand for it. Twenty or 30 years ago most health care organizations were in a reasonably strong financial position because of cost-based reimbursement and unrestricted lengths of stay. Efficiency and financial prudence were non-issues.

The present competitive health care environment has prompted many organizations to adopt a marketing-driven planning approach. Health care providers find themselves facing significant competition. In many instances, and for many subspecialties, the problem is one of supply exceeding demand. The challenge is to encourage demand for your service at the expense of your competitors. Organizations must find a differential advantage to encourage buyers to use their services. Health care organizations today must be fiscally astute. Few have the excess financial resources to afford the mistake of offering a service that is not needed in the marketplace. A marketing-driven planning process is one tool to help minimize such mistakes.

We have described a nonmarketing-driven approach to planning as an internal-to-external methodology.[14] That is, members inside the organization try to foretell or dictate what the market wants and how the service should best be configured to meet those wants. In contrast, a marketing-driven approach follows an external-to-internal methodology. First, there is an assessment of what the market wants, then the organization's response. Health care providers must realize that a marketing-driven planning process does not guarantee success, but it does, however, minimize the probability of failure.

■ The Strategic Marketing Process

The marketing-driven planning model just discussed is devised within the context of a more macro setting. FIGURE 1-4 shows the setting in which marketing occurs. An organization must develop a marketing strategy that is sensitive to three factors: (1) important stakeholders, (2) environmental factors, and (3) society at large.

Stakeholders

Stakeholders represent any group with which the company has, or wants to develop, a relationship. As seen in Figure 1-4, the stakeholders can represent customers. For health care organizations, these customers might be patients, physicians who refer to the organization, social workers for an adolescent chemical dependency program, payers, managed care providers with whom contracts are developed, or companies that contract for an industrial medicine program.

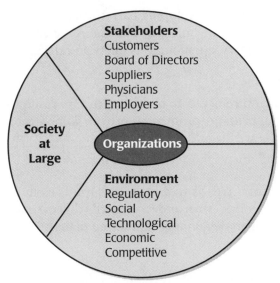

FIGURE 1-4 Environment and Marketing Strategy

Many organizations, such as hospitals or proprietary chains, also have boards of directors that serve an oversight function. Organizations develop their marketing strategy in light of the direction and values provided and communicated by this constituency. A third major stakeholder group includes suppliers. In health care, suppliers can represent companies that provide laboratory testing or maintenance services, or they again can represent physicians. For many hospitals, physicians are customers. In a group practice setting, physicians represent the shareholders or owners. In other organizations, physicians, by providing coverage of the emergency room, might actually be suppliers.

Uncontrollable Environment

Any marketing strategy is developed within the context of a broader environmental perspective. The **environment** pertains to regulatory, social, technological, economic, and competitive factors to which the organization must be sensitive when developing a strategy. These elements, which are discussed in greater detail in Chapter 3 (and briefly described below), are uncontrollable but impact marketing strategy. For example, a company cannot change the uncontrollable element that certain trends exist in society. During the past 20 years, the government has reported a dramatic increase in obesity in the United States. In 1985, only a few states were participating in the Centers for Disease Control and Prevention's Behavioral Risk Factor Surveillance System and providing obesity data. In 1991, four states had obesity prevalence rates of 15–19%, and no states had rates at or above 20%. In 2003, 15 states had obesity prevalence rates of 15–19%, 31 states had rates of 20–24%, and 4 states had rates more than 25%.[15]

However, hospitals can respond to that trend by developing bariatric surgery programs. Yet, some health insurers like Blue Cross Blue Shield of Florida as recently as February 2005 were not reimbursing for such surgery, questioning its safety and efficacy.[16]

Regulatory Factors

Regulatory factors include legal issues and requirements. In many health care communities, programs cannot be instituted without prior government approval. Some strategies, such as paying physicians for referrals, are illegal.

Social Forces

Social forces include demographic and cultural trends to which organizations must be sensitive. An aging population, a changing work ethic, and a culturally diverse marketplace are some of the issues to consider when developing marketing plans.

Technological Factors

Technological factors affect few industries more dramatically than they do health care. It is these technological forces that can change the viability of any service. Until the 1950s, the treatment of polio victims constituted a major revenue stream for many hospital facilities. As we know, this disease was all but eliminated by the technological achievement of the Salk vaccine in the 1950s.

Economic Factors

Economic factors include changes in income distribution or fiscal conditions such as borrowing rates that can determine any company's investment plans. As will be discussed in Chapter 3, the rising cost of health care has led one major customer group—corporations—to work more aggressively with their health care providers in seeking solutions to rising costs.

Competitive Forces

Competitive forces are the final uncontrollable element in any marketing plan. Strategies and programs must be developed in light of this constraint and should reflect the considerations that exist in the marketplace.

Society

Ultimately, all marketing programs and strategies are developed within the context of a broader societal perspective, a context that requires an ethically responsible decision-making process. For example, many companies have become more keenly aware of and responsible for the impact of their products and programs on the environment. The broader societal market represents all the individuals, groups, businesses, and other entities that affect, are related to, or derive benefit from the health care organization, as seen in Exhibit 1-1.

Exhibit 1-1   Organizations in the Health Care Environment

Organizations That Plan for and/or Regulate Primary and Secondary Providers

- Federal Regulating Agencies
  Health Systems Agencies (HSAs)
  Department of Health and Human Services (DHHS)
  Health Care Financing Agency (HCFA)
- State Regulating Agencies
  Public Health Departments
  State Planning Agency (CON)

- Voluntary Regulating Groups
- Joint Commission on Accreditation
  of Healthcare Organizations
  (JCAHO)
- Other Accrediting Agencies

Primary Providers (Organizations That Provide Health Services)

- Hospitals
  Voluntary (Barnes Hospital)
  Governmental (VA Hospitals)
  Investor Owned (Humana, AMI, NME)
- State Public Health Departments
- Long-Term Care Facilities
  Skilled Nursing Facilities (Beverly Enterprises)
- Intermediate Care Facilities

- HMOs and IPAs (Care America)
- Ambulatory Care Facilities
  (National Rehab Services)
- Hospices (Hospice Care, Inc.)
- Physicians' Offices
- Home Health Care Institutions
  (VNA, Upjohn Healthcare Services)

Secondary Providers (Organizations That Provide Resources)

- Educational Institutions
  Medical Schools (Johns Hopkins)
  Nursing Schools
  Health Administration Programs
- Organizations That Pay for Care (Third Party Payers)
  Government (Medicare)
  Insurance Companies (Blue Cross)
  Social Organizations (Shriners)

- Pharmaceutical and Medical
  Supply
  Drug Distributors (McKesson)
  Drug & Research (Merck, Eli Lilly)
  Medical Products (Johnson &
  Johnson, Bausch & Lomb)

Organizations That Represent Primary & Secondary Providers

- American Medical Association (AMA)
- American Hospital Association (AHA)

- State Medical Associations
- Individual Professional Associations

Individuals and Patients (Consumers)

- Independent Physicians
- Nurses
- Allied Health Professionals

- Technicians
- Patients

Source: From Ginter, P.M., Duncan, W.J., Richardson, W.D., Swayne, L.E., Analyzing the Health Care Environment: You Can't Hit What You Can't See from *Health Care Management Review*, Vol. 16, No. 4, p. 44, 1991. Used by permission of Lippincott Williams & Wilkins.

■ Target Market

At the core of the marketing program is the **target market,** the group of customers whom the organization wishes to attract. In the development of a marketing strategy, the target market is within an organization's control as a function of the effectiveness of the marketing mix developed by the health care providers.

The notion of controlling the target market, however, is an idea that is often lost on health care providers. Whom a health system attracts to its facilities and whom it targets may be two different populations. Too often in the past, health care organizations have defined their market by simply identifying who walked into their facility or used the emergency room. Health care organizations developed profiles of their patients and developed strategies based on the users. Yet the central issue to marketing strategy is to decide those users you want to attract and then determine what this group's needs are. The organization that defines a target market, such as "all consumers with incomes above $75,000 who have private insurance, and live in a particular area," can then focus its market research on identification of an appropriate strategy to meet the needs of the targeted group. Sharp Health Care of California has decided that one of its target markets will include Mexican patients. Sharp Health Care, a large health care system that includes various health care subsidiaries and five hospitals in San Diego, California, opened a hospital under the Sharp name in Mazatlan, Mexico, in December 1994. Sharp also hopes to capture referrals from this target market by an affiliation agreement with Hospital Notre Dame in Tiajuana, Mexico. To support this effort, Sharp will provide continuing medical education programs for that hospital's medical staff.[17] Determining the target market resulted in several strategies to attract this consumer population.

The subtle nature of the target market definition must be underscored when talking about health care. This aspect of marketing is not meant to imply that the organization will deny care to anyone. However, defining and going after a *particular* group of customers from a strategic marketing perspective is different from having a business strategy that is unfocused. In health care it would be immoral to deny care to a patient who appears at a facility in crisis and need, but a marketing strategy should have a defined group of individuals that it is trying to reach, appeal to, or attract. It is this group of individuals, be it an underserved population for an acquired immune deficiency syndrome awareness clinic, an upscale group of white-collar professionals for a boutique medicine practice, or a medium-to-large business for a managed care plan that might all represent a target market.

■ Organizing for Marketing

Establishing the marketing function within an organization can be accomplished in one of several ways. The two most common organizational structures for marketing are by product and by market.

Product-Oriented Organization

The product management structure, as shown in FIGURE 1-5, has been increasingly common in health care settings. In this setting, the responsibility, authority, and accountability rest with the product line manager. Nursing, pharmacy, laboratory, and other departments coordinate their services across, and in support of, the product lines. In the true **product-oriented organization**, each distinct product or related set of products has its own marketing organization.

The product manager is responsible for developing and overseeing the marketing strategy for the product or **strategic business units**, which are businesses operated as separate profit centers within a large organization. In a product management structure, individual managers commonly share staff resources, such as marketing research, as well as operational personnel, such as the sales force. The product manager approach is of value when a product has such unique requirements that it demands the commitment of a separate individual.

Product line management has two major advantages for health care organizations. First, having someone responsible for all aspects of a product line helps to refine the service area and to meet needs more easily. This structure helps combine services and

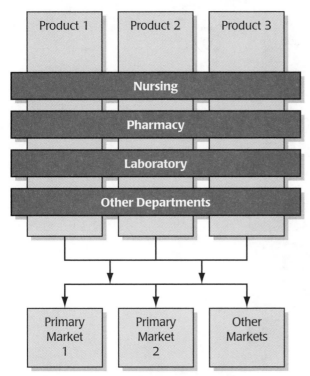

FIGURE 1-5 Product-Oriented Organization

Source: From Zelman, W.N. and Parham, D.L., Strategic, Operational, and Marketing Concerns of Product-Line Management in Health Care, *Health Care Management Review*, Vol. 15, No. 1, pp. 29–35, 1990. Used by permission of Lippincott Williams & Wilkins.

benefits for customers. Second, packaging related services into product lines helps contribute to continuous, rather than sporadic, planning.[18] A disadvantage with the product management structure in traditional businesses has been the fact that the product manager has no direct control over many operational details—the product manager must negotiate for sales force time or marketing research resources. This same limitation occurs in health care. While the product manager has the focus to develop program plans, there is no direct operational control over how the service is delivered within the facility. In many health care organizations, the product manager acts as the salesperson for the program. For health care organizations, there is another consideration that may limit the value of a product organization. If the same customer is targeted for more than one product line, significant marketing inefficiencies or customer resistance may be the result. For example, a referral physician may be unwilling to meet with four different product line representatives from one tertiary medical center.

Market-Oriented Organization

The second most common marketing structure is a **market-oriented organization** in which each distinct major market has its own marketing organization, as seen in FIGURE 1-6. A

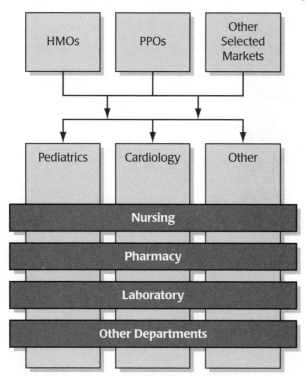

FIGURE 1-6 Market-Oriented Organization

Source: From Zelman, W.N. and Parham, D.L., Strategic, Operational, and Marketing Concerns of Product-Line Management in Health Care from *Health Care Management Review*, Vol. 15, No. 1, p. 32, 1990. Used by permission of Lippincott Williams & Wilkins.

health care organization might design a marketing organization around its major customer groups (referral physicians, corporations, managed care buyers, and other referral sources) as shown in this figure.

The value of this approach is its focus on customers who have different buying structures and purchasing requirements. For any health care organization, supporting marketing activities can be serviced by the manager of each major market group. The underlying rationale for this approach is that each major customer group has distinct needs.

For decades, IBM Corporation was organized around product lines. In 1994, the corporation concluded that customers demanded solutions to problems, not products. This forced the company to restructure around major markets and industries. In this way, IBM can develop expertise in financial services, telecommunications, or manufacturing and meet the information needs of these respective industries. Whether the solution is provided by a local area network system, a mainframe computer, or a series of independent desktop computers is irrelevant to the customer. This same analogy applies to the health care setting. Corporate expectations and demands differ from the requirements and concerns of a second major market of referral physicians. Each group of customers seeks solutions to problems rather than the purchase of specific clinical programs.

■ Requirements for Organizational Marketing Success

Many hospitals and medical groups have problems making the transition to becoming a market-oriented organization. Often, marketing has not met the expectations of filling hospital beds or generating substantial numbers of new subscribers into the MCO. The disappointment in marketing is due to a lack of appreciation of what it means to be marketing driven, and of what marketing alone can accomplish. There are four prerequisites for successful marketing, as shown in FIGURE 1-7.[19]

Pressure to Be Market-Oriented

First, there must be pressure to be market-oriented. There must be a shared view that is accepted throughout the organization concerning the need for an improved marketing

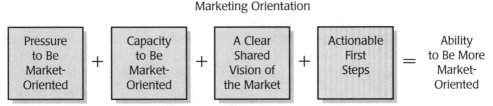

Conditions for Developing an Effective
Marketing Orientation

| Pressure to Be Market-Oriented | + | Capacity to Be Market-Oriented | + | A Clear Shared Vision of the Market | + | Actionable First Steps | = | Ability to Be More Market-Oriented |

FIGURE 1-7 Prerequisites to Marketing Success

Source: From Diamond, S.L. and Berkowitz, E.N., Effective Marketing for Health Care Providers. Reprinted with permission from the Journal of Medical Practice Management, Vol. 5, No. 3, p. 198, © 1990 Greenbranch Publishing, PO Box 208, Phoenix, MD 21131, (800) 933–3711.

program. To some extent, this represents the fourth stage in the evolution of marketing that is appearing in organizations previously mentioned, such as Sentara. Not only must senior management want to become more market-oriented, but peer pressure to understand and to respond to customer needs must be strong throughout the organization. Information and reward systems must recognize the value of a customer orientation, and department program objectives and measurement systems must be tied to progress on this goal.

Capacity to Be Market-Oriented

A second criterion for organizational marketing success is the capacity to be market-oriented. The health care organization must have enough staff members who are not only experienced and adequately trained, but also devoted to improving the organization's marketing effort. Management, staff, and clinical personnel must be receptive to ideas on how to become more market-oriented and have a marketing budget to support their efforts. Besides financial support, significant time must be devoted to improving marketing efforts and to developing an understanding of how these efforts integrate with other organizational priorities.

Shared Vision of Market

A clear, shared vision of the market is a third prerequisite to success. Many questions must be answered when developing an understanding of the marketplace: Who are the key customers and stakeholders? What are their needs? What change must the organization make in terms of its marketing mix to meet the needs of these core constituencies? How will this organization differentiate itself from other providers?

Action Plan to Respond to Market

Last, the organization must develop a clear set of actionable steps to respond to market needs. It will need a detailed marketing plan that includes the necessary strategies and tactics along each of the four Ps. This also requires well-defined mechanisms to track the progress of and address minor difficulties in implementation before they become major customer problems.

Missing any one of these elements can lead to marketing ineffectiveness. FIGURE 1-8 reveals the results of these prerequisite gaps. Without the pressure to be market-oriented, there is a "bottom of the in-box" feeling toward marketing. The words are mouthed but there is no pressure to change. Lacking the capacity to be marketing-oriented leads to frustration and anxiety. Attempting to be efficient, many health care providers have pared resources. Yet, marketing personnel and programs must be viewed as an investment to generate additional revenue, not solely as an expense item.

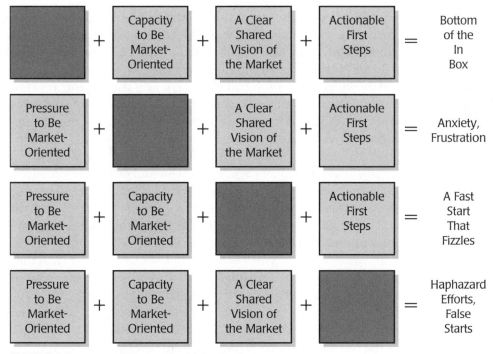

Prerequisite Gaps

| | Capacity to Be Market-Oriented | A Clear Shared Vision of the Market | Actionable First Steps | Bottom of the In Box |
| | Pressure to Be Market-Oriented | | A Clear Shared Vision of the Market | Actionable First Steps | Anxiety, Frustration |

FIGURE 1-8 **Prerequisites to Marketing Failures**

Source: From Diamond, S.L. and Berkowitz, E.N., Effective Marketing for Health Care Providers. Reprinted with permission from the *Journal of Medical Practice Management*, Vol. 5, No. 3, p. 203, © 1990 Greenbranch Publishing, PO Box 208, Phoenix, MD 21131, (800) 933–3711.

Many health care organizations' marketing efforts have suffered from a fast start that quickly fizzled because of the absence of a clear, shared vision of the market. Well-designed, effective marketing programs require an in-depth understanding of the marketplace. Many hospitals, in the 1980s, began to advertise programs before they even knew what they were advertising.[20] This same problem seems to be reoccurring now as many health organizations rush to promote their integrated delivery systems with little understanding of system definition or market requirements.

False starts, another pitfall for marketing, occur when there are no actionable, first steps in place. Effective marketing requires detailed plans that specify the tactics to be implemented within each of the four Ps. Allocated responsibilities, benchmarks for measuring performance, and timetables are specified at the planning process. With all four components in place, the contributions of the marketing function and result-ant strategy to any health care organization's success increase dramatically.

■ The Evolving Perspective of Marketing

In the past five years, there has been a dramatic shift in the thinking that has driven marketing thought. Historically, the perspective was of a transactional nature. That is, marketing, while trying to fulfill the needs and wants of the customer (see "The Dilemma of Needs and Wants") still focused on the individual sale or interaction between the patient and the provider, or the referral physician and the organization to which they may have referred. The focus of marketing efforts today is different. Rather than considering each interaction with a customer or patient as an individual transaction, the goal is on customer retention or building longer term loyalty. There is a separate chapter in this edition (Chapter 7) devoted to developing customer loyalty.

The challenge for organizations today in creating loyalty and customer retention is a significant marketing issue. Employees are recognized as a key component, not only as an internal customer as noted in Figure 1-1 but as a major link to long-term customer loyalty.[21] Table 1-2 shows the shift in paradigm between the traditional marketing focus and the emerging marketing customer relationship focus. In the traditional paradigm, the organizational focus was to complete the sale, but the structure of the organization was geared for efficient throughput. This was most easily seen in a setting such as the outpatient surgery center. Often a patient might be scheduled for a day surgical procedure at 1:00 or 2:00 PM. However, the instructions given to the individual were to show up at 7:30 in the morning. The reason is that in case another patient did not arrive for the scheduled surgery, they could fill the queue with another individual who might happen to be waiting. Although this approach was not conven-

Table 1-2	The Changing Marketing Paradigm	
Strategic Focus	**Traditional Paradigm**	**Relationship Paradigm**
Sales focus	Individual sale	Customer retention
Staff selection	Focus on clinical skill	Focus on clinical and customer service attitude
Customer service commitment	Limited commitment	Goal to exceed expectations
Management of wait time	Customer time to increase operational efficiency	Customer wait time to enhance experience
Technology access	Provided when cost justified	Considered for first mover advantage competitively
Customer key drivers	Cost and clinical effectiveness	Quality, cost, service delivery
Service system design	Developed for clinical efficiency	Designed for seamless customer service

Sources: Adapted from Robert C. Ford and Myron D. Fottler, "Creating Customer Focused Healthcare Organizations," *Health Care Management Review*, (2000), Vol. 25, No. 4, pp. 18–33; Adrian Payne, Martin Christopher, Helen Peck, and Moira Clark, *Relationship Marketing for Competitive Advantage* (Butterworth–Heinemann, 1995).

ient for the customer, it was very efficient for the organization. And, as long as the organization is focusing on a single transaction, this model works fine.

In the emerging marketing paradigm, certainly operational efficiency must be considered. Yet along with quality and efficiency, the value to the customer must be considered in terms of service delivery. As will be discussed further in Chapter 7 in developing a loyal customer, it is important to recognize the customer's value equation in health care today. Only in delivering value can patient and customer retention be achieved.

■ The Changing Health Care Marketplace

No discussion of marketing in health care can begin without an overview of the dramatic restructuring occurring in the industry today. As this chapter began, it mentioned terms that any reader of health care literature or practitioner in the field faces daily—integration, satellites, managed care. What are the implications of these changes for marketing? To appreciate the impact on marketing of the restructuring occurring within health care today, it is instructive to reexamine the traditional industry structure from which we are rapidly moving away.[22]

The Traditional Industry Structure

In communities that have not truly experienced the formation of an integrated delivery system, the health care marketplace can be considered fractionated, in that each entity operates independently. FIGURE 1-9 shows the major components of this traditional health care structure. At the top of the figure is the hospital, then physicians, followed by the community-at-large.

The focus of the hospital's marketing efforts is twofold, represented by the solid arrows. The focus primarily has been on physicians. The key to maintaining a census

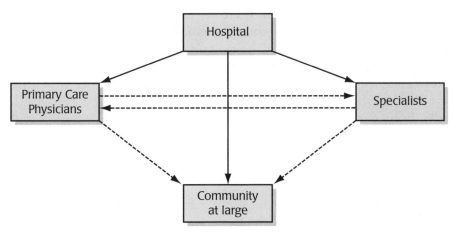

FIGURE 1-9 The Traditional Health Care Structure

within the facility is encouraging physicians to admit to one's own particular facility as opposed to a competitor's. Consider, then, what has been the typical marketing efforts by hospitals in this regard.

Most hospitals today have a physician relations staff who call on physicians to ensure they are satisfied with the facility and to determine whether the hospital can provide any additional services to meet their needs. Other hospitals have built connecting medical office buildings and rented space at attractive rates for physicians' offices, on the premise that physicians will admit to the hospital most convenient to their offices. In any case, physicians are a major focus of marketing efforts.

A second market for the hospital in the traditional industry structure is the community-at-large. Since 1975, hospitals have targeted their advertising efforts at building name recognition within the community for the facility and its programs. The rationale for this strategy is that patients may ask their physicians to refer them to a specific hospital, or they may self-select the facility when they need medical treatment.

The second level of this chart involves physicians and their marketing focus, represented by the dotted lines. Here, too, there have been two markets—other physicians and the community-at-large. Specialists focus their efforts on generating referrals from primary care physicians, although in some specialties, such as plastic surgery and dermatology, it's common to see direct appeals to the community-at-large through advertisements. Primary care physicians have historically attracted new patients in the community either through word-of-mouth, or through more formal communication strategies including advertisements or detailed telephone directory listings. This type of market structure is very similar to that faced by consumer product companies. That is, the decision to buy the service is typically made by one individual or a small group of individuals. A physician decides to admit to a particular hospital, or a family decides to become regular patients at a particular medical clinic. In this type of consumer market, mass communication is vital since there are so many people within the community who could, at any point of time, avail themselves of the medical provider's service. Similarly for the specialist, there are always a large number of primary care physicians who could refer patients to them. The comfort of this world knows that individual buyers represent only their own volume of business.

This is a somewhat simplified but macro view of the traditional health care market structure that has existed for many years, and still does in communities with little managed care or little pressure from employers to control health care costs. This world, however, is rapidly disappearing. The health care marketplace of the next decade will be defined as more of an industrial marketplace.

The Evolving Industry Structure

Today's health care marketplace is evolving in a slightly different way as seen in FIGURE 1-10. Many hospitals have aligned closely with physicians and specialists in integrated systems. In Boston, Massachusetts, one large system is Partners, formed in 1994 by the

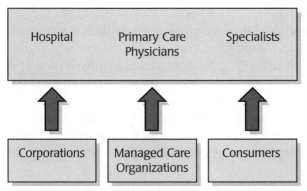

FIGURE 1-10 Evolving Health Care Marketplace

integration of the Brigham and Women's Hospital and Massachusetts General Hospital; affiliated with this organization is Partners Community Healthcare, Inc., representing 1000 internists, pediatricians, and family physicians and over 3500 specialists. Partners would represent the top box in Figure 1-10. At the new level of the figure are corporations, MCOs, and increasingly the community at large. Companies are continuously looking to control the cost of health care. In a 2001 Harris Interactive Poll of 304 human resource directors and 100 health plan managers, 59 percent reported that their health care costs are out of control.[23] Some companies are becoming directly involved in the provision of care. Quad/Graphics, one of the U.S.'s largest printing companies, provides most of its own medical care for its 12,000 employees. Beginning in 1990, it has brought most of its primary care in-house as a way to control cost. Perdue Farms, Sprint Corporation, and Pitney Bowes are also doing the same. Pitney Bowes runs it own clinic with specialists such as podiatrists and neurologists. Thus, the evolving market in the next few years may well see the corporate box loom larger or be a direct contractor or even provider of care, making this chart look far different in another edition of this book.

A second major group represented in this figure is comprised of the MCOs. As will be discussed in Chapter 3, the five largest plans (Wellpoint, The Blues, Cigna, Aetna, and United) control the bulk of commercially insured patients in the United States. As a result these MCOs can wield significant power in negotiation of contractual rates with hospitals, physicians, and ambulatory centers.

Finally, there are consumers. A significant evolving change for consumers is the growing movement toward **health savings accounts**. These plans are designed to force people to make economic trade-offs between consuming more health care services with the opportunity to accumulate tax-free dollars that are unspent in an account designated for health care. The purpose of these plans is to make individuals more sensitive to avoid unnecessary care and hopefully make them "smarter shoppers." In the same regard, the providers may be forced to be more responsive to customers with quality service and to provide proof of such quality. One forecast predicts as many as 25% of all commercially insured people are likely to enroll in such plans by 2009.[24]

These changes carry tremendous marketing implications. The hospital is still at the top of this evolving health care marketplace, but is now joined by physicians. It is one organizational entity that can bring to bear all the necessary resources to meet the health care needs of the community. In a sense, this box can be viewed as the integrated delivery system, representing the hard assets (inpatient beds, surgery centers, laboratory, rehabilitation facility, and long-term care beds), and the personnel (skilled clinicians) that can deliver the expertise, the appropriate technologies, and the setting for needed care.

At the next level are now three major buying entities or customers; companies, MCOs, and, with the emergence of health savings accounts, individuals. The consolidated MCOs represent a powerful buying constituency. Corporations also represent a price sensitive group that in some markets is deciding to take over the provision of care or shift that cost to employees. And, ultimately the end user (the patient) exists. For many years, this entity has been shielded from the cost of that care. Now, increasingly, as will be discussed more in Chapter 3, this consumer is aging. However, access to more information sources (e.g., the Internet) might allow easier shopping for price and quality to access the best, most cost-responsive, health care provider to meet the individual needs of each customer.

From a marketing perspective, the implications of this restructuring are dramatic. While the traditional health care structure was a consumer market with a large number of potential buyers (physicians who could use the facility or patients who could access the hospital), this new structure has some of these elements as consumers return with their health savings accounts. However, there are also elements of an industrial market in dealing with the large, powerful buyers like Aetna or Cigna or a Pitney Bowes or Toyota that may decide to open their own clinic. The tactics, concepts, and strategies discussed in the following chapters are critical to respond to one of the most dynamic industries that exist—health care.

■ Conclusions

Marketing has evolved over the past 30 years in health care. Originally it was viewed with great derision as little more than advertising. The narrow perspective of marketing as only advertising minimizes its contribution. Marketing really brings with it an external perspective that adds a key value in organizational planning. For marketing to be successful, however, the organization must feel a need to be market responsive, have the capacity to respond, have a clear vision, and have actionable steps. In recent years, there has even been a dramatic paradigm shift within marketing from a simple focus of individual transaction and the gaining of market share to the retention of customers and the building of loyalty. This paradigm shift has significant implications within the organization in terms of structure and for the employees. Finally, there is also a significant marketplace evolution occurring. While consolidation among managed care plans has created large, powerful buyers who must be responded to, companies are also being more proactive in dealing with costs by either directly offering medical care or shifting it to employees. Consumers will be returning as direct buyers with health savings accounts.

■ Key Terms

Marketing
Marketing Research
Four Ps
Marketing Mix
Product
Price
Place
Promotion
Need
Want

Marketing Orientation
Differential Advantage
Stakeholders
Environment
Target Market
Product-Oriented Organization
Strategic Business Units
Market-Oriented Organization
Health Savings Accounts

■ Chapter Summary

1. Marketing is a process that involves planning and execution of the four marketing mix variables: product, price, place, and promotion.
2. Effective marketing for health care organizations involves the recognition of multiple customers or markets who often have a diverse array of needs and wants.
3. A nonmarket-based approach to planning is one in which the conception of the service begins internally within the organization. Marketing-based planning is an external-to-internal process.
4. The strategic marketing process must consider the broad macro environment consisting of stakeholders, environmental factors, and society at large.
5. Health care marketing planning requires identification of the target market, which may differ from the organization's present customer base.
6. In a product-oriented organization, services are managed as separate profit centers, or strategic business units.
7. In a market-oriented organizational structure, major markets or customer groups are the focus.
8. Marketing success has four prerequisites: pressure, capacity, vision, and actionable steps.

9. The marketing paradigm is shifting from a transactional focus to a customer retention strategy.
10. The structure of the health care industry is evolving. There are three main customers: corporations, MCOs, and, with new health insurance options like health savings accounts, consumers.

■ Chapter Problems

1. Several prerequisites are necessary for marketing to occur. Identify each prerequisite in the following examples: (a) a politician running for political office, (b) a consumer seeking physical therapy, (c) a company choosing health coverage for its employees.
2. At a recent hospital planning meeting, the marketing director reports on consumer interest in a women's health center. Hearing strong interest, the planning committee endorses the concept. A group of clinicians is charged with developing the program. Upon introduction, market response does not meet expectations. A senior physician was heard to complain, "What went wrong? We did the survey." Explain the possible reasons for this program's failure.
3. An orthopedic group practice has decided to develop a pediatric sports medicine program. Identify potential target markets for this new service.
4. In developing the new pediatric sports medicine program (described above in question 3), what are some of the uncontrollable environmental factors to consider?
5. A major concern for many health care professionals is the belief that marketing "creates" needs. Explain the complexity of this issue.
6. After reviewing the volume of subscribers to the managed care plan, the executive director is dismayed. Projected enrollment is far below the forecasted level for the targeted time period. A decision is made to hire additional salespeople to market the plan more aggressively. Explain the inconsistencies between this decision and an evolutionary marketing perspective.
7. Explain the difference between existing customers, target markets, and stakeholders for an acute-care community hospital.

■ Notes

1. Peter D. Bennett, ed., *Dictionary of Marketing Terms*, 2nd ed. (Chicago: American Marketing Association, 1995).
2. P. Kotler and S. J. Levy, "Broadening the Concept of Marketing," *Journal of Marketing* 33, no. 1 (1969): 10–15.
3. This conceptualization of the four Ps was first proposed by J. McCarthy, *Basic Marketing: A Managerial Approach* (Homewood, IL: Richard D. Irwin, Inc., 1960).

4. Lee Hawkins, Jr., "GM Plans to Cut Salaried Staff: Overhaul Looms," *The Wall Street Journal* (March 21, 2005), A1, A6.

5. Gina Kolata and Reed Abelson, "A Bonus for Health Payable to the Doctor," *The New York Times* (April 15, 2005), C1, C2.

6. *Webster's New World Dictionary*, 3rd college ed. (New York: Simon and Schuster, 1994), 906.

7. Ibid., 1504.

8. K. Pallarito, "State Legislatures Enter Debate on Mom, Newborn Hospital Stays," *Modern Healthcare* 25, no. 24 (1995): 22.

9. R. F. Keith, "The Marketing Revolution," *Journal of Marketing* 24, no. 3 (January 1960): 36.

10. Ibid.

11. E. N. Berkowitz and W. Flexner, "The Market for Health Services: Is There a Non-traditional Consumer?," *Journal of Health Care Marketing* 1, no. 1 (Winter 1980–81): 25–34.

12. J. Narver and S. Slater, "The Effect of a Market Orientation on Business Profitability," *Journal of Marketing* 53, no. 4 (October 1990): 20–22.

13. This discussion is based on E. N. Berkowitz, "Marketing as a Necessary Function in Health Care Management: A Philosophical Approach," in *The Physician Executive*, ed. W. Curry (Tampa, FL: American College of Physician Executives, 1994), 221–228.

14. W. A. Flexner and E. N. Berkowitz, "Marketing Research in Health Services Planning," *Public Health Reports* 94, no. 6 (November–December 1979): 503–513.

15. Overweight and obesity: Obesity trends: U.S. obesity trends 1985–2003, Centers for Disease Control and Prevention (http://www.cdc.gov/nccdphp/dnpa/obesity/trend/maps/).

16. Mark Hagland, "Hospital Obesity Programs: Growth Potential and Controversy Meet in a Booming Service Line," *COR Healthcare Market Strategist* 5, no. 12 (December 2004): 1, 14.

17. L. Kertesz, "California-based Sharp Taps Mexican Market," *Modern Healthcare* 24, no. 35 (1994): 28.

18. E. M. Robertson, "Product Line Management Focuses on the Customer," *Health Care Competition Week* 8, no. 23 (1991): 1–2.

19. S. L. Diamond and E. N. Berkowitz, "Effective Marketing: A Road Map for Health Care Providers," *The Journal of Medical Practice Management* 5, no. 3 (Winter 1990): 197–204.

20. S. Powills, "Hospitals Calling a Marketing Time-out," *Hospitals* 60, no. 11 (June 5, 1986): 50–55.

21. Dennis C. McCarthy, *The Loyalty Link* (New York: John Wiley and Sons, 1997).

22. This discussion is drawn from an unpublished working paper, E. N. Berkowitz and M. Guthrie, "The New Health Care Paradigm" (November 1994).

23. "As Corporate Concerns about Health Care Costs Continue to Rise, Many Employers Plan to Shift More Costs to their Employees," Health Care News, *Harris Interactive* 1, no. 29, (October 10, 2001) (http://www.harrisinteractive.com/news/newsletters_healthcare.asp).

24. Paul D. Mango and Vivian E. Riefberg, "Health Savings Account: Making Patients Better Consumers," *The McKinsey Quarterly* (January 2005).

Marketing Strategy

■ Strategic Planning Process

In order to respond to the opportunities and challenges of the marketplace, most organizations engage in a process of strategic planning. **Strategic planning** has been defined as a process that describes the direction an organization will pursue within its chosen environment and guides the allocation of resources and efforts.[1] The strategic planning process is shown in FIGURE 2-1 as containing four steps. It is within the context of this strategic plan that the functional areas of marketing, finance, human resources, and operations develop their own plans, as shown in FIGURE 2-2.

To develop an effective strategic plan, an organization must first define its mission. Second, it must conduct a situational assessment of the threats and opportunities to which the organization can respond in light of its mission. At this stage, the organization must also assess its own distinctive competencies. Last, the organization must establish a set of priorities based on organizational objectives that align with the mission. Once these steps have been taken, the organization can then determine which strategies to pursue when competing in the broader market.

Defining the Organizational Mission

Organizational mission refers to the organization's fundamental purpose for existing, defining who the organization is, its values, and the customers it wishes to serve.

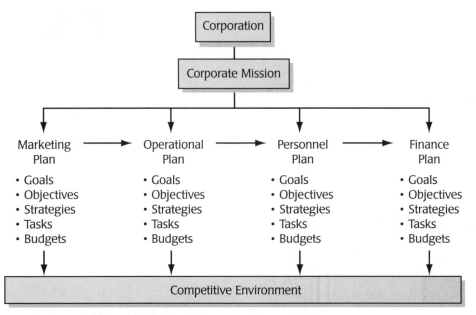

FIGURE 2-1 The Strategic Planning Process

Source: Steven G. Hillestad and Eric N. Berkowitz, *Health Care Marketing Plans: From Strategy to Action*, 1991: Jones and Bartlett Publishers, Sudbury, MA. www.jbpub.com. Reprinted with permission.

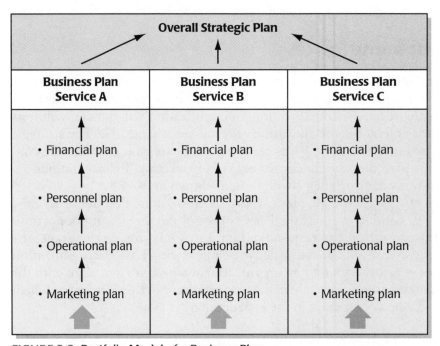

FIGURE 2-2 Portfolio Model of a Business Plan

Source: Steven G. Hillestad and Eric N. Berkowitz, *Health Care Marketing Plans: From Strategy to Action*, 2004: Jones and Bartlett Publishers, Sudbury, MA. www.jbpub.com. Reprinted with permission.

Mission statements are established to set the tone for the organization and provide the management with a purposely broad set of directions for how it should develop further business strategies. EXHIBIT 2-1 shows two alternative mission statements: one

Exhibit 2-1

Commonwealth Orthopaedics & Rehabilitation, PC

Mission Statement

Commonwealth Orthopaedics & Rehabilitation, PC, an orthopaedic surgery group practice, provides comprehensive, high quality, cost effective care to patients with injuries and diseases of the musculoskeletal system.

We act with the best interest of our patients in mind, strive to provide the best medical care available, and treat them with respect, compassion, and confidentiality.

We attempt to minimize the inconveniences of treatment to our patients by providing prompt courteous service. To this end, we offer, as part of our practice, outpatient ambulatory surgery and physical therapy.

We promote quality medical care in the community through participation in hospital medical staff functions, benchmarking with similar organizations and participation with local and national medical societies. We participate with the local medical educational institutions to prepare new healthcare professionals for our community.

We keep the health and well-being of our patient as our top priority.

Source: Mission Statement for Commonwealth Orthopaedics & Rehabilitation from website www.c-o-r.com. Reprinted by permission.

SwedishAmerican

Our Mission

Through excellence in healthcare, and compassionate service, we care for our community.

Our Vision

Our vision is to develop a fully integrated healthcare delivery network that will continuously set the standard for quality of care and service, accept responsibility for building a healthier population, provide regional access, improve resource utilization through collaboration with key stakeholders, and manage patient care and our resources in such a way that we create value for our patients and return an investment to our community. SwedishAmerican recognizes its responsibility to all the people of our community, regardless of their ability to pay for care. Within the capacity of our financial and medical resources, we pledge to use the resources available to us to foster our charitable, medical, and educational purposes.

Our Values

SwedishAmerican believes that its success in fulfilling its mission and vision is highly dependent upon and a product of the culture and core values of its people and its heritage. Those values are respect for people; care for patients and families; respect for the healing professions; commitment to quality, service, creativity, and innovation; empowerment and teamwork; and financial accountability.

Source: Mission statement of SwedishAmerican Health System from www.swedishamerican.org. Used by permission.

for Commonwealth Orthopaedics & Rehabilitation PC of Alexandria, Virginia; and the other for SwedishAmerican Health System of Rockford, Illinois. These two mission statements reflect the significant changes that health care providers face today. Commonwealth Ortho is one of the largest orthopedic groups in the United States today. As its mission statement reflects, while narrowly defined within the area of orthopedics and rehabilitation, this group has great depth in its specialization. Moreover, it is responding to the challenges (to be discussed further in Chapter 3) of benchmarking to quality as well as ongoing education. SwedishAmerican is a large health system, with Swedish Hospital as its major organization, that is focused on establishing an integrated health system. SwedishAmerican Health System has a partnership between the physicians on the medical staff and the hospital.

Organizations can establish missions that are either broad or narrow, but it's important to establish a mission with the greatest likelihood of success in a competitive marketplace. FIGURE 2-3 shows the range of possibilities regarding a health mission statement.

An effective mission statement should clearly articulate most of the following components:

1. The basic product or service, primary market, and technology to be used in delivering the product or service
2. Organizational goals, such as growth, profitability, stability, or survival, stated in a strategic sense
3. Organizational philosophy—the code of behavior that guides the organization's operation

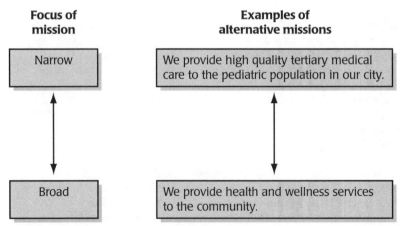

Focus of mission

Narrow

Broad

Examples of alternative missions

We provide high quality tertiary medical care to the pediatric population in our city.

We provide health and wellness services to the community.

FIGURE 2-3 Strategic Mission Options

Source: Steven G. Hillestad and Eric N. Berkowitz, *Health Care Marketing Plans: From Strategy to Action*, 2004: Jones and Bartlett Publishers, Sudbury, MA. www.jbpub.com. Reprinted with permission.

4. Organizational self-concept—a self-evaluation based on a realistic determination of its strengths and weaknesses
5. Public image—how those outside the organization view the particular entity[2]

Essential to a successful mission statement is the recognition of what the business is and what the customer wants. Levitt described the marketing myopia of some organizations whose definition of their mission failed to recognize the threats and opportunities in the external marketplace. For many years, the railroads described themselves as "railroad companies." In fact, the marketplace was not so interested in railroads as much as it was in transporting goods quickly and saving time. This led other firms such as air transportation companies to supplant the service that could have been provided by a diversified "railroad" company.[3] The health care industry has suffered a great deal of myopia in the past regarding organizational mission. A modern health care organization today must decide whether providing high-quality medicine or improving societal or community health status should be the organizational goal. If community wellness becomes the mission, this might lead to the recognition of different trends in the environment and necessitate different responses from the organization. In this greater recognition of health care as opposed to medical care, Riverside Health System in Newport News, Virginia has broadened its focus. Once a four-hospital, nonprofit system, Riverside now also operates five profitable wellness centers. And Springfield Hospital (part of the Crozer-Keystone Health System, of Media, Pennsylvania) built a 170,000-square-foot athletic club called the Healthplex Sport Club in 1996. It is a state-of-the art health and fitness facility and helps transitional patients from the hospital with a variety of wellness programs (http://www.crozer.org/CKHS/Left+Nav/Healthplex/Wellness/).[4,5]

Situational Assessment

The **situational assessment** is an analysis of the organization's environment and of the organization itself. This process is referred to as the **SWOT analysis** (so named because it examines the Strengths and Weaknesses of the organization, as well as the Opportunities and Threats relevant to the organization's future strategy).

One aspect of this SWOT analysis involves assessing the environment. It is at this stage in the process where the organization must consider the economic, competitive, regulatory, social, and technological changes occurring in the marketplace. Scanning these dimensions of the environment yields insight into the opportunities and threats that exist, to which the organization must respond in its overall strategic plan and in subsequent functional plans.

In reviewing each of these environmental areas, the organization must ask: (1) What are the changes and trends? (2) How will these changes affect the organization's businesses? and (3) What opportunities do these changes present? While these changes will be discussed in greater detail in Chapter 3, consider one demographic change—the aging marketplace—and its impact on company strategy.

For many years, the Gerber Products Company of Fremont, Michigan, defined its business as "Babies are our business, our only business." This was a great mission in the early 1950s when the United States was witnessing a rapidly growing birthrate. An aging population, however, as shown in FIGURE 2-4, might necessitate some revisions to that mission. A review of this environmental position might lead Gerber to make some basic strategic changes.

As the population ages, Gerber must consider this trend and decide what implications it holds for its business. In what ways must the company respond, and what opportunities does it present? Does an aging population suggest a need for food that is easily digestible, such as baby food? Will an aging population result in a greater number of widows and widowers who will avail themselves of easily prepared food in single-sized servings? What impact will this trend of an aging population have on the future growth of a health care organization whose strength lies in pediatrics?

One other example of demographic change—the competition—highlights its role in corporate marketing strategy. Analyzing business opportunities in the 1990s, a Wisconsin health insurance firm found a market that was a direct result of the waiting time for elective surgery in Canada. Wisconsin-based American Medical Services

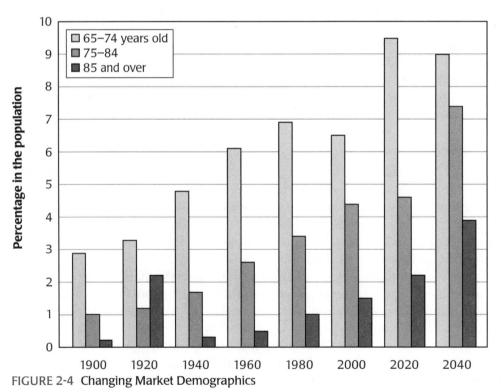

FIGURE 2-4 Changing Market Demographics

Source: Administration on Aging. Washington, DC: U.S. Department of Health and Human Services.
http://www.aoa.gov/prof/Statistics/online_stat_data/AgePop2050.asp.

offered a policy that covers the cost of travel for Canadians treated in the United States. The $450 policy pays part of the patient's travel costs, plus food and lodging for a family member. Coverage begins once the policyholder has to wait more than 45 days for the surgery in Canada.[6] With this situational analysis, it is important for the organization to consider the barriers that exist in the marketplace. In analyzing any business plan, an organization must consider the **barriers to entry**, which are the conditions that a company must overcome in order to pursue a business opportunity. Barriers to entry might be regulatory, technological, financial, or strategic. In health care, for example, the regulatory process in many states has provided a strong barrier to entry. To enter certain businesses that require the addition of resources and capital allocations, hospitals must obtain various forms of regulatory approval.

One of the fastest growing segments of the health care industry is subacute care. This level of care is designed for those patients who are sufficiently stabilized to no longer require acute-care services. Subacute care can be provided in a free-standing nursing home or a skilled nursing facility, rather than a hospital. Since these nursing facilities face fewer regulatory hurdles than hospitals do, the barriers to entry are often low. Hence, this new segment of health care is projected to grow from a $1 billion business in 1994 to a $10 billion segment of the industry by the year 2000.[7] Acquisition of some technology might be a barrier to entry, or the cost of such technological acquisition could represent an effective barrier. Image alone can also be an effective strategic barrier. A competitor may have established a strong reputation and marketplace position regarding a particular service that poses a real challenge—and forms a barrier—for a competing health care organization wanting to enter the market for that service.

In the same regard, the organization must also consider the **barriers to exit,** or the costs of leaving a particular business line. In health care, many services require a large commitment of fixed assets or specialized personnel. This fact alone can make it difficult to move away from a business in spite of the environmental overview provided. This, in fact, might be a weakness highlighted with a SWOT analysis.

For the SWOT to be successful, an organization must be able and willing to do the following:

1. Turn the focus of the SWOT analysis away from the organization's products and toward its business processes that meet customer needs.
2. Capitalize on its strengths by delivering better value to customers than the competition.
3. Turn any weakness into strength by investing strategically in key areas.[8]

These steps serve as a catalyst for corporate strategy, as suggested by FIGURE 2-5. As seen in this representation, strengths that have no matching opportunities are of little value. A liability exists when a weakness is matched by a competitive threat. Capabilities to capitalize on marketplace potential exist when one can match organizational strengths to market opportunities.

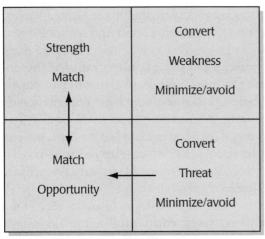

Strength Match	Convert Weakness Minimize/avoid
Match Opportunity	Convert Threat Minimize/avoid

FIGURE 2-5 Four-Cell SWOT Matrix

Differential Advantage

Within this situational analysis, an organization must also consider its own strengths and weaknesses. At this point, an organization should assess what it does that is better than the competition and gives it a differential advantage, which has been defined in Chapter 1 as the incremental benefits of a product relative to competing products that are important to the buyer as perceived by the buyer. This analysis and specification of the differential advantage are based on the core competencies of the firm that are critical to success.[9]

Criteria for a Good Differential Advantage

There are four important criteria that are the hallmarks of a good differential advantage.

1. *Importance*—First a differential advantage must be important to the buyer. There are myriad processes and elements that are essential in the delivery of high quality care, but if they are not important to the buyer it is not a differential advantage. For example, one hospital may have a more stringent quality assurance or credentialing procedure than another. The clinicians may recognize that this is a key in providing a certain standard of care, but again, if the buyer does not value or understand the importance, it cannot be a differential advantage.
2. *Perceived*—A second hallmark is related closely to the first. A good differential advantage must be perceived by the buyer. Consider the previous example concerning the credentialing procedure. If the buyer, in this case the patient, does not perceive the value of a more stringent credentialing procedure, it cannot be used as a point of difference from the competition. Herein lies an important

role of promotion from a marketing perspective. When an organization has elements that it considers the market would view as important, the requirement then is to ensure that these advantages are perceived by the buyer.

3. *Uniqueness*—A third important component of a differential advantage is that it must be unique from other providers. This aspect of uniqueness is particularly challenging in health care. Often a medical group might state that it perceives its differential advantage to be that all the physicians in the group are board eligible or board certified. However, when an analysis is done of the second closest competing medical group, this group also has all physicians who are board certified or board eligible. They both have the board eligibility aspect as strength, but because it is not unique, there is not an operational differential advantage.

4. *Sustainable*—It is the dimension of uniqueness that leads to the fourth major criterion of a good differential advantage—sustainable. When seeking a differential advantage, it is essential that the organization consider focusing on aspects of the operation or business that are sustainable for some period of time. To a large degree it is this last criterion that has often led to the "marketing" function receiving the greatest criticism from clinicians.

Too often, as was noted in Chapter 1, marketing has been defined as advertising. Thus organizations often get involved in an ad war game. One hospital places a billboard on the highway touting its concern for patients by saying "We care!" Soon, the second hospital in the community runs a similar billboard proclaiming, "We care more!" The first hospital retaliates "Not as much as us!" And, both competitors become involved in a never-ending advertising war that has limited sustainability. While there are few things that can be done in most service businesses that will be totally immune from competitor imitation, the need is to focus on the most difficult challenges in service delivery. Easy improvements like valet parking for elderly patients should be considered part of ongoing process improvement; it is the more difficult operational challenges that can lead to a differential advantage that has some protection from quick competitive imitation. In health care, few examples may be more tangible than something like electronic medical records. The Veteran's Administration was one of the first health care organizations and systems to implement such an approach. These electronic medical record systems are expensive. The cost prevents many smaller organizations from easily copying. And, the second real hurdle for implementation is cultural, training clinicians to use them and input the data properly. But, if one organization can get this accomplished, it will be a significant amount of time, and thus sustainability, before other competitors also provide such a program.

Sources of a Differential Advantage

There are three areas in which an organization can seek a differential advantage: (1) product, (2) market, or (3) cost.[10] As shown in Table 2-1, a product-based

Table 2-1	Sources of a Differential Advantage		
Product-based	**Market-based**	**Cost-based**	
Technological capability	Targeted segment	Operational efficiency	
Clinical expertise	Narrow product line	Expense control	
Name/image	Geographic focus	Experience curve	
Distribution network		Government subsidy	

differential advantage is one in which the company has a unique technological capability or clinical expertise that allows it to establish a competitive position. In health care, the establishment of a product-based differential advantage is difficult. To some extent one might argue that M.D. Anderson in Houston has a differential advantage that is product based with its specialized focus in cancer care. The pace of technological change is such that the advantage goes to competitors who have the resources to acquire a new technology. A distribution network that improves access, however, can be a differential advantage.

A market-based differential advantage is available to those who focus on a particular market segment. For example, in the Boston metropolitan area, Children's Hospital has been recognized as a leader in pediatric care. While other competitors also provide pediatric service, the differential advantage rests with Children's Hospital and its narrow market focus.

The third area in which to establish a differential advantage is cost. An organization that is highly efficient, either through the use of technology or with tight management control of expenses, can achieve this advantage. Increasingly in health care, as the marketplace focuses on the cost of care, a cost differential advantage is becoming a strong competitive position. Kaiser Permanente has traditionally tried to be a health care organization that is efficient and priced to be a cost advantage relative to competing managed care alternatives. The challenge for the organization, however, is that it must strive for large market share in order to receive the margin lost from a cost leadership position. Establishing a differential position in this area is closely tied to the pricing strategies the organization pursues in the market. This issue is discussed in greater detail in Chapter 9.

Each of these respective sources of differential advantage has its own set of inherent weaknesses. In a product-based approach, the challenge is to maintain the product advantage in the face of competitors who take a low-cost position. As low-cost providers enter the market, the consumers must still value the product differential advantage. There is also the risk that the marketplace changes its preferences and no longer values the product's differential advantage. A more realistic possibility is that there are a large number of imitators, which minimizes any perceived differentiation in product.

For a market-based position, competitors might target smaller groups or submarkets to establish a differential advantage. Or, cost factors could eliminate an advantageous position within the market. In health care, the cost position may be the most difficult to maintain. Technology has a dramatic impact on the cost position of any provider. Exclusive focus on cost can also lead to a failure to recognize market needs or new service opportunities that might present themselves.

■ The Visible Value Challenge of a Differential Advantage

Ultimately, a differential advantage must be important to the buyer—the first criterion cited in the previous discussion. Organizations then must recognize that in marketing there is a related concept of visible and invisible value. **Invisible value** is the value that the producer builds into its product or service. **Visible value** is the value that is seen by the customer. In most industries, organizations can typically charge only for visible value.

Consider the challenge for some businesses outside of health care. A hotel chain might proclaim that it provides clean hotel rooms. Unfortunately, cleanliness is an attribute that is often only noted in the absence thereof. How then does the hotel chain make its cleanliness advantage a visible value? Notes are placed in the room from the chambermaid who cleaned the area, lids are on top of the glasses in the bathroom, toilet tissue is folded, and a paper strip is placed across the toilet seat. Consider the challenge for Intel, the maker of processing chips. How many people would recognize one if they saw it? How could you differentiate it from others? Why doesn't Intel place a little sticker on its computers that proclaims "Intel inside"?

So, too, the issue of visible value remains for health care organizations. How does a health care facility demonstrate its staff is up-to-date in training? Is there a display board in the lobby indicating the number of continuing medical education hours the nurses and physicians have obtained at a particular point in the year? Are there pamphlets with biographical sketches of the staff in a notebook in the lobby as well as on the Webpage? Making value visible is essential in delivering a differential advantage that will affect buyer preference.

The Cleveland Clinic has begun to try to make its quality advantage visible to the customer both on its Web page as well as in its facility. EXHIBIT 2-2 is the portal to comprehensive data on all clinical services and quality information at the Cleveland Clinic. The Web site for the Cleveland Clinic Foundation also provides further information on its patient satisfaction scores (http://www.clevelandclinic.org/quality/). This site provides explanations about the meaning of board certification, provides suggestions for how the patient should judge quality, and shows how the Cleveland Clinic compares to other similar facilities. This effort is a major step in making the clinical value of this facility visible to the market.

Exhibit 2-2   The Cleveland Clinic

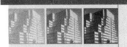

Quality
Measures

THE CLEVELAND CLINIC

‡| Select a Department/Disease

HOW WE MEASURE UP

:: At a Glance Measures

:: Innovations

:: Outcomes
  (FOR PHYSICIANS / PROVIDERS)

:: Quality Indicators

CHOOSING QUALITY

:: About This Site

:: How to Choose

:: Web Site Survey

:: Why Patients Choose
   The Cleveland Clinic

ADDITIONAL INFORMATION

:: Appointments

:: Contact Us

:: e-Cleveland Clinic

:: Health Information

:: Patient Safety Video

:: Physician Directory

:: The Quality Institute

Search
Quality Measures

Search
The Cleveland Clinic

:: AT A GLANCE MEASURES

How much experience your doctors and hospital have with respect to treating a certain condition is a good indicator of how well you'll do under their care, particularly when you need sophisticated care for a complex condition. According to a report published in the *Annals of Internal Medicine* (Sept. 17, 2002), the majority of studies find a lower patient mortality (death) rate for a given procedure when the hospital or physician has high-volume experience performing that procedure. In other words, the more experience, the better the results.

Remember, though, that experience is just one quality indicator you should use to judge if a doctor or hospital is better for you than another. We recommend you combine information from more than one quality indicator. For example, you can be confident of your choice if you find that the hospital specializes in treating your condition and reports a low mortality rate, and that the physician is certified and has extensive training and experience in treating your condition.

***U.S. News & World Report* Ranks The Cleveland Clinic 4th Among the Nation's 6,000+ Hospitals in 2005**
The Cleveland Clinic is once again ranked No. 4 in the United States according *U.S. News & World Report*. Overall, the magazine ranked 16 specialties at the Clinic among the nation's best and deemed 11 of those specialties to be among the Top 10 in the United States. *U.S. News & World Report* ranked The Cleveland Clinic Heart Center as the nation's No. 1 cardiac care center for the 11th year in a row. Both the Glickman Urological Institute and the Digestive Disease Center ranked number two in the nation. Other specialties ranking in the Top 10 were ear, nose and throat; gynecology; endocrinology; kidney disease; neurology and neurosurgery; orthopaedics; rheumatology; and pulmonology. Geriatrics, ophthalmology, psychiatry and rehabilitation were also ranked nationally. In addition, the Cleveland Clinic Taussig Cancer Center is Ohio's highest-ranked cancer center, according to the "America's Best Hospitals" survey. The Taussig Cancer Center leapt from No. 30 to No. 14 in the magazine's annual rankings, moving ahead of all other cancer centers in Ohio.

In other national recognition:

• The Cleveland Clinic was named one of the nation's top 100 hospitals by health data consultants Solucient in a survey that recognized medical and operations excellence.

• 81 Cleveland Clinic physicians were named in the 2005 edition of "America's Top Doctors." The Cleveland Clinic was one of the best-represented hospitals in the directory.

• 195 Cleveland Clinic physicians were named in "The Best Doctors in America," a survey of 30,000 physicians nationwide. This was the most of any hospital in Ohio and among the largest number of any hospital in America.

The Cleveland Clinic Foundation.

Organizational Objectives

The third step in the strategic planning process is the establishment of **organizational objectives,** which are the long-term performance targets the company hopes to achieve. These might include sales, market leadership position, or market share terms. In setting these objectives, it is valuable that, as much as possible, they be stated quantitatively and in realistic terms. General Electric Company (GE), for example, had an organizational objective that related to market share. The company would operate only in business lines in which it could be the number one or number two company in terms of market share. Similarly, a national managed care organization (HMO) might set an organizational objective to compete only in market areas in which it could be the dominant plan in terms of number of subscribers. The organizational objectives set the broad targets for the operating units.

■ Organizational Strategy

Once it has progressed through the previous planning stages, the organization can then begin to formulate its broad strategies. For any organization, these can include either *growth market strategies* or *consolidation strategies*. With growth market strategies, the organization is attempting to gain more sales from an existing business line or attempting to penetrate new markets. An alternative growth perspective might lead the firm to develop a new product or service that can generate sales from existing customers to new buyers. An organization that implements a consolidation strategy is paring either the services it offers or the markets it serves.

Growth Market Strategies

EXHIBIT 2-3 shows four broad strategies that can guide an organization's growth; they reflect the internal organization and the external market conditions. Internal capabilities and services are represented by the product dimension. External market factors, a reflection of the situational analysis, are represented by the market dimension. Using this product/market matrix as a guide, there are four broad strategies to consider.[11]

Market Penetration

The **market penetration** strategy involves increasing the sales of present products and services in present markets. This a useful approach when the current market is strong and growing. Fulfillment of this strategy might involve attracting new customers or converting nonusers. For example, a managed care product might attempt to win over subscribers from a competing health plan, or to convert fee-for-service customers to a prepaid plan. A health care organization also might attempt to increase its business from existing customers. A managed care plan might try to increase the number of employee subscribers within corporations and other businesses that offer the plan to their employees.

Exhibit 2-3   Product/Market Opportunity Matrix

Product/Market	Present	New
Present	Market penetration strategy	Market development strategy
New	Product development strategy	Diversification strategy

Source: Reprinted by permission of *Harvard Business Review*. Product/Market Opportunity Matrix from "Strategies for Diversification" by H. I. Ansoff, September–October 1957. Copyright © 1957 by the Harvard Business School Publishing Corporation; all rights reserved.

Another way to fulfill a market penetration strategy is through more intensive efforts to distribute the product or service, or through more aggressive promotion. Or, the managed care plan can price itself more competitively to attract more customers.

Market Development

A second growth strategy involves initiating sales of existing products and services in new markets, a **market development** strategy. This strategy is followed when existing markets are stagnant in terms of growth and market share gains would be difficult to achieve because of strong, dominant competitors. This approach is followed by relocating a service to regions where it has not previously been offered. There are several variations to this strategy.

A health care organization might enter new geographical markets. For example, a hospital in San Antonio, Texas, might establish a clinic in Mexico to attract consumers who might ultimately be referred to the hospital for inpatient tertiary care. Joslin Clinic, renowned for its diabetes treatment and management, undertook a market development strategy by offering its program to other hospitals in New England and then throughout the United States. Now, it is pursuing its strategy globally.

Alternatively, a health plan can follow a market development strategy of appealing to new market segments that it has been unable to attract before. Many HMOs have established senior programs to enroll more elderly subscribers, such as the Harvard Community Health Plan's First Seniority health care plan in Massachusetts.

Product Development

A third organizational growth strategy is **product development**, which involves providing new products to existing markets. In this situation, a health system has a strong customer base and seeks to retain these customers by offering new services or quality improvements. Organizations pursue this strategy to meet changing customer needs, to take advantage of new technologies, or to meet the needs of some specific segment of the market. This situation is becoming increasingly typical in the health care industry. Many well-known organizations that first entered the marketplace as fee-for-service, multi-specialty group practices, such as the Carle Clinic in Champaign-Urbana, Illinois, and the Fallon Clinic in Worcester, Massachusetts, have developed their own managed care products in the form of HMOs. This strategy is a response to changing market conditions, and it provides loyal users with another option for receiving care from member physicians. This strategy is ultimately a reaction to a changing competitive marketplace.

In pursuing this strategy, health care organizations will often engage in **vertical integration,** which involves incorporating related services or products previously developed or offered by others to the marketplace. There are two forms of integration strategies. A health care system can use **backward integration,** which entails becoming its own supplier. Increasingly, for example, hospitals have established their own physician–hospital organization (PHO). These entities offer a managed care product to the market as the PHO accepts risk. SwedishAmerican Health System of Rockford, Illinois, actively pursued risk contracts for its new entity. With **forward integration** a company offers new services or products usually closer to the customer than existing services. Many of these have been previously provided by other intermediaries. PRU-CARE of Orlando has its own providers who staff an HMO at multiple locations in the community. Prudential, which acted solely as an insurance firm, has integrated forward by now providing care directly. Each of these strategies is discussed in greater depth in Chapter 10.

Diversification

The fourth growth strategy, **diversification,** entails developing new products or services for new markets. This strategy is followed when the growth in existing markets is slowing or when environmental changes—be they societal, technological, economic, regulatory, or competitive—make it risky to remain in present markets. The University of Pennsylvania Medical Center (UPMC) finds that the market is nearly saturated in the western Pennsylvania marketplace. Its name is now on 16 hospitals, several cancer centers, and over 400 outpatient sites. In order to look for more opportunities for growth, it is reaching out to new markets by taking a global perspective. In 2004, UPMC opened a 70-bed organ transplant hospital in Palermo, Italy, in partnership with the government. The medical center is also in talks with the governments of Ireland, Saudi Arabia, and the United Arab Emirates, as well as the City of Las Vegas, for similar partnership arrangements.[12] Diversification strategies are currently being followed by innumerable health care providers. Hospitals have diversified into long-term care facilities, influenced by several factors such as reimbursement, utilization, and network referrals. Table 2-2 shows several factors influencing diversification and some of their benefits.

Strategic Alliances

For many organizations, it is often difficult—in terms of resources or for strategic reasons—to enter new markets. In such instances, many companies following a

Table 2-2   Factors Influencing Long-Term Care Diversification

LTC Option	Market Variables	Risk	Reimbursement Climate	Advantages	Disadvantages
Nursing homes	% of elderly in population, affluence of elderly, competition	High (construction or purchase costs required)	Depends on state	Earlier hospital discharge, referral network, ancillary charges, economies of scale	Reimbursement is often low, requires a great deal of attention
Retirement housing, life care, CRCs	Affluence of elderly	High (need good market survey)	Not applicable	Ties residents to hospital	Very costly to build
Domiciliaries, assisted living, personal care	% of elderly in population, affluence of elderly	High because of construction costs	Not applicable	Referrals, ties residents to hospital, economies of scale	Target market is usually small
Home health care	Degree of market saturation	Medium (low capital intensity)	Good	Flexible staffing, referral network	Potential market saturation
Wellness programs, health promotion	Not applicable except to determine if other hospitals are doing this	Low	Not applicable	Good will, referral network	Poor financial return
Outpatient rehabilitation	% of elderly in population, proximity to industries	Medium (purchase of equipment, employment of staff)	Excellent	Referral network, flexible staffing (if existing therapists can be used)	Potential market saturation

Source: From Giardinia, C.W., Fotter, M.D., Shewchuk, R.W., and Hill, D.B., The Case for Diversification into Long-Term Care from *Health Care Management Review,* Vol. 15, No. 1, p. 79, 1990. Used by permission of Lippincott Williams & Wilkins.

diversification strategy have established **strategic alliances** or formal arrangements with other companies to operate in a particular market.[13] Strategic alliances assume many forms. Some strategic alliances involve the establishment of **joint venture businesses**, which are new corporate entities in which both partners hold an equity position. There might be natural strategic alliances—for example, between obstetricians and pediatricians—but one might consider alliances with former competitors. For example, it has been suggested that creative relationships between nurse practitioners and primary care physicians can maximize the use of physician extenders to generate revenue for the practice.[14] Other strategic alliances can simply be formal agreements that give each partner some access to the distinctive strengths of the other firm. JC Penney in Plano, Texas, has formed such an alliance with Presbyterian Health Systems. Penney opened a 6000-square-foot urgent care and occupational medicine facility. The company asked Presbyterian to staff and operate the center with a physician and nurse and to provide medical referrals when necessary.[15]

Hoffman-LaRoche and Millennium Pharmaceutical is a strategic alliance formed in the early 1990s within the pharmaceutical industry. Millennium is a small biotechnology firm that has a differential advantage because of its expertise in genetics research. Hoffman-LaRoche is a large pharmaceutical company that holds a differential advantage in its marketing capabilities and regulatory process knowledge. The two firms have formed a strategic alliance to develop gene-based drugs to treat chronic obesity and adult onset diabetes. In order to enter the Asian market, Sterling Winthrop Inc. of New York, a manufacturer of pharmaceutical preparations, established a strategic alliance with a Chinese partner, Shanghai Melyou Pharmaceutical Company. Marketers at Shanghai Melyou will promote Sterling Winthrop's drugs, but brand managers at Sterling Winthrop will monitor these activities closely to ensure they meet with its worldwide plans.[16]

Consolidation Strategies

Occasionally, when examining marketplace considerations, an organization might establish strategies for **consolidation**, or focusing business on a smaller set of markets, products, or services. There are several ways to accomplish this objective.

Divestment

Selling off a business or product line is called **divestment**. This strategy is often followed when an organization believes there is a weak fit between its major core business and a particular product line. The lack of fit may be due to the management resources required or the result of a product whose market differs from the core market being pursued by the company. Often, divestment is the result of an unsuccessful diversification growth strategy. In the late 1980s, Hospital Corporation of America of Nashville, Tennessee, divested itself of its psychiatric hospital business in order to concentrate on the acute-care business.

Pruning

A second consolidation strategy occurs when a firm **prunes** or reduces the number of products or services it offers to the market. The company continues to serve the market, but does so with a reduced set of products. IBM remains in the personal computer (PC) business. However, in 1984, it decided not to pursue the low-end user and it dropped its junior PC model, which was not well accepted. This approach is useful when certain segments of the market are too costly or too small to service.

Retrenchment

In a **retrenchment** strategy a company decides to withdraw from certain markets. This strategy might be considered the opposite of the market development growth strategy. A clinic might decide to close a primary care satellite in a neighboring community. Organizations follow this kind of strategy when certain market areas do not perform well or meet overall corporate objectives.

Harvesting

A fourth consolidation strategy, **harvesting,** involves gradually withdrawing support from a product until there is little or no market demand. In these instances, an organization continues to support a product, but at a decreasing level. A business would follow this strategy as long as the service had some level of profitability, or had a loyal customer base that generated additional revenues through purchases of other services.

■ Determining Organizational Strategy

Several alternative models have been proposed to help companies develop their organizational strategies. Two well-known approaches are the Boston Consulting Group (BCG) matrix and the GE matrix. Each of these models has received widespread recognition as useful conceptualizations for formulating organizational strategic direction.

The BCG Matrix

BCG, a well-known management consulting firm, developed a strategy based on market growth rate and relative market share to focus company strategies in firms with multiple product lines.[17] FIGURE 2-6 represents the **BCG matrix.** In this model, the underlying assumption is that cash flow and profitability are closely related to sales volume. Products or strategic business units are then placed within this matrix according to their position on two dimensions. **Market growth rate** refers to the rate of sales growth in the market, while **relative market share** is the ratio of a product's share of business within the market compared to that of its largest competitor. This second measure is an indicator of market dominance. If the share equals that of the largest com-

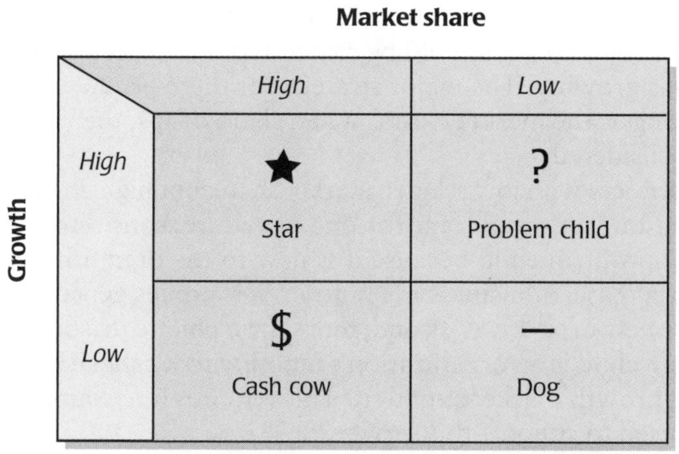

Market share

FIGURE 2-6 The BCG Matrix

Source: Bruce Henderson, *Henderson on Corporate Strategy* (Boston: Abt Books, 1979).

petitor, the measure would be 1.0. An administrator can then classify the organization's product lines into one of these four quadrants.

In examining the position of businesses in this matrix, it is important to consider the issue of control. A company cannot directly control the market growth rate. This rate is determined by uncontrollable, variable environmental forces. For example, pediatrics may be a declining business, but there is little direct control a provider can have over the overall growth rate of the number of children. A company does have direct control of its relative market share, however, which is a reflection of the success of the organization's strategy, particularly its marketing strategy relative to competitors. A company that places a service in the quadrants representing lower share must reexamine its internal strategy and its implementation.

Products and services are represented in the matrix as one of the following: stars, cash cows, problem children, or dogs. *Stars* are products with high market share and high growth rate. An organization is doing well with these products (represented by their high relative market share), and their future potential is still strong as reflected in the high growth rate. From a cash perspective the revenues generated by these business lines should be reinvested back into services that need additional investment in personnel or facilities in order to capitalize on the market growth rate. Growth strategies are the primary focus of products placed within this quadrant.

Cash cows are products that have a high market share but a low growth rate. These might be seen as mature businesses, but this maturity is not due to any controllable factor. Placing a service in the cash cow position means that, even though the market is maturing, a company has been able to retain a strong share position. These businesses typically generate a substantial amount of cash; in fact, they usually represent the greatest source of cash flow. There is no need to invest in new facilities or other fixed assets. Monies from these product lines should be reinvested or redirected into services whose market position is growing. The major strategy for these products focuses on maintaining share as long as the market exists. When share drops, then consolidation strategies might be considered.

Problem children represent services with low relative market share, but high growth rate. A product could be placed into this quadrant for one of two reasons. First, a product might be classified as a problem child because it is new to the organization and has low market share. In that case, a business needs to invest monies generated by cash cows in marketing of the new product. A second, more problematic reason for a product to be labeled a problem child is an organization's inability to establish market dominance in the midst of a growth market situation. This requires a reexamination of the strategy and tactics used to support this service.

Dogs represent those products with low share and low growth. These services typically drain an organization's cash and become targets for consolidation strategy. The simplest recommendation is to drop the product or get out of the market. In health care, however, an organization must often keep one service (such as rehabilitation services) in order to deliver other services (such as orthopedics) to the market. It is important to recognize the dog only because of its resource implications.

The broad nature of the BCG matrix often makes it too limiting for significant strategy formulation. Yet, in health care organizations, it can serve as a valuable conceptual framework to engender strategy discussions. A major source of organizational conflict occurs when everybody views their clinical service in a different market position requiring a different level of resource commitment. The BCG framework is a useful tool for focusing management attention on broad marketplace considerations and for getting participants to discuss the issues of market growth and the requirements for market dominance in a particular clinical setting.

The BCG matrix is also a useful tool for helping a medical organization assess its internal strengths and future direction. Depending on the distribution of services within the matrix, an audit might reveal an organization that needs to redirect resources to generate more new products or services. For example, if a health care organization has a large number of cash cows (60%), a reasonable number of stars (25%), a few dogs (5%), and only 10% problem children, it might indicate that the program directors of mature services have succeeded in keeping the cash within their own operations. Little revenue, therefore, has been redirected to generate new opportunities at the low-share, high-growth potential position. Similarly, a business with a large number of problem children relative to the number of cash cows might need to prioritize which problems it will invest in to gain share. To move a service from the problem child to star position often requires redirecting the marketing mix and infusing financial and management resources in new areas. If too many services are vying for these resources, investment must be prioritized to ensure that at least some services receive the needed support to become successful market competitors.

The GE Matrix

The BCG matrix is limited by the consideration of only two dimensions. Yet, for most products and services, these considerations often require a multidimensional evaluation. Table 2-3 shows the considerations used in the **GE matrix**, a multidimensional model for focusing corporate strategy in organizations with multiple product lines based on the dimensions of market attractiveness and business strength.

Table 2-3	General Electric Business Screen		
	Business Strength		
	Strong	Average	Weak
High	Premium—Invest for Growth: • Provide maximum investment • Diversify worldwide • Consolidate position • Accept moderate near-term profits • Seek to dominate	Selective—Invest for Growth: • Invest heavily in selected segments • Share ceiling • Seek attractive new segments to apply strengths	Protect/Refocus—Selectively Invest for Earnings: • Defend strengths • Refocus to attractive segments • Evaluate industry revitalization • Monitor for harvest or divestment timing • Consider acquisitions
Medium	Challenge—Invest for Growth: • Build selectively on strengths • Define implications of leadership • Avoid vulnerability —fill weaknesses	Prime—Selectively Invest for Earnings: • Segment market • Make contingency plans for vulnerability	Restructure—Harvest or Divest • Provide no unessential commitment • Position for divestment *or* • Shift to more attractive segment
Low	Opportunistic—Selectively Invest for Earnings: • Ride market and maintain overall position • Seek niches, specialization • Seek opportunity to increase strength (for example through acquisition) • Invest at maintenance levels	Opportunistic—Preserve for Harvest: • Act to preserve or boost cash flow • Seek opportunistic sale *or* • Seek opportunistic rationalization to increase strengths • Prune product lines • Minimize investment	Harvest or Divest: • Exit from market or prune product line • Determine timing so as to maximize present value • Concentrate on competitor's cash generators

Source: Reprinted by permission of the publisher from *Strategic Market Planning*, page 88, by B. A. Rausch, © 1982 American Management Association. Published by American Management Association, New York, New York. www.amanet.org.

Market attractiveness is an index comprised of the following nine elements:

1. overall market size
2. annual market growth rate
3. historical profit margin
4. competitive intensity
5. technological requirements
6. inflationary vulnerability
7. energy requirements
8. environmental impact
9. social/political/legal issues

Business strength is an index comprised of the following elements:

1. market share
2. share growth
3. product quality
4. brand reputation
5. distribution network
6. promotional effectiveness
7. production capacity
8. production efficiency
9. unit costs
10. supply costs
11. research and development (R & D) performance
12. management talent

Each of these factors within both dimensions is given a weighting of importance. A product is rated on each factor and then multiplied by the weighting. Every product is assigned a value for marketing attractiveness and business strength. Calculation of the value for a product leads to its positioning within the matrix, which includes its relevant strategic direction as well.

The GE matrix has nine cells representing three broad zones of strategic corporate action. The three cells at the lower right represent businesses that are low in attractiveness and low in business strength. As suggested within the chart, these represent services for which consolidation strategies must be considered. Services that fall within the cells on the diagonal from lower left to upper right are either weak or average in attractiveness and in business strength. These are businesses where selective growth strategies or some harvesting might be appropriate. Finally, services within the cells in the upper left represent businesses with the most promise. Growth strategies need to be pursued.

The advantage of the GE matrix compared to the BCG model is that it provides consideration of multiple factors. Like the BCG model, however, it ultimately places the services along a two-dimensional framework. Also, many of the elements used within the composition of the matrix values are often considered within the BCG discussion of growth rate. The specification is helpful, yet can pose a challenge for managers considering both models simultaneously.

■ Analyzing the Competitive Market

Within the context of strategic planning, companies must analyze the competition. Firms must assess not only the existing competition but also potential competition. Porter has developed a widely accepted conceptual model that considers factors affecting the competitive intensity within an industry.[18] As shown in FIGURE 2-7, competitive intensity is affected by four major forces: (1) the threat of new entrants, (2) bargaining

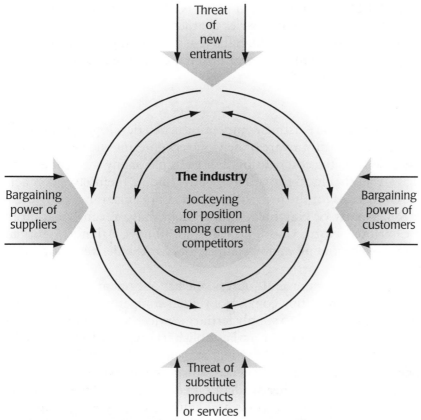

FIGURE 2-7 Forces Impacting Competitive Intensity

power of suppliers, (3) bargaining power of customers, and (4) the threat of substitute products or services.

Existing Competitors

In analyzing the competitive environment, it is important to first look at the existing competitors. This analysis provides a perspective on the cost of competing and on the bases around which the competition will occur. A major focus of the competitive analysis is also to assess the degree to which competition is cost-based.

Competition is intense among existing competitors when the product is relatively standardized and the competitors are relatively numerous and similar in size. This frequently describes the market for hospitals and medical groups in major metropolitan areas. Competition can also be intense when the cost of switching providers is relatively low. In health care, this is a major factor that managed care companies face. For many employers, the cost of switching health plans is often not a large obstacle. Competition also tends to be intense in industries characterized by overcapacity and among firms still in the market because of a high fixed-asset position. These latter two issues define the competitive setting for inpatient hospital care in the 1990s.

New Entrants

While it is essential to consider the existing competition when developing a strategic plan, an organization must be keenly aware of new players entering the marketplace. As the market changes, so does the competition. For example, many medical groups that once competed against other local providers are now finding themselves competing against insurance companies for the provision of care. Large insurance providers, such as Aetna Life & Casualty of Hartford, Connecticut, have recently acquired provider groups in Charlotte, North Carolina; Chicago, Illinois; Atlanta, Georgia; and Dallas, Texas, and are becoming major competitors for the delivery of care in many local markets.

New competitors can come from several sources, such as a segment or market that is underserved. Occasionally, competition comes from either competitors or customers. The academic medical group that used to supply tertiary services to a community hospital might integrate to a lower level of care and establish its own academic group of family practitioners. Many academic medical centers, such as George Washington University in Washington, D.C., actively compete against other providers by offering their own health maintenance plans. Other academic medical centers, such as the one at the University of Minnesota in Minneapolis and University of Michigan in Ann Arbor, have established faculty practice plans as vehicles to attract, process, and organize for patient revenue activities. Similarly, an employer that had purchased outside medical services might hire its own medical staff and conduct employee health programs in-house.

Threat of Substitution

A second major source of competition is found in the threat of substitution. In traditional businesses, this threat exists when one product class can be substituted for another. For example, plastic can be a major threat to steel as the tensile strength of the product increases.

In health care, the threat of substitution most often occurs due to technological change. Technology can eliminate a particular business line in a short period of time. FIGURE 2-8 shows how each successive new generation of diagnostic imaging technology affected the usage of preceding technologies in a particular area. The source of suppliers of this technology has also continually changed. Each new technological advance has provided increased performance in terms of scanning and imaging capabilities. The new technology moves the existing product into a mature phase of its life cycle.

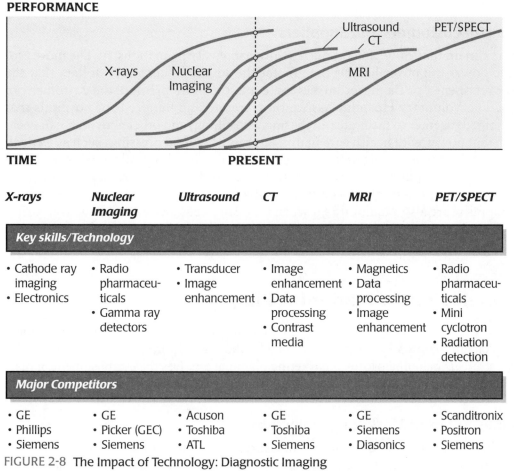

X-rays	Nuclear Imaging	Ultrasound	CT	MRI	PET/SPECT
Key skills/Technology					
• Cathode ray imaging • Electronics	• Radio pharmaceuticals • Gamma ray detectors	• Transducer • Image enhancement	• Image enhancement • Data processing • Contrast media	• Magnetics • Data processing • Image enhancement	• Radio pharmaceuticals • Mini cyclotron • Radiation detection
Major Competitors					
• GE • Phillips • Siemens	• GE • Picker (GEC) • Siemens	• Acuson • Toshiba • ATL	• GE • Toshiba • Siemens	• GE • Siemens • Diasonics	• Scanditronix • Positron • Siemens

FIGURE 2-8 The Impact of Technology: Diagnostic Imaging

Source: Reprinted from *Healthcare Forum Journal*, by permission, September/October 1989, Copyright © 1989, by Health Forum, Inc.

As can be seen in this figure, there is an ever-decreasing time before new technology with higher performance capabilities appears. Several warning signs have been identified by McKinsey et al., indicating when a technology may be nearing obsolescence and supplanted by a competing new technology:

1. Greater efforts are needed to produce even small performance improvements.
2. R&D shifts away from product improvement toward process improvement.
3. Sales growth comes from minor product modifications that serve new segments rather than from quality improvements that improve penetration across all segments.
4. There are wide differences in R&D spending among competitors, with minor differences on resultant market shares.
5. Some market leaders begin to lose share to small competitors in selected market segments. This shift may indicate that smaller competitors are being more productive with a new emerging technology.[19]

Powerful Customers and Suppliers

Buyers can dramatically affect the competitive intensity in an industry. The more economic power the buyer has, or the greater the source of customer dollars that the buyer represents, or the fewer buyers there are, the more pressure the customer can exert. The Voluntary Hospital Association, comprising hundreds of hospitals that have joined together to facilitate purchasing, consulting, and other activities, can wield significant power with health care manufacturers of wound dressings such as Kendall or 3M, because this organization represents all its member hospitals. Buyers can wield power when they purchase a relatively standard product, or when they can integrate backwards and provide a service for themselves.

Suppliers are also a major threat when they can integrate forward to deliver a service. They also can exert great power when other sources of supply are few, or when it would be very costly for an organization to shift suppliers.

■ Developing the Marketing Plan

After an organization develops a strategic plan, it can then formulate a marketing plan to implement the broad strategies identified by the top corporate management. Similar to the strategic planning process, marketing planning involves the establishment of marketing objectives, formulation of marketing strategies, and development of an action plan.

Establishment of Marketing Objectives

Marketing objectives are quantitative measures of accomplishment by which the success of marketing strategies can be measured. Marketing objectives might include retention, new sales growth, and market leadership in the form of a share gain.

Marketing Strategy Formulation

The next step is the formulation of marketing strategies. This aspect of strategic market planning involves determining the target market, specifying the market strategy, and developing the tactical plans for the four Ps.

Determining the Target Market

As noted in the previous chapter, the basic first step in this process is the identification of the *target market*, specifying whom the organization is trying to attract. Selection of the target market involves assessing the organization's own strengths, the competitive intensity for the target market, the cost of capturing market share, and the potential financial gain in attracting the targeted group.

In selecting the target market, organizations have several options, as presented in FIGURE 2-9. They can treat the entire market as one homogeneous group of customers, or they can divide the market into segments or subgroups that are homogeneous within a particular dimension. The concept of segmenting a market is described in more detail in Chapter 6.

Treating the entire market as one target market and appealing to the broadest group is referred to as **mass marketing**. Customers are viewed as relatively undifferentiated in what they desire. This strategy tries to satisfy the greatest number of buyers with a single product. Historically, most hospitals in the United States have followed a mass market strategy in their own local areas. The advantage of this approach is that the largest number of people can be targeted. The size of the market alone can increase the likelihood of attracting customers. The disadvantage of this marketing strategy is that it leaves the organization susceptible to new competitors who might tailor a marketing strategy that is more closely aligned with the needs of particular subgroups.

Figure 2-9 shows the possibilities of a segmented strategy. An organization might consider targeting all possible segments or a number of different segments. This approach is

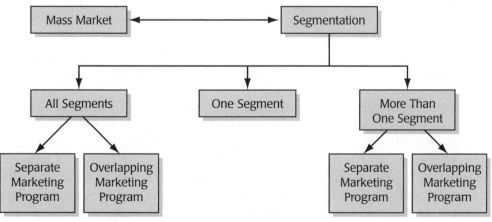

FIGURE 2-9 Segmentation Alternatives

referred to as **multisegment marketing,** in which a distinct marketing strategy might be developed for each group. A hospital might target two segments within the female population. One program might address issues and concerns for women of childbearing age, while a second program targets older women, offering education and resources regarding menopause, breast cancer screening, and osteoporosis. Or, a company can recognize differences in market segments yet have an overlapping strategy that uses similar parts of the marketing mix for all groups, but different strategies for particular groups. For example, a medical group practice might have one main office where all services are delivered. Yet, the group has decided to target two different groups: higher income executives and elderly consumers with third-party insurance. While they are offering the same product and services and using the same distribution strategy, they employ different promotional strategies for each group. The group practice might advertise to executives in the metropolitan edition of *The Wall Street Journal*. At the same time, however, the group will send a representative to senior citizens clubs to speak about the health needs and concerns of older consumers.

Another option for some organizations is to pursue only a subset of market segments or just one market segment. Targeting only one segment of the market is referred to as the **market concentration strategy**. In selecting only one segment, an organization must be able to defend its choice in the face of competition. For example, in Boston there are a small but growing number of custom care or boutique style medical practices. Targeted to the group of consumers who are willing to pay additional out-of pocket dollars for more personalized, almost concierge-style, medical care,[20] these types of groups are following a market concentration strategy. In any market there are only a limited number of such people willing to pay an additional fee that might be as high as $7500 or more for families. An organization's entire future may be based on its ability to solidify its market-share position within this particular group. This strategy does have the advantage of sometimes providing opportunities for efficiencies in production, distribution, or promotion, because a company can tailor its efforts to one segment's requirements.

Specifying Market Strategies

In developing marketing plans, a company must decide which one of several market positions it will take. The options are to be a market leader, market challenger, market follower, or a market niche.[21]

Within a single industry, one organization usually tries to be the **market leader**— the firm that has the largest market share and dominates the competitors in a given market. This leader dictates the pricing strategies of its competitors and is the first to introduce new products. The market leader defends its position against all new entries and will seek to expand the market or expand its current market share. A health care study conducted in 1992 found that hospital return on investment was significantly related to market share. Hospitals that sought and attained large market share had higher profitability than those that did not.[22]

A second market position is that of being the **market challenger**—the firm that attempts to confront the market leader. These companies tend to be smaller than the market leaders, but aggressive in their strategy formulation. They attack the market leader, either through directly vying for the leader's customers, or by trying to attract customers or market segments where the market leader is weak.

A market challenger can follow several approaches that might involve any one or more of the marketing mix elements, such as price cutting, less costly product alternatives, an improved distribution strategy, or a novel promotional approach.

A **market follower** is a business that competes in the marketplace by following the market leader rather than by attacking it directly. These companies try to maintain existing customers and attract new ones. In industries where there is little product differentiation and high price sensitivity, a follower strategy is often useful. By implementing this approach, an organization tries to prevent aggressive price competition. It will gain new customers by offering a quality service at a good value.

A final market position that a firm may try to create is that of a **market niche**, which it achieves by following a strategy of targeting a narrow segment or segments in a large market with specialized products or services. This is a common approach for many small, successful companies. This approach is so common, in fact, that *Forbes* magazine has labeled its listing of the 200 best small companies as its "Niche List."[23] An interesting niche strategy is being developed by Helian Health Group of Monterey, California. This company has set up inns licensed to provide acute care. These small facilities are targeted to handle surgery and recovery for less cost than what is incurred in traditional facilities. California data indicate this recovery center concept can save 28% on the cost of recovery from an abdominal hysterectomy and 60% on recovery from a cholecystectomy.[24]

Niche strategies are becoming more common in health care, especially among large academic medical centers that historically focused upon the highest level of tertiary care. Yet the movement of technology and the existence of well-trained physicians in a community make that a difficult niche to defend. Consider the situation faced by the University of Minnesota's medical center in Minneapolis. This institution has a history of being the center of significant medical advances. In 1952, it was the site where the first successful open heart surgery was performed, and, in 1977, it pioneered the first full-body CT scanner. While both of these technologies have great market potential, they are available at several facilities in the Minneapolis–St. Paul market. At one time, the University of Minnesota's medical center dominated the transplant surgery niche and was recognized as a world leader in bone marrow transplants. In 1995, five other hospitals in the Twin Cities were performing the identical procedure.[25]

Development of an Action Plan

Once the target market has been selected and the broad strategy determined, an organization can specify the tactical components of the marketing plan. These tactics address each of the marketing mix elements. The tactical plan identifies actions to be taken regarding each aspect of the marketing mix. This plan will address the advertising strategy, pricing strategy, distribution issues, and the nature of the product in terms of quality, range of options, and so on.

Evaluating the Plan

The final aspect of the marketing plan involves evaluating its results. The monitoring and evaluation stage is described in greater detail in Chapter 14. Ultimately, the success of monitoring depends on the initial quantitative objectives used in the plan's development.

While each health care organization's marketing plan will vary to some degree, an outline of a basic marketing plan is provided in EXHIBIT 2-4 as a guide.

Exhibit 2-4 Marketing Plan Outline of Fidelity Bank, Philadelphia

Marketing Plan Outline

For each major bank service:

I. MANAGEMENT SUMMARY

What is our marketing plan for this service in brief?

This is a one-page summary of the basic factors involving the marketing of the service next year along with the results expected from implementing the plan. It is intended as a brief guide for management.

II. ECONOMIC PROJECTIONS

What factors in the overall economy will affect the marketing of this service next year, and how?

This section will comprise a summary of the specific economic factors that will affect the marketing of this service during the coming year. These might include employment, personal income, business expectations, inflationary (or deflationary) pressures, etc.

III. THE MARKET—qualitative

Who or what kinds of organization could conceivably be considered prospects for this service?

This section will define the qualitative nature of our market. It will include demographic information, industrial profiles, business profiles, etc., for all people or organizations that could be customers for this service.

IV. THE MARKET—quantitative

What is the potential market for this service?

This section will apply specific quantitative measures to this bank service. Here we want to include numbers of potential customers, dollar volume of business, our current share of the market—any specific measures that will outline our total target for the service and where we stand competitively now.

Exhibit 2-4 (*Continued*)

V. TREND ANALYSIS

Based on the history of this service, where do we appear to be headed?

This section is a review of the past history of this service. Ideally, we should include quarterly figures for the last five years showing dollar volume, accounts opened, accounts closed, share of market, and all other applicable historical data.

VI. COMPETITION

Who are our competitors for this service, and how do we stand competitively?

This section should define our current competition, both bank and nonbank. It should be a thoughtful analysis outlining who our competitors are, how successful they are, why they have (or have not) been successful, and what actions they might be expected to take regarding this service during the coming year.

VII. PROBLEMS AND OPPORTUNITIES

Internally and externally, are there problems inhibiting the marketing of this service, or are there opportunities we have not taken advantage of?

This section will comprise a frank commentary on both inhibiting problems and unrealized opportunities. It should include a discussion on the internal and external problems we can control, for example, by changes in policies or operational procedures. It should also point up areas of opportunity regarding this service that we are not now exploiting.

VIII. OBJECTIVES AND GOALS

Where do we want to go with this service?

This section will outline the immediate short- and long-range objectives for this service. Short-range goals should be specific, and will apply to next year. Long-range goals will necessarily be less specific and should project for the next five years. Objectives should be stated in two forms:

(1) qualitative—reasoning behind the offering of this service and what modifications or other changes we expect to make.

(2) quantitative—number of accounts, dollar volume, share of market, profit goals.

IX. ACTION PROGRAMS

Given past history, the economy, the market, competition, etc., what must we do to reach the goals we have set for this service?

This section will be a description of the specific actions we plan to take during the coming year to assure reaching the objectives we have set for the service in VIII. These would include advertising and promotion, direct mail, and brochure development. It would also include programs to be designed and implemented by line officers. The discussion should cover what is to be done, schedules for completion, methods of evaluation, and officers in charge of executing the program and measuring results.

Source: The Marketing Plan (New York: The Conference Board, 1981). The Conference Board Report No. 801, pp. 63–64.

■ Conclusions

Development of marketing strategy begins with defining an organization's mission. Planning of a firm's final marketing strategy must include an examination of the market environment as well as a SWOT analysis. Understanding the nature of the competition allows a health care organization to develop the appropriate response to face the challenges of a changing health care market.

■ Key Terms

Strategic Planning
Organizational Mission
Situational Assessment
SWOT Analysis
Barriers to Entry
Barriers to Exit
Invisible value
Visible value
Organizational Objectives
Market Penetration
Market Development
Product Development
Vertical Integration
Backward Integration
Forward Integration
Diversification
Strategic Alliances
Joint Venture Businesses

Consolidation
Divestment
Prunes
Retrenchment
Harvesting
BCG Matrix
Market Growth Rate
Relative Market Share
GE Matrix
Marketing Objectives
Mass Marketing
Multisegment Marketing
Market Concentration Strategy
Market Leader
Market Challenger
Market Follower
Market Niche

■ Chapter Summary

1. Marketing plans—along with finance, production, and human resource plans—form the core elements of an organization's strategic plan.
2. An organization's strategic plan is guided by the mission that defines its purpose for existing. The mission must recognize who the customer is and what the customer wants to buy.
3. In developing strategic plans, a SWOT analysis provides a review of internal and external factors that can affect strategic outcomes.
4. In developing strategic plans, an organization must be able to recognize the barriers to entry and exit for any new service venture.

5. Invisible value is the value a producer builds into its product or service; visible value is the value that a customer sees. Typically a company can only charge for visible value.
6. An organization can develop a differential advantage that is either product-based, market-based, or price-based.
7. There are four broad growth strategies that any organization can pursue:
   - market development
   - market penetration
   - product development
   - diversification
8. The BCG matrix and GE matrix are conceptualizations that can aid an organization in the review of its service portfolio. Both models encompass market and competitive considerations.
9. In any industry, the level of competitive intensity is affected by the threat of new entrants, the bargaining power of both suppliers and customers, and the threat of substitute products and services.
10. In developing a marketing plan, organizations can pursue a mass marketing or a market concentration strategy.

■ Chapter Problems

1. At a strategic planning retreat of a six-person general surgery group, the senior partner begins by stating, "Our mission is to perform the highest quality invasive surgery procedures in the community." In what ways might this view of the organization's mission suffer from the myopia that afflicted the railroads in an earlier era?
2. Children's Hospital, in Boston, Massachusetts, has long been considered an outstanding medical center specializing in the diagnosis and treatment of pediatric problems. This facility is linked academically to the Harvard University Medical School. Conduct a brief SWOT analysis for Children's Hospital in light of the present health care environment.
3. Describe the possible barriers to entry and exit for: (a) a physician wanting to establish a solo practice office in internal medicine, (b) a company offering a health club facility in the same building where employees work, and (c) a tertiary hospital developing a coronary bypass program.
4. You have recently been hired as the senior marketing officer for a new HMO. Two other HMOs have been operating for more than two years in the same community. The first HMO is a closed-panel medical group with three satellite offices. The second plan is an independent practice association with a panel of 125 physicians equally divided along primary care and specialty lines with 20 different locations. Both plans offer dental coverage. As the third entrant into

the market, where can you turn to establish a differential advantage? Provide some examples.

5. Retin–A is a topical ointment originally developed for the treatment of severe cases of acne and related skin disorders. An observed side benefit resulting from use of this product is its beneficial effect on aging skin. If the manufacturer of this product decided to pursue the latter market, what type of a growth strategy would it be pursuing?

6. Since 1982, there has been a steady decline in the number of hospital inpatient days. How might an acute-care community hospital implement the consolidation strategies of: (a) divestment, (b) retrenchment, and (c) harvesting?

7. Two large multi-specialty medical groups have recently asked you to conduct audits using the BCG matrix. For the first group, your analysis reveals the following distribution of services: Cash cows—65%; stars—10%; problem children—20%; dogs—5%. In the second group, the distribution is: Cash cows—20%; stars—60%; problem children—15%; dogs—5%. Provide your analysis to each group.

■ Notes

1. P. D. Bennett, ed. *Dictionary of Marketing Terms* (Chicago, IL: American Marketing Association, 1988), 195.

2. J. A. Pearce, II, "The Company Mission as a Strategic Tool," *Sloan Management Review* 23, no. 3 (1982): 15–24.

3. T. Levitt, "Marketing Myopia," *Harvard Business Review* 38, no. 4 (1960): 45–56.

4. K. Pallarito, "Hospitals Strengthen Networks through New Fitness Facilities," *Modern Healthcare* 24, no. 50 (1994): 45.

5. "Springfield Hospital Fitness Center 'Pumps Up' Ambulatory Care," *Inside Ambulatory Care* 2, no. 3 (1995): 1, 5.

6. J. R. Rose, "Competition Has No Borders," *Medical Economics* 70, no. 14 (July 26, 1993): 13.

7. A. Waldman, "Subacute Care: Spreading the Word," *Healthcare Management Report* 12, no. 8 (1994): 6–9.

8. G. Stalk, P. Evans, and L. E. Shulman, "Competing on Capabilities: The New Rules of Corporate Strategy," *Harvard Business Review* 70, no. 2 (1992): 57–69.

9. M. A. Hitt and R. D. Ireland, "Corporate Distinctive Competence, Strategy, and Performance," *Strategic Management Journal* 6, no. 3 (1985): 273–293.

10. M. E. Porter, *Competitive Strategy: Techniques for Analyzing Industries and Competitors* (New York: Free Press, 1980).

11. This framework was originally presented by H. I. Ansoff, *Corporate Strategy* (New York: McGraw-Hill, 1965).

12. Cinda Becker, "Spanning the Globe," *Modern Healthcare* 35, no. 15 (April 11, 2005): 17.

13. For a useful reading on strategic alliances see P. Lorange and J. Roos, *Strategic Alliances: Formulation, Implementation, and Evolution* (Cambridge, MA: Blackwell Scientific Publications, 1992).

14. Roberta Clarke and Therese O. Sucher, "Benchmarking for the Competitive Marketplace," *Journal of Ambulatory Care Management* 22, no. 3 (July 1999): 72–78.

15. P. J. Henkel, "Delivering Corporate Health Services," *Modern Healthcare* 23, no. 23 (1993): 24–27.

16. "Kodak Unit's Entry in China," *The Wall Street Journal* 3 (September 1993): A4.

17. Boston Consulting Group, *Perspectives on Experience* (Boston: 1972). See also B. D. Henderson, "The Experience Curve Reviewed: The Growth Share Matrix of the Product Portfolio," in *Perspectives no. 135* (Boston, MA: The Boston Consulting Group, 1973).

18. Porter, *Competitive Strategy*.

19. R. N. Foster, *Innovation: The Attacker's Advantage* (New York: Summit Books, 1986), 162.

20. Liz Kowalczyk, "Custom Medicine Raises Care, Concerns," *Boston Globe* 262, no. 35 (August 2002): 1, A29.

21. P. Kotler, *Marketing Management: Analysis, Planning, and Control*, 8th ed. (Englewood Cliffs, NJ: Prentice Hall, 1994), 381–407.

22. W. O. Cleverly and R. K. Harvey, "Critical Strategies for Successful Rural Hospitals," *Healthcare Management Review* 17, no. 1 (Winter 1992): 27–33.

23. S. Kirchen and M. Schifrin, "Niche List," *Forbes* 138, no. 10 (November 3, 1986): 160–161.

24. R. L. Cohen, "Recovery Inns: A Concept Whose Time Has Come," *Healthcare Management Report* 11, no. 5 (1993): 18.

25. L. Page, "Playing Catch-up," *American Medical News* 37, no. 29 (1994): 3, 7.

The Environment of Marketing Strategy

After reading this chapter you should be able to:

- Understand the impact of the five environmental forces on organizational strategy

- Explain how social and economic forces affect marketing strategy

- Describe the impact of technology on health care organizations' survival and competitive environment

- Know the major regulatory requirements that must be followed when formulating health care marketing strategy

Marketing strategy is formulated in response to consumer needs. As discussed in Chapter 1, consumers can be individuals or organizations. Yet, marketing strategy must be formulated in response to the environmental conditions that affect the market. An effective marketing organization must continually scan the environment to assess and identify trends that its marketing strategy must consider. An organization must focus its environmental scan on five major environmental forces: economic, technological, social, competitive, and regulatory. As shown in FIGURE 3-1, environmental scanning is conducted to assess the trends in each of these five areas for their potential impact on the organization's target market. In this way, the health care organization can appropriately adjust its marketing mix strategy.

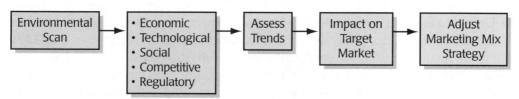

FIGURE 3-1 The Environmental Scan

This chapter will present a brief overview of each of these environmental factors and their potential implications for health care marketing.

■ Economic Factors

For any organization, the prevailing major macroeconomic conditions must be a major concern. Whether the marketplace is experiencing inflationary or recessionary conditions affects the willingness and ability of consumers to pay. **Inflation** is the decline in buying power when price levels rise faster than income. The cost of borrowing increases during an inflationary period. A health care provider who might find the opportunity to offer new services is constrained by the higher cost of capital.

Inflation and Health Care

Health care costs have been on a steady rise since the 1980s. Increasingly, as shown in Figure 3-2, health care is consuming a growing percentage of the United States' Gross Domestic National Product. According to forecasts, this trend will continue as far out as 2013, rising to slightly more than 18%. It is this growing cost of health care that is putting pressure on corporations, as well as federal, state, and local governments to examine alternative ways in which to cover the cost of care for employees and others in their communities, such as government employees, school teachers, or union members. In the 1980s and through the early 1990s, the response by some companies was to turn to health maintenance organizations (HMOs) as a mechanism to counteract the rapid rise in health care costs. The data in FIGURE 3-2 show that this approach did little in and of itself to slow the growing expense of health care.

Consumer Income

There are three dimensions to any consumer's income: (1) gross income, (2) discretionary income, and (3) disposable income. **Gross income** is the total amount of money earned by a person or family in one year. Figure 3-3 shows the change in median consumer income from 1970 to 1992. While the typical family earned $29,760 in 1970, by 2002 that figure had risen to $42,409.[1] As can be seen in the chart, differences exist among ethnic and racial groups. The gross income of African Americans and Hispanics lags significantly behind Caucasians. Disconcertingly, African Americans in the United States in absolute dollars have seen their incomes remain at the same level. Adjusted for inflation, they are far below what their dollars purchased in 1970 (with a gross income in 2002, according to the data in FIGURE 3-3, of $29,026).

Disposable income is the amount of money a consumer has left for food, clothing, and shelter after paying taxes. During the 1990s, many politicians felt that taxes were rising faster than wages for the middle-income class. The end result was a

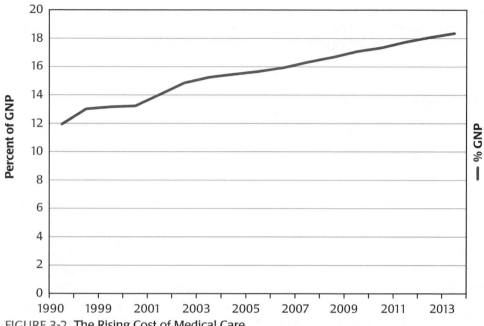

FIGURE 3-2 The Rising Cost of Medical Care

Source: http://www.cms.hhs.gov/statistics/nhe/projections-2003/t1.asp#navigation.

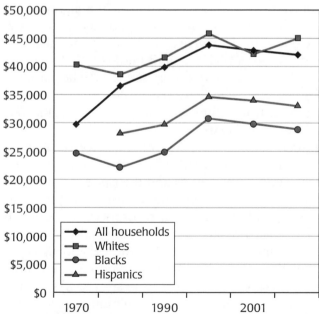

FIGURE 3-3 Consumer Income: Looking Below the Average

Sources: 2000 Statistical Abstract of the United States, U.S. Census Bureau, p. 470; 2004–2005 Statistical Abstract of the United States, U.S. Census Bureau, p. 441.

decline in disposable income. The last component of income is **discretionary income**, which is the income left after paying for taxes and necessities. Discretionary income is what the consumer uses for entertainment, recreation, or luxuries.

■ Technological Factors

Few industries are more greatly affected by technology than health care. **Technology** refers to the innovations or inventions from applied science and research. As new technology enters the market, existing products or services are pushed out. The impact of technology in health care is threefold. In the short term, new technology results in increasing costs. Each new generation of imaging device has required hospitals to upgrade their equipment. Yet, in the same regard, technology can also contribute to a decrease in cost. Consider the technological changes affecting one of the top 10 surgeries performed in hospitals—hysterectomy. The conventional abdominal hysterectomy involves a three- to four-day hospital stay and costs approximately $7000, excluding the anesthesiologist's charge.[2] Increasingly, this procedure is being performed as an outpatient vaginal surgery and can cost almost three thousand dollars less than when the procedure is done abdominally.[3]

The third competitive consideration for technology is that as each new generation of equipment enters the market, the preceding generation or model becomes cheaper. This factor allows smaller competitors to offer a service by acquiring the slightly older technology or a less expensive version of the new technology. As noted in Chapter 2, academic medical centers such as the one at the University of Minnesota are now facing the competitive realities of the widespread availability of technology. No longer are these facilities the exclusive providers of sophisticated tertiary services.[4] The marginal potential market for the hospital with the new technology depends heavily on whether the new-generation equipment offers significant improvement to the preceding version and is sufficient to capture or shift market share.

Technology may well have a dramatic impact on how care is delivered or managed in the physician's office. **Telemedicine,** the Internet, and wireless communication will dramatically change the interface between providers and their patients into this century. The electronic medical record, increasingly common with such systems as EPIC in many health care organizations, is allowing for the transportability of a patient's record to multiple physicians across sites. Smart cards will store patients' records on a wallet size credit card for access by emergency personnel to access and swipe information. In the next-generation cell phones, it is highly likely that blood pressure monitoring and other vital signs can be sent remotely to a physician's office. As today's physician carries a wireless palm to access pharmaceutical information or send information within a hospital, so too will a patient do so for transmitting vital signs to a physician. Europe is moving ahead quickly. In 1993 a high capacity telemedicine center was established in Tromsø, Norway, which is north of Oslo. Norwegians in remote locations now have access to specialists they never had before. In May 2005, the Wales government committed 2.7 million pounds ($4.95 million U.S. dollars) over the next three years for further development of telehealth. That amount may pale in this country, but it is a significant expenditure in a country the size of Wales.[5]

Technology is having the greatest impact in terms of how consumers are behaving. In 1998 more than 40 million Americans searched online for health care information and spent $1 billion online on health care products.[6] Behaviorally all age groups are being affected. In 2002, 24% of young adults between the ages of 15 and 24 reported getting a "lot" of information on the Web with 50% of them reporting looking up "specific diseases," 44% sexual health matters, and 32%[7] issues about weight loss or gain. The use of the Web by adults is also growing at a dramatic rate. A study by Solucient reported that 45% of adults turn to the Internet for numerous health-related purposes, including personal health research, prescription medication purchases, or details on hospitals and health plans. In contrast, only 16% of adults refer to their physicians for health-related information. Another 10% consult a pharmacist or newspapers and magazines, while 5% confer directly with their local hospital. However, the study also found significant disparities among adult health care consumers using the Web, particularly when compared by age and income. Upper income, married couples between the ages of 25–35 were nearly 80% more likely to use the Web for health care purposes than adults age 55–64 and 150% more likely than adults age 65 and over. Nearly 57% of households earning more than $100,000 seek health care information on the Internet and are nearly 60% more likely to use the Internet for this purpose than households earning less than $50,000.[8]

It is also important to recognize that seniors too are becoming more wired and turning to the Internet. A recent study reported that the number of seniors who went online increased 47% between 2000 and 2004. Twenty-two percent of seniors (over 65) reported having access to the Internet. This percentage represented 8 million consumers. It was also reported that 66% of these wired seniors looked for health information online at some point and that this itself was an increase of 13% from 2000. The percentage increase of seniors going online for health information represented a 25% growth rate in turning to the Internet for health care information. These seniors searched for information about medical treatments and procedures, prescriptions, and experimental treatments.[9]

▪ Social Factors

The social dimension of the environment includes the demographic characteristics of the population, its culture, and its values. Income, also a factor, was reviewed in the previous section, "Economic Factors."

Demographics

Demographics are statistics that describe members of a population in terms of who they are, where they live, and the types of jobs they have.

The Population

The population of the United States is changing in two major ways. Population growth in the country is declining and our population is aging. Between 1990 and 2000, the number of Americans over the age of 65 increased from 31 million to over 34 million, while the oldest over the age of 85 increased from 3 to 4 million in that same time period. The percentage of people in this age group has remained fairly constant at 12.5% of the general population.[10]

However, as FIGURE 3-4 shows, Americans who are now between 45 and 64 years of age will continue to grow older in the next 10 to 15 years and will become the elderly population requiring the health care system in ever-increasing numbers.

Health care organizations are becoming more attentive to this group. Senior care programs, adult day-care centers, Alzheimer's clinics, and long-term care facilities are potentially growing business opportunities in light of this aging marketplace. With

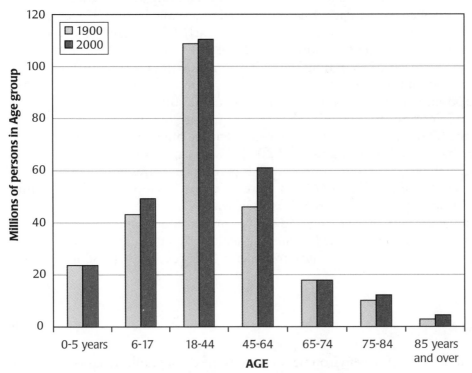

FIGURE 3-4 **Changes in Distribution in the U.S. Population 1900–2000**

Source: Health Care in America: Trends in Utilization (U.S. Department of Health and Human Services, Centers for Disease Control and Prevention, 2004).

Alzheimer's disease alone, the predicted increase in patients is dramatic. Presently, 3.8 million Americans are diagnosed with this illness. The number of people with this illness is expected to grow to between 7.98 and 12.95 million people in the U.S. by 2050, a twofold to fourfold increase from present levels, given the number of people forecasted to be living over the age of 85.[11] The mature household headed by people over the age of 55 is becoming a statistically more significant group. The 2000 census counted approximately 60 million people over the age of 55; the number in this age group is expected to double by the year 2030.[12] And, as the population has aged, the number of skilled nursing facilities has risen from 5155 in 1980 to 14,193 in 1999 and the number of nursing home beds has increased from 1,624,000 in 1985 to 1,965,000 in 1999.[13]

Baby Boomers
The next group that looms large for health care providers are those Americans who were born between 1946 and 1964—250 million Americans referred to as the **baby boomers**. This segment of the population is in middle-age and accounted for 11.3% of the population in 1993. These consumers are now increasingly involved in the health care decisions for their aging parents as they play the role of decision maker and, often, caregiver. Companies are beginning to realize the role being assumed by their employees. A 1993 survey of almost 2000 employees of Transamerica Life Companies of San Francisco found that the firm lost 1600 workdays, or about $250,000, because of employees taking time off from work to care for elderly relatives. These data, coupled with the fact that the percentage of elderly living with their children declined from 7.5% in 1980 to 4.8% in 1991, suggest a growing market for elder care services and residential facilities.[14] Within a 10–15-year period, this large group will become major users of more intensive health care services themselves.

The baby boomer generation also represents an interesting market segment in terms of its own health care needs. In fact, the Centers for Disease Control and Prevention is already reporting an increase in visits by this age group. In 2001, 53% of patients visiting a physician were over the age of 45, compared to only 42% in 1992. And, while the total number of people over the age of 45 rose by 11% in the last decade, the number of physician visits rose 26%. The leading diagnoses for these boomers were hypertension, joint disorders, and diabetes. Diabetes diagnoses increased a dramatic 63% from 1992 to 2001.[15] A study conducted in 1991 by David M. Eisenberg et al. of Harvard University Medical School in Boston found that more than one-third of Americans had turned to alternative medicine therapies. The use of such nonwestern medicinal approaches was most likely among well-educated, white, baby boomers who live in western states.[16,17]

The Family
Few elements of the American demographic profile have changed more than those representing the family. In the 1950s, 70% of U.S. households consisted of a stay-at-home mother, a working father, and one or more children. Today only 25% of all families would have a similar profile. In today's society, almost a quarter of all people live as

singles, while slightly more (28%) live as couples without children. The fastest growing household units are single parents, or unrelated people living together.[18–20] In the United States, many first marriages have ended in divorce and individuals have re-formed family units. There is the rise of the **blended family**, which is the joining of two households through remarriage or living together in the same household.

Geographic Shifts

Not only is the U.S. population changing in terms of age and family structure, but it is also moving. The past 20 years have seen a stagnant level of growth in the Northeast region of the United States and substantial shift in the population to the South and the West. FIGURE 3-5 shows the net migration across the regions in the United States from 1990 through 1999.

To help analyze geographic markets, the federal government has created a three-tiered description of communities that reflect their population density. Data are gathered and reported according to the following classifications:

1. *Metropolitan Statistical Areas.* These include cities having a population of at least 50,000, or an urbanized area with a total metropolitan population of at least 100,000.

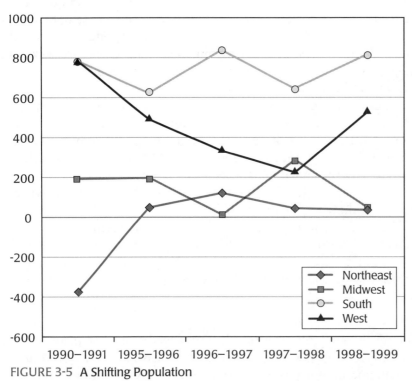

FIGURE 3-5 A Shifting Population

Source: 2004–2005 Statistical Abstract of the United States, U.S. Census Bureau, p. 28.

2. *Primary Metropolitan Statistical Area* (PMSA). The second largest category is an area that has a total population of more than one million. It must also include counties that have a total population of at least 100,000, have a population that is at least 60% urban, and have fewer than 50% of its residents commuting outside the county for employment.
3. *Consolidated Metropolitan Statistical Area.* This is the largest geographical categorization in terms of geographical area and market size. It is comprised of PMSAs that total at least one million people.

Racial and Ethnic Distinctions

The face of the United States is rapidly changing. Increasingly, African Americans, Hispanics, and Asians are representing a larger percentage of the population. This demographic shift is particularly noticeable in the major metropolitan areas and in some parts of the southwest. In 2000, the U.S. Census Bureau reported that 60% of the population was white, 12.8% was African American, 11.8% was Hispanic, 3% was Asian and Pacific Islander, and 1% was Native American. The Bureau predicts that by the year 2050, the composition of the population will be 53% white, 21% Hispanic, 15% African American, 10% Asian and Pacific Islander, and 1.2% Native Americans.[21] Almost one third of all Americans under age 35 are now minorities.[22] Of greater significance may well be the median age difference between these racial and ethnic groups. The median age for whites is projected to be 37.9, for blacks 31.5, and for Hispanics only 27 years of age. In some metropolitan areas there is a heavy concentration of certain ethnic and racial groups. Eighteen percent of all Hispanic Americans live in Los Angeles, where in 2005 this city elected a Hispanic mayor. Health care marketers must recognize and respond to the changing American population. Further discussion about appealing to these market segments is presented in Chapter 6 on market segmentation.

Culture

A second dimension of the social environment is the **culture**, which incorporates the values, customs, and conforming rules passed from one generation to the next. Several cultural changes are occurring in the marketplace, which health care marketers must heed.

The Roles of Women and Men

A significant cultural change that has occurred over the past 20 years is the large number of women who are pursuing higher education and working outside the home. Women are working in larger numbers than ever before. Of the 116 million women over the age of 16, 68 million are in the labor force for a work force participation rate of 59.2%. And, the higher a woman's educational level, the greater the likelihood she will be a labor force participant. Of the 64.7 million women working in the United States in 2004, 74% worked full-time with 38% of these in management or professional occupations.[23] They are also heading households in greater numbers. In 1970, slightly more than 20% of U.S. households were headed by women, yet that number will grow to 30% by the year 2000.[24]

As women work outside the home in greater numbers, organizations must respond to their needs. Pediatric hours may need to be extended to evenings or weekends for appointments. And, as will be discussed in Chapter 4 on buyer behavior, the educated woman who works outside the home plays a different role in terms of household decision making. In these instances, health care organizations are beginning to appreciate the woman's role in the health care decision process. And, women have been found to be more active users of today's technology, the Web, when it comes to health care information. A study conducted by Datamonitor, a multinational survey firm, reported that 44% of all female respondents searched the Web for health information compared to 32% of men. The survey included 4531 adults from France, Germany, the United States, Spain, and the United Kingdom.[25] Women have always been important to health care providers from a utilization perspective. The average number of annual encounters for females in 1998 was 1.4 times higher for women than for males. And as the population continues to age, society will continue to become more female dominated. In 2000, U.S. women outnumbered men by 6 million.[26]

Changing Providers

The increasing number of women working outside the home has changed the face of medicine, itself. FIGURE 3-6 shows the increasing percentage of women represented in health care professions. Interestingly, the percentage of women in the traditional profession of nursing is declining as shown in Figure 3-6. But the percentage of female physicians is increasing significantly from 26.5% in 1980 to 43.9% in 1999–2000. In 2004, for the second consecutive year, women outnumbered men in applying to medical school with slightly more than 50% of all applications. However, of the entering class of 16,638 students, slightly less than half (8229) were female.[27] Many health care organizations recognize the importance of having clinicians who are sensitive to and representative of the market they serve. Attracting female practitioners is an important priority for many medical groups in their recruiting efforts.

Changing Attitudes

Attitudinal shifts in health care are a constant factor. Since the 1990s a major shift in the United States has been toward a greater concern for health and fitness, diet, and alternative medicines—all ways for Americans to be more proactive regarding health. According to a 1998 survey in the *Journal of the American Medical Association*, about 42% of American health care consumers have used at least one complementary or alternative medicine approach. And, a later survey by the American Hospital Association in 2000–2001 showed that hospitals were responsive to this changing consumer behavior. Of 5800 surveyed hospitals, 23% reported offering some type of hospital-based complementary or alternative medicine service. From 1998 to 2002 the number of hospitals offering complementary or alternative medicine doubled from 7.9% to

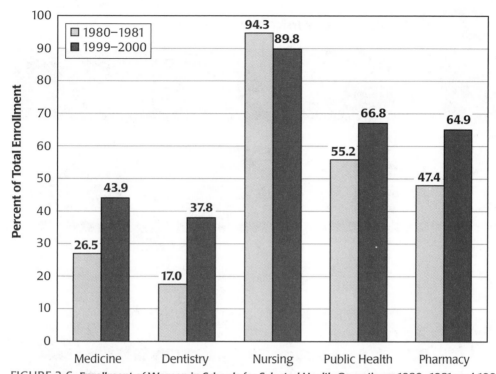

FIGURE 3-6 Enrollment of Women in Schools for Selected Health Operations, 1980–1981 and 1999–2000

Source: U.S. Department of Health and Human Services, Health Resources and Services Administration, Maternal and Child Health Bureau. Women's Health USA 2002. Rockville, Maryland: U.S. Department of Health and Human Services, 2002.

16.6% with the primary services being offered as massage therapy (47%), stress management (40%), yoga (37%), and relaxation techniques (32%).[28] The Center for East-West Medicine at UCLA is an example of this approach.[29] Hospitals have also begun to respond with a changing product line. According to the Association of Hospital Health and Fitness, the number of fitness centers affiliated with hospitals and physician groups has doubled since 1991 to a total of 221 such facilities in 1994.[30]

A second shift among consumers has been aided by technology. Individuals are becoming more active in searching for information on their health care provider, hospital, or organization. Companies like COMPARE YOUR CARE (http://www.compareyourcare.org/) are providing an opportunity for consumers to become more active in evaluating their physicians' approach relative to what might be considered good standards of care. One of the more visible organizations to help consumers understand "quality" information is Healthgrades (http://www.healthgrades.com), where a consumer is able to get specific information on a physician or a hospital. EXHIBIT 3-1 shows a sample of Healthgrades information regarding hospitals on a particular procedure.

The number of organizations trying to provide greater information to respond to this shifting attitude of evaluation is growing. These responses are occurring from the

Exhibit 3-1 Health Grades Information Ranking

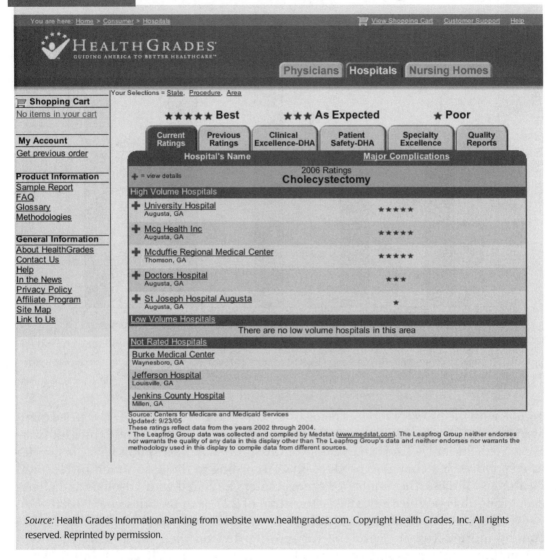

Source: Health Grades Information Ranking from website www.healthgrades.com. Copyright Health Grades, Inc. All rights reserved. Reprinted by permission.

organizations themselves, such as the Dartmouth Hitchcock Medical Center, which has a "Quality Reports" link on its Web site concerning the organization's quality evaluations from external sources (http://www.dhmc.org) to external organizations like URAC (www.URAC.com) that develops standards for managed care organizations regarding medical management, patient satisfaction in conjunction with J. D. Powers, and even Web site content. And, in January 2004, Healthgrades released a study indicating that 40% of U.S. consumers considered a hospital's quality rating when selecting a facility.[31]

■ Competitive Factors

A fourth major component of the environment pertains to the competition, the alternative providers of the health care service. There are four basic structural forms of competition that can be arrayed on a continuum as shown in Table 3-1: pure competition, monopolistic competition, oligopoly, and monopoly.

At one end of the spectrum lies **pure competition**, a situation in which every company has the same product. This might be the case of a number of solo-practice, primary care internists who all work in a small community that has no managed care plans. The competitive advantage is difficult to establish, but it is often based on distribution. Whose office is more conveniently located, or who offers extended hours needed by the patient might be the difference in attracting more patients. Other aspects of marketing are of little relevance in this competitive setting.

The second point on the continuum is **monopolistic competition** in which many sellers compete and have substitutable products. Such a situation might exist in a community where two alternative managed care plans are available. Many of the community's physicians participate on the panels of both competing plans. In this case, small price changes might lead to a consumer shift from one plan to the other.

A third competitive market structure is **oligopoly**, where a few companies control a majority of the industry sales. This is the structure that has dominated the airline industry over the past two decades. This situation is what truly exits in the commercially incurred population in the United States in the early part of the 21st century. The five largest plans are Wellpoint (including their acquisition of Anthem), the other Blue Cross and Blue Shield plans, United Health Group, Aetna, and Cigna. In 2002–2003, in only two states (Nevada and New Mexico), less than 50% of the population belonged to one of these five plans, And, in this same time period, Wellpoint and the Blues held the largest market share in every state except Nevada and California.[32] This situation might be considered an oligopolistic market condition. In health care, greater consolidation has been occurring among the top insurance companies over the past few years. In 2002, Trigon Healthcare and Anthem joined together as Anthem; in early 2004 this plan merged with Wellpoint. This joining together of two large insurers covered 28 million people in 13 states. United Health began to acquire other plans in 2003, such as Mid Atlantic Medical Services, Oxford Health Plans, and

Table 3-1	The Continuum of Competition		
Pure Competition	Monopolistic Competition	Oligopoly	Monopoly
Many sellers	Many sellers	Few, large sellers	One seller
Substitutable products	Substitutable product	Similar product	Unique product
Little differentiation	Price a key	Little price cutting	Regulatory oversight

Definity Health in 2004; then Pacificare acquired American Medical Security Group. These insurers are added to the growing giants of insurers Aetna and Cigna.[33] At the beginning of 2005, few individuals in health care believed that the consolidation among health insurers was over. Some oligopolistic markets are considered differentiated, in which buyers perceive a difference among the few competitors. The automobile industry can be viewed as a differentiated oligopoly. The few major manufacturers try to protect their differentiation by focusing on the product component of the marketing mix.

The final position on the continuum is **monopoly**, in which there is only one firm that sells a product. This is quite common for certain natural resources such as water and energy. Usually, government agencies have been established to offer the service or to review the rates and service levels. In health care, monopolies have often been created through a patent, which gives the manufacturer exclusive right to the manufacturing and selling of a product. Because of the high cost of research and development in the pharmaceutical industry, patent protection is a valuable reward, and an incentive to help recoup costs. At the same time, as is true with many monopolies, it often has led to the appearance, or actuality, of abuse. Critics have charged that pharmaceutical companies price their patented drugs too high.

Health Care Competition

The nature of competition within health care is a function of who is defining the competitive set. In recent years the industry has evolved from one dominated by HMOs and a payment under a capitated system to a return to more of a fee-for-service mode. With the growing pressures of cost as was noted earlier, buyers are still looking for ways to bring these costs under control. At the same point, the competition within the industry is intensifying as there is consolidation from within each segment, and it is also broadening as there is growing global competition. Although there is a wide array of different provider organizations, consider the changes that have occurred within two segments: hospitals and the managed care organizations.

Hospitals

The environment of the traditional acute-care hospital has changed dramatically in the past 10 to 15 years. The environment has not been kind to the acute-care community hospital. From 1990 to 2003 the number of hospitals in the United States declined 6.4%, while the number of beds actually declined 9.8%. However, although the number of beds is declining, FIGURE 3-7 does show a dramatic turnaround in the early part of the early 2000 decade—inpatient hospital admissions have begun to increase. To a large degree, this might well be attributable to an aging population as noted earlier in this chapter. At the same time, the number of outpatient surgeries rose 30.5%; correspondingly, inpatient surgeries increased only 1.1% in that same time period.[34] The proprietary hospital segment has also undergone continual shifting. One can look at the history of Hospital Corporation of America (HCA) to see the shifting fortunes of pro-

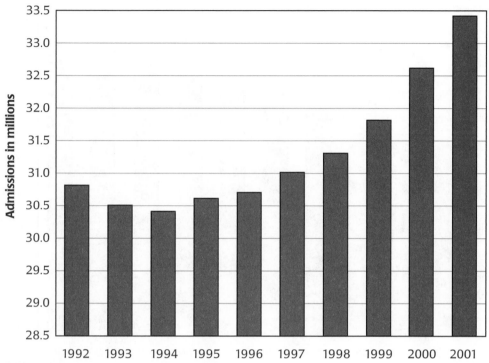

FIGURE 3-7 Change in Hospital Admissions

Source: American Hospital Association Statistics 2003.

prietary systems. In the early 1980s, HCA acquired General Care Corporation, General Health Services, Hospital Affiliates International, and Health Care Corporation. In 1993, HCA merged with Humana and at its peak in 1994 the company owned or managed 350 hospitals along with a 145 outpatient surgery centers and was a $20 billion dollar company. In 2004 HCA had 191 hospitals that are locally managed and 82 outpatient surgery centers.[35] Tenet, which owned or operated 100 acute-care hospitals as of February 2004, is also facing a changing competitive market. As not-for-profits become more competitive, Tenet is selling hospitals in markets such as Massachusetts where it finds it cannot be a market leader.[36]

Ambulatory surgery center (ASC) volume has grown dramatically. In 1980, three million procedures were done in ASCs; by 1995 that number had climbed to 27 million.[37] FIGURE 3-8 shows the dramatic growth that has occurred into the early part of the 21st century despite the rise in inpatient hospital admissions.

Managed Care Providers

The prepaid segment of health care shifted dramatically in the latter part of the 1990s as can be seen in FIGURE 3-9, which shows the percentage growth rate of HMO enrollment through the decade of the 1990s. After several years of a steady rise in growth,

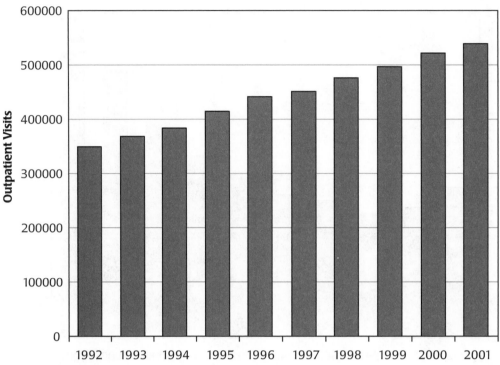

FIGURE 3-8 Growing Trend in Outpatient Surgical Visits

Source: Data from *Modern Healthcare* (December 23, 2002).

HMO enrollment peaked at 81.5 million members in 1998, but by the first half of 1999, it lost half a million members. In the early part of the 21st century, the managed care segment of the health care marketplace has moved into the stage of consolidation. As noted in the discussion of oligopolistic market conditions, there was greater consolidation occurring among the top insurance companies during the past several years.

International Competition

The recent years in health care have seen the competitive landscape shift to one of global competition for those patients who have the financial resources to seek care where needed. In the post 9/11 world, the United States dramatically tightened entry visas for international visitors. Major medical centers such as the Mayo Clinic, the Cleveland Clinic, M.D. Anderson, and others experienced a significant decline in volume because of the difficulty of accessing that care from international patients. Other hospitals, mostly in Asia, have risen to provide very effective competition that competes on quality, price, and amenity levels. Hospitals in Thailand had over 300,000 patients from around the world in 2002, while more than 10,000 international patients were reported to check into Indian hospitals.[38] One of the largest in Asia is The Parkway Group Inc. Its subsidiaries include Parkway Group Healthcare, which owns a network of regional hospitals in

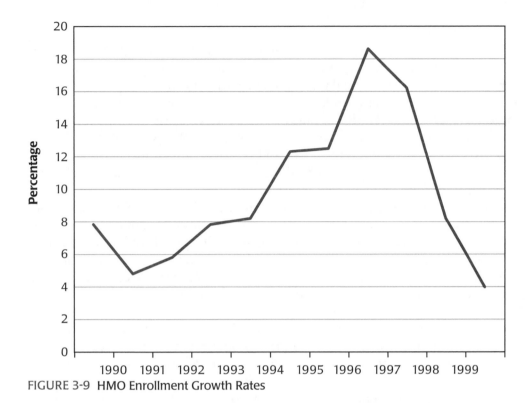

FIGURE 3-9 HMO Enrollment Growth Rates

Malaysia, India, and Brunei. Parkway Hospitals of Singapore owns three private hospitals in Singapore: East Shore, Gleneagles, and Mount Elizabeth Hospitals. Checking the Web site for Parkway Hospitals, one also notices a very competitive pricing package that is also offered to Citibank customers (http://www.pgh.com.sg/citibank_pkg.jsp).

■ Regulatory Factors

The final aspect of the environment to consider is the regulatory component. **Regulation** consists of the rules or restrictions placed on companies by federal or state governments. Within health care, there is a wide array of regulations pertaining to the delivery of care. In this section, we will review those aspects of major federal legislation that have an impact on the marketing mix.

Competition

There are several key regulations protecting competition that have been in place more than a century. Initiated in the late 1800s in the face of monopolies, they continue to be applied today with increasing frequency in health care.

Antitrust Legislation

Two major antitrust laws are the Sherman Antitrust Act (1890) and the Clayton Act (1914). The **Sherman Antitrust Act** forbids any contracts, combinations, or conspiracies in the restraint of trade. Actual monopolies or attempts to monopolize any part of trade or commerce are also forbidden. The **Clayton Act** supplemented the Sherman Antitrust Act by forbidding certain actions that were likely to lessen competition, even if no actual damages had occurred. In 1950, the Clayton Act was amended by the **Antimerger Act**, which broadened the power of the federal government under Section 7 of the Clayton Act to prevent intercorporate acquisitions that would substantially reduce competition.

This issue of mergers is increasingly a factor in health care. In 1994, for example, Minneapolis Children's Medical Center announced a merger with Children's Hospital in St. Paul. This merger of the two facilities would result in the hospitals controlling 88% of the pediatric inpatient care market in Minneapolis–St. Paul. As a result, the state attorney general filed a suit saying it would violate Section 7 of the Clayton Act. The state agreed to withdraw the suit only after the two institutions agreed to several conditions, such as the provision that they would acquire no other hospital; nor would they manage the inpatient pediatric care of another facility. The newly merged facility also cannot enter into an agreement with a physician that would prevent him or her from also practicing at another hospital.[39] Similarly, the Federal Trade Commission (FTC) intervened in Punta Gorda, Florida, a town north of Fort Meyers. Columbia/HCA proposed to buy a hospital in that community. The FTC denied the acquisition because it would have given the corporation control of two of the three hospitals in the local market.[40]

With the increasing formulation of networks and mergers throughout health care, the federal government released new guidelines on September 27, 1993, clarifying six antitrust "safety zones":

1. The FTC and the Department of Justice will not challenge any merger between two general acute-care hospitals in which one has averaged fewer than 100 licensed beds and an average daily census of less than 40 patients for the past three years. An additional requirement is that the hospital must be more than five years old.
2. No joint venture will be challenged regarding an agreement among hospitals to purchase, operate, or market the services of high-tech or other expensive medical equipment, providing the number of hospitals are needed to support the cost of the service. A joint venture will not be challenged that includes additional hospitals if these hospitals could not support the cost of the equipment.
3. The agencies will provide a "rule of reason" in the antitrust review of joint ventures that fall outside the antitrust "safety zones." The concern is whether the joint ventures will reduce competition. Even if the result is such, the examination will consider whether procompetitive efficiencies are produced to outweigh this concern.

4. The agency will not challenge the collective provision of medical data by physicians that may improve the purchasers' resolution of mode, quality, or efficiency of treatment issues.
5. The agencies will not challenge hospital participation in written surveys of price for hospital services, wages, or benefits for personnel. The survey must, however, be administered by a third party and contain data more than three months old. A minimum of five hospitals must report the data. No one hospital's data can represent more than 25% of the information.
6. The agencies will not challenge any joint purchase agreement among health care providers as long as two conditions are met: (a) the purchase accounts for less than 35% of the total sales of the product purchased in the relevant market, and (b) the cost of the product and service purchased jointly accounts for less than 20% of the total revenue from all products and services sold by each joint venture participant.[41]

In recognition of this 20% requirement, the FTC and the Department of Justice applied the "rule of reason" and cleared a venture by a group of Denver-area cardiologists whose proposed Rocky Mountain Cardiovascular Affiliates would have represented 22% of the cardiologists within the market.[42] The federal government strove to protect competition further with passage of the **Robinson-Patman Act** (1935). This law makes it illegal to discriminate in prices between different buyers of the same product, where the effect may be to lessen competition and create a monopoly.

In July 2004 the FTC and the Department of Justice issued a major report entitled "Improving Health Care Competition." This report was a comprehensive look at all sectors of the health care industry, physicians and physician groups, hospitals, insurance and other third party programs, and pharmaceuticals. The report made the observation that the federal government had been unsuccessful in its recent challenges against hospital mergers. However, it also noted that where there is less competition, health care prices tend to be higher. The sentiment in the report tended to indicate the government intends to continue to want in the coming years to instill a competitive marketplace in the health care arena. The major recommendations of this report in which marketers may find themselves being guided out are:

1. Private payers, governments, and providers should continue experiments to improve incentives for providers to lower costs and enhance quality and for consumers to seek lower prices and better quality.
   a. Private payers, governments, and providers should improve measures of price and quality.
   b. Private payers, governments, and providers should furnish more information on prices and quality and consumers in ways that they find useful and relevant, and continue to experiment with financing structures that will give consumers incentives to use such information.

c. Private payers, governments, and providers should experiment further with payment methods for aligning providers' incentives with consumers' interests in low prices, quality improvements, and innovation.
2. States should decrease barrier to entry into provider markets.
   a. States with Certificate of Need programs should consider whether these programs best serve their citizens' health care needs.
   b. States should consider adopting the recommendation of the Institute of Medicine to broaden the membership of state licensure boards.
3. Governments should reexamine the role of subsidies in health care markets in light of their potential inefficiencies and potential to distort competition.
4. Governments should not enact legislation to permit independent physicians to bargain collectively.
5. States should consider the potential costs and benefits of regulating pharmacy benefit manager transparency.
6. Governments should reconsider whether current mandates best serve their citizens' health care needs. When deciding whether to mandate particular benefits, governments should consider that such mandates are likely to reduce competition, restrict choice, raise the cost of health insurance, and increase the number of uninsured Americans.[43]

This report and these recommendations have significant implications for health care marketing because they address issues of quality, choice, and innovation.

Product Legislation

In terms of the marketing mix, several laws have also been passed that affect the product and, in varying instances, protect the company or the market. As mentioned earlier, a major form of federal legislative protection is the granting of a patent.

A second major law protecting companies is the **Lanham Act**, which provides for the registration of a company's trademarks—in other words, its brand name. When this law was initially passed, it provided trademark protection to the first user of the trademark. Then, in 1988, the trademark law was updated with the **Trademark Law Revision Act**, which granted a company trademark protection prior to actual use.

A trademark is a valuable asset for a company (more on the value of brand names is described in Chapter 8), but the trademark law does not give a company ownership of the trademark. A company can lose its trademark if the name becomes so generic that it applies to the entire product class. "Aspirin," for example, used to be a company's trademark, so too was "elevator." Now companies such as Xerox and FedEx, both registered trademarks, work to protect against any trademark infringement, but also to ensure that their names are not used as nouns or verbs—which would classify them as generic terms. When you think you are xeroxing a memo, the Xerox Company will tell you that you are photocopying.

Pricing

In health care there are several regulations related to issues of reimbursement. At the macro level, issues of price fixing and price discounting were addressed by the Sherman Act. Although this law did not specifically outlaw price fixing, the courts have ruled that price fixing, *per se*, is illegal and will restrain trade. In terms of discounting, the law allows for discounts to be offered to buyers, providing cost savings can be demonstrated in dealing with a particular buyer. Promotional allowances can also be granted differentially to buyers, but they must be offered on an equal proportionate basis to each buyer based on volume purchased.

Distribution

In this third aspect of the marketing mix, the government has three major areas of concern. The first pertains to **exclusive dealing**, in which a buyer is required to handle only the products of one manufacturer but not a competitor. This requirement is considered a violation of the Clayton Act.

A second area of concern pertains to **requirement contracts**, in which a buyer is required to purchase all or part of its needs for a product from one seller for a defined period of time. The justice system has examined each instance of a requirement contract separately. A third area involves **tying arrangements**, where the seller of a product requires that the purchaser also buy another item. These arrangements are considered illegal when they result in restraining trade in the tied product.

In health care an increasingly important area of government regulatory investigation pertains to vertical integration. Although not specifically illegal, the courts evaluate issues of vertical integration with regard to the Clayton Act to ensure that the result of this activity neither lessens competition nor creates a monopoly. This issue of vertical integration is becoming more important as hospitals establish integrated delivery systems and acquire primary care practices.

Within health care, there is a separate set of regulations pertaining to the issue of patient referrals. In 1991, the Health Care Financing Administration (now known as Centers for Medicare and Medicaid Services [CMS]) published regulations for the Ethics in Patient Referrals Act, referred to as "Stark I" (for the congressman who sponsored the legislation). This law prohibited physician referrals to entities in which they held a financial interest. This law was broadened in the Omnibus Budget Reconciliation Act of 1993. The new law, known as **Stark II**, also prohibits physician referrals to entities in which they hold a financial interest and applies to both Medicare and Medicaid. Effective January 1, 1995, no physician or physician family member who has a financial interest in an entity may refer a patient to that entity for health services. This law puts restrictions not only on the physician but also on the entity to which the patient is referred. That organization cannot present a claim or a bill to any individual or third party for reimbursement. While there are degrees of interpretation and exceptions to this legislation, it greatly determines the strategies used to control the channel of distribution for patient referrals.[44]

On July 26, 2004, some technical corrections went into effect regarding Stark II. The details of these changes get to be subtle but pertain to the following sections of the Stark rule:

- methods for establishing physician compensation that will be deemed to be consistent with fair market value
- an accommodation for percentage and other formula-based physician compensation methodologies
- CMS's decision to adopt a very narrow interpretation of the statutory exception for "hospital remuneration unrelated to designated health services"
- a new bright-line definition of "same building" for purposes of the in-office ancillary services exception
- a physician recruitment incentives exception that permits certain incentives to residents and interns already practicing in the hospital's service area, and incentives to physicians recruited to existing medical practices
- a new physician retention incentive exception
- a new exception for unavoidable and temporary lapses in compliance.[45]

Promotion

The last element of the marketing mix—promotion—is also subject to various government regulations. The majority of promotional activities are closely monitored and regulated by the **Federal Trade Commission Act of 1914**. This law, which created the FTC, forbids deceptive or misleading advertising and unfair business practices. The FTC has the power to issue cease and desist orders, and it can order any company to conduct **corrective advertising**, a means of communication by which the company must correct misimpressions formed in the marketplace.

In 1975, the issue of advertising for professional services underwent a dramatic turnaround. At this time, the U.S. Supreme Court ruled that professional associations were subject to antitrust laws, which were designed to protect competition. In order to comply with this judicial view, the American Medical Association (AMA) and other professional medical and legal associations loosened their restrictions that prohibited their members from advertising. Later U.S. Supreme Court decisions in 1980 and 1982 ruled that restricting advertising was illegal, and since then, advertising has become very common in both the health and the legal professions.

In 1993, the federal government also put into effect the Medicare and Medicaid antikickback law, which affects certain promotional programs. The government recently investigated programs that give physicians frequent flyer miles each time they complete a questionnaire for new patients prescribed the company's product. According to government requirements, a payment or gift may be considered illegal under the kickback law if: (1) it is made to a person who is in a position to generate business for the paying party, (2) it is related to the volume of business generated, (3) it is of greater than nominal value and exceeds free-market value, or (4) it is unrelated to any service other than the referral of a patient.

The HIPAA Challenge[46]

The most significant regulatory change to occur in the past decade may well be the Health Insurance Portability and Accountability Act (**HIPAA**), which was signed into law on August 21, 1996. Overall, this legislation was to facilitate health insurance portability, protect patient security and privacy of information, and further reduce health care fraud and abuse. It is mostly in the areas of protecting the patient privacy that marketing is affected by the passage of this legislation. The law went into effect in April 2003. HIPAA requires all health care providers to have patient consent for access to their medical records or information. For the individual physician's office, this entails logistical as well as operational changes. For example, the physician who uses an outside vendor for cleaning the facility after hours will need to ensure that all medical records are locked. A physician who sends out information on a patient will need to obtain prior approval that such information can be transmitted.

For marketers, it is necessary to ensure that all marketing actions are compliant with HIPAA regulations. This regulation might have the greatest impact on database management programs. Data will need to be aggregated so that medical information cannot be attached to names and addresses of individual patients.[47] Patient identifiable information cannot be used to send them marketing materials. Organizations must create a system that allows patients to opt out of marketing activities tied to their personal information.

HIPAA does allow for certain marketing activities in which the health care organization can use patient data without the person's prior approval. One of the interesting implications of HIPAA is the use of patient data for marketing and fundraising activities. Under the regulations a health care organization must have written authorization to use patient information for purposes that are not related to the treatment or payment of their care. Under the privacy rule, however, certain marketing and fundraising activities have been allowed without patient authorization. But, this opportunity to use patient data is only in support of several limited fundraising and marketing activities.

Health care organizations and the institutionally related foundations (foundations that qualify as nonprofit charitable foundations under section 501(c)(3) of the Internal Revenue Code and that have in their charter statement of charitable purposes an explicit linkage to the health care organization) may use or disclose an individual's demographic information and/or the dates that the individual received treatment without obtaining written authorization.

These uses and disclosures are permissible in the following instances:

1. The covered entity's notice of privacy practices states that individuals may be contacted for the purpose of raising funds.

2. Any and all fundraising materials include instructions on how to opt-out of future communications.
3. The covered entity makes reasonable efforts to ensure those individuals' opt-out requests are honored.

The use or disclosure of patient health information (PHI) for marketing purposes is permissible without an authorization in three instances:

1. First, health care organizations are permitted to use or disclose patient information without authorization to make marketing communications in face-to-face encounters. These communications may include discussion of any services or products, including the services or products of a third party.
2. Second, patient information may be used or disclosed without authorization to make marketing communications involving products or services of nominal value. This would allow for the distribution of calendars, pens, and other merchandise that is generally considered to be of a promotional nature.
3. Finally, no authorization is required for marketing communications about health-related products or services of the health care organization, if the communication:
   - Identifies the covered entity as the party making the communication
   - Discloses any direct or indirect remuneration received by the covered entity for making the communication
   - Contains instructions on how to opt-out of similar future communications
   - Explains why the individual has been targeted for the communication in those instances where PHI was used to target the communication to particular individuals based upon their health status or condition

This third type of marketing communication is restricted to uses by covered entities or disclosures to their business associates pursuant to a business associate agreement.[48]

Under HIPAA it is important for marketing professionals and providers to recognize that patients have certain basic "rights." These are:

1. The right to written notice of information practices of health care plans and providers
2. The right to inspect and copy their protected health information
3. The right to request an amendment or correction
4. The right to an accounting of disclosures for purposes other than treatment, payment, or health care operations

Health care organizations are allowed to maintain communication relationships with patients, using protected health information without patient consent unless it falls within the definition of marketing as defined by the revisions of HIPAA. Any marketing communication requires prior authorization. With certain stated exclusions, marketing is defined by HIPAA as follows:

- "To make a communication about a product or service that encourages recipients of the communication to purchase or use the product or service . . ." and
- "An arrangement between a covered entity and any other entity whereby the covered entity discloses [PHI] to the other entity, in exchange for direct or indirect remuneration, for the other entity or its affiliate to make a communication about its own product or service that encourages recipients of the communication to purchase or use that product or service."[49]

The following three types of communications were exempted from the definition of marketing:

- Communications describing a health-related product or service that is offered by the provider or included in its plan of benefits
- Communications describing the individual's treatment
- Communications for case management or care coordination for the individual or directions/recommendations for alternative treatments, providers, or settings of care[50]

Ongoing Federal Monitoring

Beyond the HIPAA challenges, the Department of Justice and the FTC have six areas in which they provide rather close supervision of the health care industry. These pertain to (1) mergers, (2) hospital joint ventures involving high technology, (3) physicians' provision of information to purchasers of health care services, (4) hospital participation in exchanges of price and cost information, (5) health care providers' joint purchasing arrangements, and (6) physician network joint ventures. In terms of mergers, the FTC has stated that the agencies will not challenge any merger between two general acute-care hospitals where one of the hospitals (1) has an average of fewer than 100 licensed beds over the three most recent years, and (2) has an average daily inpatient census of fewer than 40 patients over the three most recent years, absent extraordinary circumstances. This antitrust safety zone will not apply if that hospital is less than five years old. Rules and concerns around joint ventures are extremely detailed and entail definitions of the relevant market and the technology itself that is under consideration. A detailed explanation of the issues and concerns is provided by the Department of Justice and the FTC in their material entitled "Department of Justice and Federal Trade Commission Statements of Antitrust Enforcement Policy in Health Care."[51]

Self-Regulation

In response to this more active government role, the medical and health professions are stepping up their self-policing efforts. The AMA has developed a set of guidelines that were adopted by the Pharmaceutical Research and Manufacturers of America

(PhRMA), a pharmaceutical manufacturers' trade group headquartered in Washington, D.C. (www.phrma.org). The PhRMA's members produce almost 90% of all the brand-name drugs in the United States. These guidelines restrict drug company gifts to physicians to those that have only nominal value or those with direct educational or patient benefit. The PhRMA also publishes a 700-page book detailing government and private-sector standards on drug promotion.[52]

Marketing plans and strategies are developed in the context of, and in response to, the broader macroenvironment. While the environment cannot be controlled, organizations must recognize ongoing trends and factors that will likely affect their market success. Because the environmental factors are dynamic, a health care organization must maintain a continual monitoring process and adjust its marketing plans accordingly.

■ Key Terms

Inflation	Regulation
Gross Income	Sherman Antitrust Act
Disposable Income	Clayton Act
Discretionary Income	Antimerger Act
Technology	Robinson-Patman Act
Telemedicine	Lanham Act
Demographics	Trademark Law Revision Act
Baby Boomers	Exclusive Dealing
Blended Family	Requirement Contracts
Culture	Tying Arrangements
Pure Competition	Stark II
Monopolistic Competition	Federal Trade Commission Act of 1914
Oligopoly	Corrective Advertising
Monopoly	HIPAA

■ Chapter Summary

1. Marketing strategy must be developed in response to and in concert with the broader macroenvironment. Economic, technological, social, competitive, and regulatory forces can all determine the effectiveness of any organization's marketing program.

2. In recent years, the rise in the cost of medical care has dramatically outstripped the rise in cost of consumer goods. This increase has caused employers and other health care buyers to take more aggressive actions to control their health care expenses.

3. Health care is a technologically driven industry. New technological advances dramatically affect the institutions and providers who deliver health care and

determine how that care is delivered. The Internet and wireless will dramatically affect how patients interact with their health care providers.

4. The changing demographics of the U.S. population represent significant opportunities for health care providers. Older consumers—a fast-growing segment—are major utilizers of health care services and products. Baby boomers are often attracted to alternative medical approaches.

5. Changing marketplace demographics, related to gender, ethnicity, and race require health care providers to be more responsive to the needs and concerns of women, Hispanics, and African Americans. In many metropolitan areas, Hispanics and African Americans represent a significant proportion of the market.

6. The competitive market can be defined as either a pure competition, a monopolistic competition, an oligopoly, or a monopoly. The differences represent the number of sellers in the marketplace.

7. The prior movement to managed care is now returning to a fee-for-service market. While there is consolidation among hospitals, inpatient admissions are rising and outpatient surgeries continue to grow. The five largest managed care plans control the bulk of the commercially insured population in the United States.

8. A wide variety of federal and state regulations exist that affect each aspect of the marketing mix. In recent years, major federal regulatory attention in health care has been paid to mergers and acquisitions of hospitals and providers by competitors. The government has provided some guidelines pertaining to health care mergers and acquisitions.

9. The issue of provider referrals has also come under scrutiny of federal regulators. While the laws are not exact, in general, it is illegal for physicians to refer to a facility in which they have a financial interest.

10. HIPAA regulations, which were passed to primarily affect the portability of patients' insurance, also impact the marketing activities and communications that can be conducted without a patient's consent.

■ Chapter Problems

1. The major online computer services such as America Online Inc. and WebMD provide health news and medical and health forums where users can access medical libraries, exchange messages, and discuss health problems. In what ways might the growing use of these services by consumers affect future strategies for: (a) family practitioners and (b) specialists?

2. What environmental factors would you suggest account for: (a) the rapid growth of NordicTrack, a premium-priced home fitness equipment company that formerly sold only through direct mail and has now opened retail stores in shopping malls, and (b) the success of after-hours clinics and urgent care facilities in many metropolitan areas?

3. Assume you were hired to design a managed care organization plan targeted to baby boomers in San Antonio, Texas, a city with a large Hispanic population. How would you make this service offering unique to respond to the major trends discussed within this chapter?

4. The U.S. Justice Department settled a case involving ClassiCare Network, a joint venture of eight Long Island hospitals. The joint venture was to act as the "exclusive bargaining agent" in negotiations with all HMOs regarding hospital discounts. The agreement reached with the hospitals barred this arrangement. On what grounds and rules was the Justice Department action based?

5. A primary care medical group has a list of patients who had once used the group on a regular basis as their primary source of care. However, in scanning their records, these patients had not been in for an appointment in the past two years. The senior partner wants to send them an informational flyer about the practice and a refrigerator magnet that has the group's telephone number and after-hours service number. As the marketing director for the practice, evaluate this approach in light of the HIPAA regulations. Can it be implemented?

■ Notes

1. 2004–2005 Statistical Abstract of the United States, U.S. Census Bureau, 443.

2. "Hospital Stays for Hysterectomy Are Dwindling," *Health Technology Trends* 5, no. 9 (1993): 7.

3. Donald I. Galen, Arnold Jacobson, Louis N. Weckstein, "Outpatient Laparoscopic Hysterectomy: A Review of 50 Patients," *Journal of the American Association of Gynecologic Laparoscopists* 1, no. 3 (May 1994).

4. L. Page, "Playing Catch-up," *American Medical News* 37, no. 29 (1994): 3, 7–8.

5. "Surgeons Raise the Bar with Telemedicine," *Advanced Imaging Pro* (June 30, 2005). (http://www.advancedimagingpro.com).

6. Andrew Cudmore and Paula Bobrowski, "Working the Web," *Marketing Health Services* 23, no. 3 (Fall 2003): 37–41.

7. Victoria Rideout, "Generation Rx.com," *Marketing Health Services* 22, no. 1 (Spring 2002): 26–30.

8. "Nearly Half of U.S. Adults Turn to Web for Health Care Needs," *U.S. Newswire, Inc.*, July 15, 2003.

9. Susan Fox, "Older Americans and the Internet," *Pew Internet and American Life Project* (March 25, 2004).

10. "Health Care in America: Trends in Utilization," U.S. Department of Health and Human Services, Centers for Disease Control, DHHS Up. no. 2004-1031 (January 2004), p. 8.

11. "Alzheimer's Rates to Double Despite Advances: Growing Number of Elderly Means More Cases," WRAL.com (May 29, 2002) (http://www.wral.com/health/1485249/detail.html).

12. George Moschis, Danny N. Bellenger, and Carolyn Folkman Cursai, "Before Targeting the Elderly Market, Find Out How They Make Their Healthcare Choices," *Marketing Health Services* 23, no. 4 (Winter 2003): 17–21.

13. Gregg A. Warshaw, Elizabeth J. Bragg, and Ruth W. Shaull, "Geriatric Medicine Training and Practice in the United States at the Beginning of the 21st Century," The Association of Geriatric Academic Programs (July 2002).

14. P. Braus, "When Mom Needs Help," *American Demographics* 16, no. 3 (1994): 38–46.

15. "Aging Baby Boomers Flocking to Doctors: High Blood Pressure Is Leading Diagnosis" (http://usgovinfo.about.com/cs/healthmedical/a/aasickboomers.htm).

16. S. Mitchell, "Healing Without Doctors," *American Demographics* 15, no. 7 (1993): 46–49.

17. D.M. Eisenberg et al., "Unconventional Medicine in the United States," *The New England Journal of Medicine* 328, no. 4 (1993): 246–252.

18. Ken Bryson and Lynn Casper, "Household and Family Characteristics: March 1997," U.S. Department of Commerce (April 1998).

19. U.S. Census Bureau, "Current Population Survey" (March 1998).

20. Peter Francese, "America at Mid-decade," *American Demographics* (February 1995): 23–29.

21. J. R. Evans and Barry Berman, *Marketing* (New York: MacMillan & Co., 1994), 228.

22. "The Trend You Can't Ignore," *American Demographics* 16, no. 7 (1994): 2.

23. "Quick States 2004," U.S. Department of Labor, Women's Bureau (http://www.dol.gov/wb/stats/main.htm).

24. D. Crispell, "Workers in 2000," *American Demographics* 14, no. 9 (1992): 27–28.

25. "Women Dominate the Web," *Marketing Health Services* 22, no. 4 (Winter 2002): 9.

26. MHS Staff, "Women's Health: Marketing Challenges in the 21st Century," *Marketing Health Services* 20, no. 2 (Fall 2000): 4–11.

27. "Women Outnumber Men Applying To Medical School," *Psychiatric News* 39, no. 23 (December 3, 2004): 46.

28. Lenn Ann Runy, "Providing Alternatives," *Hospitals and Health Networks* 78, no. 1 (January 2004): 30.

29. Elayne Howard and Karen Gillespie, "A Break from Tradition," *Marketing Health Services* 23, no. 2 (Summer 2003): 14–19.

30. K. Pallarito, "Hospitals Strengthen Networks Through New Fitness Facilities," *Modern Healthcare* 24, no. 50 (1994): 44–46.

31. Laura Landro, "Consumers Need Health-care Data," *The Wall Street Journal* (January 29, 2004): D3.

32. James C. Robinson, "Consolidation and Transformation of Competition in Health Insurance," *Health Affairs* 23, no. 6 (2004): 11–24.

33. David Carpenter, "Health Care's New Behemoths," *Hospital's and Health Networks* 79, no. 1 (January 2005): 38–46.

34. "Profile of U.S. Community Hospitals," *Hospitals and Health Networks* 78, no. 2 (February 2005): 32.

35. http://www.hcahealthcare.com.

36. Charles Stein, "Profits Elude For-profit Hospitals," *The Boston Globe* (February 15, 2004): E1, E3.

37. John Bian and Michael Morrissey, "Market Determinants, Ambulatory Surgery Centers, and Hospital Outpatient Surgery Volume," presentation (June 28, 2005).

38. "Sand, Sun, and Surgery," *Business Week* (February 16, 2004): 48.

39. "Minnesota Hospitals Make Antitrust Pact," *Modern Healthcare* 24, no. 32 (1994): 34.

40. Robert Tomsho, "Giant Hospital Chain Uses Tough Tactics to Push Fast Growth," *The Wall Street Journal* (July 12, 1994): A1, A6.

41. "New Guidelines from the FTC and Justice Department," *Hospitals and Health Networks* 67, no. 23 (1993): 28.

42. "Justice Dept., FTC Offer More Antitrust Guidance," *Modern Healthcare* 24, no. 40 (1994): 34.

43. "Improving Health Care Competition": A Report by the Federal Trade Commission and the Department of Justice (July 2004).

44. H. J. Swibel and M. J. Zaremski, "Surfing Stark II: Prohibition Against Self-referrals," *Physician Executive* 21, no. 2 (1995): 11–15.

45. "Phase II of the Final Stark Regulations," McDermett, Will & Emery (April 19, 2004), http://www.mwe.com/index.cfm/fuseaction/publications.nldetail/object_id/081a59b2-7f74-4bc9-aaf5-7012b8110bfc.cfm.

46. A portion of this discussion was drawn from Steven Hillestad and Eric N. Berkowitz, *Health Care Marketing Strategy: From Planning to Action* (Sudbury, MA: Jones and Bartlett Publishers, 2004), Chapter 3.

47. Nancy Paddison and James Hallick, "HIPAA Privacy Regulations Can Guide, Strengthen Marketing Efforts," *Healthcare Marketing Report* 19, no. 11 (November 2001): 16–19.

48. "How Fundraising and Marketing Fit into HIPAA Privacy," *HIPAA Advisory*, http://www.hipaadvisory.com/action/advisor/HIPAAdvisor20.htm.

49. http://www.solucient.com/hipaa/hipaa_marketing.shtml.

50. Solucient, op. cit.

51. http://www.ftc.gov/reports/hlth3s.htm.

52. D. M. Gianelli, "Drug Makers Warned: Some Promotions are Kickbacks," *American Medical News* 37, no. 33 (1994): 9.

Understanding the Consumer

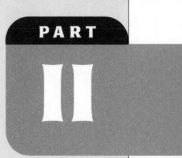

Buyer Behavior

The basic purpose of marketing is to meet the needs of consumers. Central to effective marketing strategy then, is to understand how consumers make the decision to buy a product, select a doctor, or join a health plan. As this chapter will discuss in detail, a variety of factors affect the consumer's decision-making process.

■ Decision-Making Model

The **consumer decision-making process** can be represented in six stages (as shown in FIGURE 4-1): (1) problem recognition, (2) internal search, (3) external search, (4) alternative evaluation, (5) purchase, and (6) post-purchase evaluation.[1]

Problem Recognition

The stage of *problem recognition* is where the consumer perceives a difference between the desired and actual state and is motivated to try to close this gap.[2] For example, a consumer begins to notice that he always has difficulty getting an appointment with his primary care physician. This recognition might motivate the individual to explore alternative sources of medical care and seek another physician.

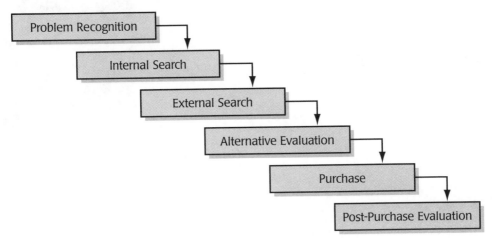

FIGURE 4-1 Consumer Decision-Making Process

It is critical for an organization to develop marketing strategies to aid the problem recognition stage. For example, an advertisement showing long waiting lines at a competing health plan's office might suggest that consumers need to explore alternatives to using that health plan. Marketing strategy attempts to influence the desired state by trying to alter perceptions of the existing state.

Internal Search

After recognizing the existence of a problem, the consumer often engages in an *internal information search* seeking a solution to the perceived problem. In this example, the individual will try to determine whether he knows of, or remembers, other possible primary care physicians, either those whom he heard about or those he recalls seeing. In traditional industries that manufacture frequently purchased products, such as toothpaste or soft drinks, the internal search process is often sufficient for the consumer to make a decision. When internal search does not produce an alternative to solve the recognized problem, the consumer may engage in external search.

External Search

An *external information search* involves seeking information from one or more sources when internal search is insufficient.[3] These sources can be media in the form of advertisements, personal sources such as friends or salespersons, public sources such as government data, or rating organizations such as the Consumers Union, which publishes *Consumer Reports*.[4] Increasingly, an important external source for search as shown in Chapter 3 for consumers of all ages is the Internet. EXHIBIT 4-1 shows a sample of data being collected by the department of Health and Human Services that can be accessed by consumers on the government's Web site. With this tool,

Exhibit 4-1 External Information on Hospital Quality Clinical Practices

Quality Measure Click on a measure name to compare all hospitals in a graph	Percentage for Baystate Medical Center	Percentage for Beth Israel Deaconess Medical Center	Percentage for Brockton Hospital	Percentage for Massachusetts General Hospital
Percent of Heart Attack Patients Given ACE inhibitor for LVSD if appropriate	92% of 130 patients[2]	80% of 120 patients	100% of 17 patients[1]	77% of 70 patients
Percent of Heart Attack Patients Given Aspirin at Arrival if appropriate	99% of 350 patients[2]	98% of 129 patients	99% of 106 patients	99% of 191 patients
Percent of Heart Attack Patients Given Beta Blocker at arrival if appropriate	98% of 278 patients[2]	96% of 131 patients	94% of 88 patients	98% of 179 patients
Percent of Heart Attack Patients Given Beta Blocker at Discharge if appropriate	99% of 505 patients[2]	97% of 413 patients	94% of 66 patients	99% of 525 patients

Source: http://www.hospitalcompare.hhs.gov/.

consumers can search by hospital name, or by geographic information to examine how hospitals compare on certain medical conditions against a national standard on heart attack, heart failure, and pneumonia. The Internet plays an important and influential role in patients' searches for information. Results from the December 2003 Pulse Healthcare Survey found that almost 8.5% of all U.S. households that sought information to judge the quality of care used the Internet to do so.[5] How information is presented, however, is critical for marketers. It has been found that if consumers do not comprehend the information, they dismiss it as unimportant.[6]

Table 4-1 shows the external search information sources used by consumers in seeking primary care assistance. Yet, in a 1991 study, women preferred physicians as their primary information source.[7]

Table 4-1	External Search Sources for Primary Care				
	Provider Used				
Information Source	Internist (N = 66)	Family Practitioner (N = 174)	OB/GYN (N = 32)	General Practitioner (N = 192)	All Respondents (N = 464)
Friends	19.7	21.4	34.8	26.4	23.4
Family	25.8	27.6	25.0	27.0	26.5
Phone call to provider	16.7	18.4	15.6	9.4	14.1
Observation of office when passing by	3.4	9.8	9.7	3.7	6.4
Another doctor	33.3	17.8	25.0	16.2	19.5
Heard doctor speak (PTA, church, etc.)	7.0	6.0	13.8	4.9	6.3
Nonphysician medical professional (nurse, paramedic, etc.)	7.0	14.4	33.3	14.3	14.7
Employer provides care through this doctor or practice	6.1	6.3	15.6	4.7	6.0

Source: Reprinted from Stewart, D.W., Hickson, G.B., Peachman, C., Koslow, S., and Altemeier, W., Information Search and Decision Making in the Selection of Family Health Care, *Journal of Health Care Marketing*, Vol. 9, No. 2, pp. 29–39, with permission of American Marketing Association, © 1989.

Alternative Evaluation

The fourth stage of the consumer decision-making process is *alternative evaluation*, where the consumer compares the various choices that may best meet the individual's need. In this stage, the consumer determines the criteria for judging the alternative products or services. These are termed the **evaluative criteria**. Evaluative criteria can differ in terms of type, number, and importance. Consumers can use tangible and intangible criteria. Tangible criteria might include the cost of joining a particular health maintenance organization (HMO). While many consumers have seen tangible rating criteria regarding hospitals, health plans, and physicians, a Harris poll found few people (one percent or less of adults) have changed providers or health plans as a result. Furthermore, a comparison of 2001 and 2002 data finds no evidence that these evaluations are growing in influence.[8] An intangible criterion might be the way a particular physician's office feels when you walk in for an appointment.

The number of criteria used to evaluate alternatives can also vary. As to be expected, fewer criteria are used for simple products like toothpaste or laundry soap.[9] An evoked set of alternatives representing those that meet the consumer's evaluative criteria are determined.[10] In forming the evoked set, the consumer selects a subset of possibilities from which to make the final choice.

Research has found that, when evaluating alternatives, the consumer typically has a set of attributes that are important and will use each attribute to evaluate the alternatives. In this type of model, developed originally by Fishbein, the consumer selects the alternatives that have the highest evaluation of desired attributes.[11] An example of this process is shown in EXHIBIT 4-2. Based on the calculations shown in this exhibit, the consumer would have the most favorable attitude toward the Johnson Clinic. This outcome is determined by multiplying the importance of the three attributes used to compare the clinics (hours for appointments, range of services, and office location) by the belief held by the consumer regarding how much each clinic meets his or her needs regarding these attributes.

Purchase

At this stage the consumer makes the *purchase*, selecting one brand or alternative over the others. The decision at this stage may involve final determinations as to when to purchase or, in the case of certain products, how much to purchase.

Exhibit 4-2 — Fishbein Choice Model

$$\text{Attitude} = \sum_{i=1}^{n} \text{Belief} \times \text{Importance}$$

1. Rate the importance of each factor on a scale of '1' Very Unimportant to '5' Very Important in choosing a doctor:

Hours for appointments	5
Range of services	3
Office location	7

2. Please rate each group listed below on a scale of '1' Doesn't meet my needs to '5' Does meet my needs on each dimension:

	Hours for appointments	Range of services	Office location
Group Health	7	8	2
Johnson Medical	5	6	9
Sutter Clinic	8	4	6

    Based on these ratings, the Fishbein model would calculate a consumer rating for each group as follows:

Group Health	5×7 (hrs) $+ 3 \times 8$ (services) $+ 7 \times 2$ (location) $=$	73
Johnson Medical	$5 \times 5 + 3 \times 6 + 7 \times 9$	$= 106$
Sutter Clinic	$5 \times 8 + 3 \times 4 + 7 \times 7$	$= 101$

    The consumer is most favorably disposed to Johnson and would choose that group.

Post-Purchase Evaluation

Be aware that the consumer's decision-making process does not end at the stage of purchase decision. Upon choosing a particular product or service, the consumer spends some time evaluating that choice. Favorable evaluations might ultimately lead the consumer to repurchase or endorse the product or service.[12] The importance of the *post-purchase evaluation* has led many health care organizations to measure the satisfaction of their patients or their referral sources. Satisfaction is measured, then, as a confirmation or disconfirmation of the consumer's expectations regarding the performance of the chosen product or service. Consumers can use data obtained from customer satisfaction measurement surveys as part of their internal search information when making subsequent purchase decisions.

Measuring Post-Purchase Satisfaction

By measuring consumer post-purchase satisfaction, a health care organization can focus management attention on areas of service that need improvement. In the post-purchase evaluation, the organization should measure two elements: (1) it should rate how important a particular aspect of the service encounter was in terms of overall consumer satisfaction, and (2) the organization should measure whether consumer (or patient) expectations were confirmed or disconfirmed. For example, a consumer post-evaluation satisfaction survey might contain the following questions:

A. How important were the following factors in your overall satisfaction?

	Very important				*Very unimportant*
Quality of food	1	2	3	4	5
Admitting process	1	2	3	4	5
Nursing attentiveness	1	2	3	4	5

B. Please indicate how well each of the following aspects of your hospital stay met your expectations?

	Much better than expected		*About as I expected*		*Must worse than expected*
Quality of food	1	2	3	4	5
Admitting process	1	2	3	4	5
Nursing attentiveness	1	2	3	4	5

The outcomes of these post-purchase evaluations will determine the direction for management action, as shown in FIGURE 4-2. Areas that hold low importance, yet exceed expectations, may present opportunities for management to shift resources into more essential aspects of the service encounter. Areas of high importance in which expectations are exceeded present opportunities to leverage with important markets.

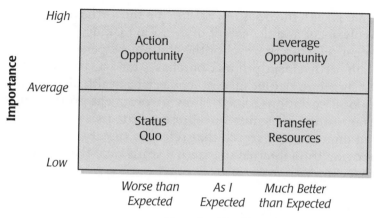

FIGURE 4-2 Action Opportunities for Post-Purchase Evaluation

A promotional program should reinforce the fact that the organization is meeting customer needs. Status quo areas are those of low importance, where expectations are minimally met but not exceeded. Dimensions of the service encounter requiring management attention and action are those factors rated as very important by customers where their expectations were not met. The importance of this framework can tie directly to future efforts in building long-term customer retention. This issue will be discussed in depth in Chapter 7.

Cognitive Dissonance

When a consumer is choosing between two or more relatively equal alternatives, a choice will occasionally lead to the creation of *cognitive dissonance*, a mental state of anxiety brought on because the consumer is unsure of the chosen alternative.[13] For example, an employee might suffer great cognitive dissonance in choosing between two managed care plans. Often when dissonance occurs, consumers will again engage in search behavior to reduce the dissonance. One of two outcomes can result. In some cases, consumers will try to reinforce the correctness of their own decisions; in other cases, they will denigrate the alternatives not chosen. For health care organizations, this aspect of post-purchase evaluation signals the need to communicate with the buyer or user of a service shortly after the encounter has occurred or the contract has been signed. Post-purchase communication in the form of a letter, newsletter, or phone call can reinforce the consumer's belief that the correct choice was made by choosing the provider that he or she selected.

Alternative Decision-Making Sequences

Not every situation in which the consumer is required to make a choice involves the sequence of steps shown in Figure 4-1. There are several alternative decision situations that modify the model previously described. Decision making varies as a function of how involved the consumer is with the decision. EXHIBIT 4-3 shows the matrix that represents the degree of involvement and the extent of decision making.

In this model, **involvement** refers to the level of the consumer's personal investment in the purchase.[14] High involvement product purchases tend to be those that represent risk (selection of a surgeon), significant cost (choice of a health plan), or social implications (the clubs or associations joined). Low involvement product purchases are not very important to the consumer or represent little risk or cost. The matrix also shows a second dimension of search that refers to the degree of effort the consumer expends in moving from internal to external search and the extensiveness of that external search.

Routine Decision Making

The **routine decision-making** situation involves repetitive purchasing. In these instances, there is often little difference between competing market alternatives. As can be seen in Exhibit 4-3, routine decision making can involve both high and low involvement. In the case of high involvement, the consumer engages in little extended decision making in frequently choosing to use his primary care physician. The consumer has developed loyalty to the provider. In product marketing, this situation is referred to as **brand loyalty**, in which the consumer regularly chooses the same product or service to fulfill a recognized need.

Complex Decision Making

Complex decision making involves situations in which there is high involvement and extended search. This scenario might well arise in health care situations. A consumer facing major surgery might decide to consult with a couple of physicians for their recommendations. The patient might also research any available data on mortality and morbidity statistics as they apply to particular hospitals and physicians. The individ-

Exhibit 4-3   Consumer Decision Making and Involvement

Decision making/ involvement	High	Low
Extended	complex (health insurance plan selection)	variety seeking (over the counter pharmaceuticals)
Routine	brand loyalty (primary care physician)	inertia (bandaid selection)

Source: Adapted from Henry Assael, *Consumer Behavior and Marketing Action* (Cincinnati, OH: Southwestern College Publishing, 1995), 5th ed., 152.

ual might also ask friends or family for their insights as to places to go for treatment. Obviously in such situations, risk is high and extended search becomes warranted.

Limited Decision Making

Limited decision making involves extended search in low-involvement situations. In traditional product marketing, this occurs when the consumer seeks variety or engages in impulse purchasing. In health care, this situation often occurs when consumers buy over-the-counter pharmaceutical products. The consumer is not particularly tied to one brand and sees little real risk in choosing an alternative. After using one particular cold remedy, an individual might decide to explore alternatives to seek a more effective brand.

■ Psychological Influences on Decision Making

There are a variety of personal, psychological factors that affect a consumer's decision-making process. To market effectively to consumers, it is useful to understand these elements: motivation, attitudes, lifestyles, learning, and perception.

Motivation

Motivation encompasses the goals or needs that propel a consumer to action. At any point in time, an individual can have multiple needs that result in some course of action.

One of the more well-known models regarding motivation is Maslow's Hierarchy of Needs shown in FIGURE 4-3.[15] Maslow developed this framework to help

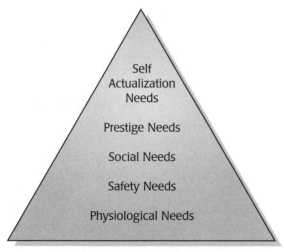

FIGURE 4-3 Maslow's Hierarchy of Needs

explain individual behavior and the differences among individuals regarding their behavior. According to Maslow, the differences in behavior might best be explained by understanding where an individual is in terms of this hierarchy. The needs at the lower end of the pyramid (e.g., physiological, safety) are the most basic. As a consumer begins to satisfy these needs, higher-order needs such as self-esteem or self-actualization begin to be addressed.

For a marketer, this framework is particularly useful in considering the positioning of products or services. A smoke detector can be positioned as meeting safety needs. Many health care plans highlight their ability to meet the safety needs of a family's loved ones. Wellness programs and smoking cessation clinics might be best positioned as responding to needs of self-esteem or self-actualization, rather than safety.

Attitudes

Attitudes and values affect a consumer's decision-making process. **Attitudes** represent a consumer's enduring cognitive evaluations, feelings, or action tendencies toward some person, object, or idea.[16] As discussed in the alternative-evaluation stage, the Fishbein model of attitude formation (shown in Exhibit 4-2) has attitudes being formed as a function of the importance of the attributes and the evaluation that the person or object contains some amount of that particular characteristic.

Since attitudes are predispositions to act in a certain way, marketers have often focused on the measurement of attitudes. Measuring consumer attitudes toward a product or service is not necessarily a measure of purchase intention. A consumer may have a favorable attitude toward the Mayo Clinic but may not seek treatment there for a variety of reasons, such as travel inconvenience, the proximity of other favorably evaluated clinics, or insurance restrictions.

While attitudes represent customers' predispositions, attitudes can be changed to some degree with varying marketing strategies.[17] Because attitudes are comprised of attributes, changing attitudes involves trying to shift the way consumers evaluate certain aspects of these attributes. One approach involves trying to shift consumers' evaluations of how much a particular brand of product or service possesses a particular attribute. For example, if pediatric coverage and availability were deemed important by managed care organization (MCO) subscribers, the MCO would tout the availability of its large panel of pediatric clinicians ready to meet subscriber needs. A second tactic involves changing the level of importance attached to a particular attribute. That same MCO might decide that its linkage with an academic medical center is a valuable component of its program. The market positioning might tout the backup expertise available in the rare instances when needed. A third strategy to change attitudes would involve helping consumers to develop an appreciation for other attributes to consider when evaluating alternatives.

Lifestyle

Lifestyle is an important aspect affecting a consumer's decision-making process. **Lifestyle** is the manner in which people live as demonstrated by how they spend their time, what they think, and the interests they have.[18] In the 1980s, for example, the term "yuppies" was popularized to describe a group of young, urban professionals who were characterized by a certain upscale, ambitious, and materialistic lifestyle and behavior. BMW automobiles, Chardonnay wine, and Burberry raincoats were some of the hallmarks of a particular lifestyle.

In marketing, lifestyle profiles of consumers are often developed through the use of AIO statements.[19] AIO refers to attitudes, interests, and opinions. A sample of AIO statements that might be used to define a health-conscious consumer is shown in EXHIBIT 4-4. These types of questions used in lifestyle analysis have also been referred to as psychographics.

VALS

One of the most commercially popular forms of lifestyle analysis is the VALS2™ system. VALS stands for Value And Life Styles, a program developed by SRI International, a Menlo Park, California, research and development company.[20] This classification scheme categorizes consumers into one of eight different basic lifestyle groups: innovators, thinkers, believers, achievers, strivers, experiencers, makers, and survivors. FIGURE 4-4 shows a breakdown of these profiles. These profiles define people based on their self-orientation and their resources. Resources are defined not just in financial terms, but refers to the full range of psychological, physical, demographic, and material means or capacities consumers have to draw upon. Resources include

Exhibit 4-4   Sample AIO Questions

1. I enjoy exercising whenever I get the chance.

2. It is important to watch your caloric intake.

3. In recent years too much attention has been paid to cholesterol levels.

4. When I exercise daily, I feel better.

5. Most of the stories on holistic medicine make me suspicious about the benefits.

6. I get nervous when my physician isn't fit.

7. I'm not sure exercising regularly really helps.

8. I like to read stories about nutrition and fitness.

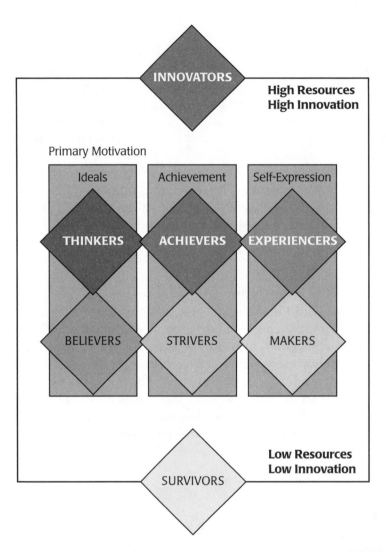

Innovators
Take-charge
Sophisticated
Curious

Thinkers
Reflective
Informed
Content

Achievers
Goal oriented
Brand conscious
Conventional

Experiencers
Trend setting
Impulsive
Variety seeking

Survivors
Nostalgic
Constrained
Cautious

Believers
Literal
Loyal
Moralistic

Strivers
Contemporary
Imitative
Style conscious

Makers
Responsible
Practical
Self-sufficient

FIGURE 4-4 The VALS Profile

Source: SRI Consulting Business Intelligence www.sric-bi.com/VALS. Used by permission.

education, income, self-confidence, health, and eagerness to buy. Self-orientation can take three primary directions:

- *Principle-oriented*—These people are guided in their choices by their beliefs and principles rather than by feelings, events, or desires.
- *Status-oriented*—These individuals are heavily influenced by the actions, approval, and opinions of others.
- *Action-oriented*—These people desire social or physical activity, variety, and risk taking.

VALS2™ has proven especially useful for understanding consumer preferences in media, electronics, travel and lodging, recreational activities, automotive purchases, home furnishings, and clothing.

PRIZM

A similar lifestyle program called PRIZM (Potential Rating Index by Zip Market) is commercially marketed by Claritas PRIZM of New York, a marketing consulting firm. This program examines census data and consumer lifestyle by zip code to develop a geodemographic profile. The company has developed approximately 66 different lifestyle profiles of neighborhoods that can be applied to any ZIP code. A marketer can then target specific appeals to certain areas and use more targeted media in each area. As Claritas mentions on its Web site (http://www.claritas.com/), the principle behind this segmentation scheme is the concept of "birds of a feather flock together." That is, similar groups of people cluster together in similar residential areas. Thus, it is useful for targeting site locations for satellite clinics or assisted living facilities as is done by one national proprietary company in this spectrum of health care. Unlike the VALS2™ approach, PRIZM is not based on attitudes. The foundation of PRIZM is demographics combined with consumption and media data. The PRIZM method is discussed in greater detail in Chapter 6 with a description of some neighborhood profiles.

Learning

Learning involves the changes in a person's behavior as a result of past experiences. Learning occurs as a result of a drive, stimulus, cues, responses, and reinforcement. The drive is a threat that motivates the individual. The stimulus is the object or factor that can reduce the drive. Related to stimuli are the cues, which are aspects calling attention to the stimuli. Response is the act of satisfying the drive. And finally, there is reinforcement, which is the reward.

Marketers can use learning theory as the foundation for a marketing plan to help the consumer enter the decision-making stage of problem recognition. A consumer has a drive or need for safety. The stimulus might be an advertisement touting the complete services and easy accessibility of Advocate Health Care's integrated health care system. The cue might occur when a consumer drives by several facilities and sees Advocate's name on the buildings. The response is the consumer's purchase of the Advocate Associate preferred provider organization plan, with appropriate reinforcement following in the form of satisfied use.

Learning theory also includes two other aspects that are useful in marketing. Learning facilitates generalizations among stimuli. *Generalizations* are the extensions of past reinforced behavior to other stimuli. A female patient who has had a positive experience in the birthing center of a hospital might generalize that positive level of care to other clinical programs in the same facility.

A second aspect of learning is referred to as *discrimination*, the ability to determine differences between stimuli. A consumer who has had an unsatisfactory experience during one inpatient stay might, from this past reinforcement, be able to discriminate better when having a similar experience (stimulus) with another provider.

Perception

A final psychological aspect affecting decision making is **perception**, the process by which individuals organize, select, and interpret information.[21] Consumers tend to change and reorganize information so that it is consistent with their past experiences and knowledge.

On any given day, consumers are exposed to a vast array of advertisements and messages. Not all of these messages are attended to or processed, because the perception process is selective. The process of selectivity can occur at several stages of the communication process.

Selective exposure is when the consumer pays attention to a particular set of advertisements. As discussed earlier in terms of dissonance, an individual who recently selected a particular health plan may pay attention to advertisements for only that plan to help them reinforce their choice. *Selective comprehension* is the interpreting of information in a way that is consistent with past attitudes, beliefs, and knowledge. This aspect of perception is important for marketers to understand. A message sent by the advertiser may be perceived in a very different fashion by the intended audience. A hospital, for example, may decide to use an advertisement with humor as the primary appeal. To the intended audience, this message might imply that the hospital is not serious enough about the issue to have faith in this facility as a place for care. Later, in Chapter 12, pretesting will be discussed as one way to overcome or assess this potential problem.

A third aspect of selective perception is that of *selective retention*. Consumers only retain a fraction of the material to which they are exposed. In advertising, the recognition of selective retention has given rise to media strategies that use repetition to reinforce past advertisements. Selective retention is a concern for marketers as consumers move through the stages of internal and external search. An interesting dictum regarding the problem of selective retention, which remains as true today as it was when first published over 100 years ago, is shown in EXHIBIT 4-5.

Perceived Risk

Within the area of perception is the concept of *perceived risk*, which can be defined as the concerns or anxieties a consumer anticipates regarding a product or service purchase. Purchases represent risk.[22] Several types of perceived risks have been identified in marketing, which are relevant in the health care decision process. Financial, performance, and physical risks are obvious concerns. For certain services, such as mental health or sexual dysfunction clinics, there may also be perceived social risks. For the marketer of such services, strategies must be developed to reduce the perceived risk. A mental health clinic might underscore for patients that mental health

Exhibit 4-5   Hints to Intended Advertisers

The first time a man looks at an advertisement, he does not see it.

The second time he does not notice it.

The third time he is conscious of its existence.

The fourth time he faintly remembers having seen it.

The fifth time he reads it.

The sixth time he turns up his nose at it.

The seventh time he reads it through and says, "Oh, bother!"

The eighth time he says, "Here's that confounded thing again!"

The ninth time he wonders if it amounts to anything.

The tenth time he thinks he will ask his neighbor it he has tried it.

The eleventh time he wonders how the advertiser makes it pay.

The twelfth time he thinks perhaps it may be worth something.

The thirteenth time he thinks it must be a good thing.

The fourteenth time he remembers he has wanted such a thing for a long time.

The fifteenth time he is tantalized because he can not afford to buy it.

The sixteenth time he thinks he will buy it someday.

The seventeenth time he makes a memorandum of it.

The eighteenth time he swears at his poverty.

The nineteenth time he counts his money very carefully.

The twentieth time he sees it, he buys the article, or instructs his wife to do so.

Source: Thomas Smith, *Hints to Intending Advertisers*, London, 1885.

is not a problem to hide; or in a different strategy, the clinic might stress its procedures for confidentiality.

Behavioral researchers have found that there are certain characteristics that affect the degree to which a person reacts to perceived risk. A greater willingness to accept risk has been found among those who have higher self-confidence, higher self-esteem, lower anxiety, and *lower familiarity with the problem*.[23]

■ Sociocultural Influences

Sociocultural factors in addition to psychological influences can also affect consumer decision making. These sociocultural elements include family life cycle, social class, reference groups, and culture.

Family Life Cycle

Consumers' decision making and purchase behavior change over the course of their lives. The **family life cycle** describes the stages the typical consumer passes through from childhood through death of a spouse.[24] The stages of the traditional family life cycle are represented in EXHIBIT 4-6. In each stage, different conditions lead to a focus on different types of purchases.[25] For example, even though single individuals are represented in several stages (bachelor stage, empty nest I, solitary survivor, and retired), the focus of purchases varies dramatically. For marketers, consideration of just marital status would be too restrictive with regard to the implication for purchases.

Modified Life Cycle

The typical family structure of the past seems less and less applicable to today's market.[26] Many consumers remain single by choice throughout their entire lives, and growing numbers of married couples enter into divorce. The traditional life cycle depiction is becoming less relevant; a modernized view of the family life cycle, or *modified life cycle*, reflects these ever more common variations of the life cycle. In this revised version (as seen in FIGURE 4-5), singles are people who are single, separated, divorced, and widowed.[27]

Family Decision Making

Within the traditional family life cycle, historical decision-making patterns have emerged. Early in the formation of the family unit there is a tendency for a large amount of shared decision making as the household is established. Over time, however, *family decision making* has become specialized into either husband- or wife-dominant. Men have traditionally dominated decisions to purchase automobiles, life insurance, and investments. Women have dominated decisions to buy appliances and home furnishings. In health care, women often were the primary decision makers re-

Exhibit 4-6   The Traditional Family Life Cycle

Stage	Characteristics
1. Bachelor stage; young single people not living at home	Few financial burdens. Fashion opinion leaders. Recreation oriented. Buy: Basic kitchen equipment, basic furniture, cars, equipment for the mating game, vacations.
2. Newly married couples; young, no children	Better off financially than they will be in the near future. Highest purchase rate and highest average purchase of durables. Buy: Cars, refrigerators, stoves, sensible and durable furniture, vacations.
3. Full nest I; youngest child under six	Home purchasing at peak. Liquid assets low. Dissatisfied with financial position and amount of money saved. Interested in new products. Like advertised products. Buy: Washers, dryers, TV, baby food, chest rubs and cough medicines, vitamins, dolls, wagons, sleds, skates.
4. Full nest II; youngest child six or over six	Financial position better. Some wives work. Less influenced by advertising. Buy larger-sized packages, multiple-unit deals. Buy: Many foods, cleaning materials, bicycles, music lessons, pianos.
5. Full nest III; older married couples with dependent children	Financial position still better. More wives work. Some children get jobs. Hard to influence with advertising. High average purchase of durables. Buy: New, more tasteful furniture, auto travel, nonnecessary appliances, boats, dental services, magazines.
6. Empty nest I; older married couples, no children living with them, head in labor force	Home ownership at peak. Most satisfied with financial position and money saved. Interested in travel, recreation, self-education. Make gifts and contributions. Not interested in new products. Buy: Vacations, luxuries, home improvements.
7. Empty nest II; older married couples, no children living at home, head retired.	Drastic cut in income. Keep home. Buy: Medical appliances, medical care, products which aid health, sleep, and digestion.
8. Solitary survivor, in labor force	Income still good but likely to sell home.
9. Solitary survivor, retired	Same medical and product needs as other retired group; drastic cut in income. Special need for attention, affection, and security.

Source: Reprinted from Wells, W.D., and Gubar, G., Life Cycle Concept in Marketing Research, *Journal of Marketing Research*, November 1962, p. 362, with permission of American Marketing Association, © 1962.

FAMILY LIFE CYCLE FLOWS

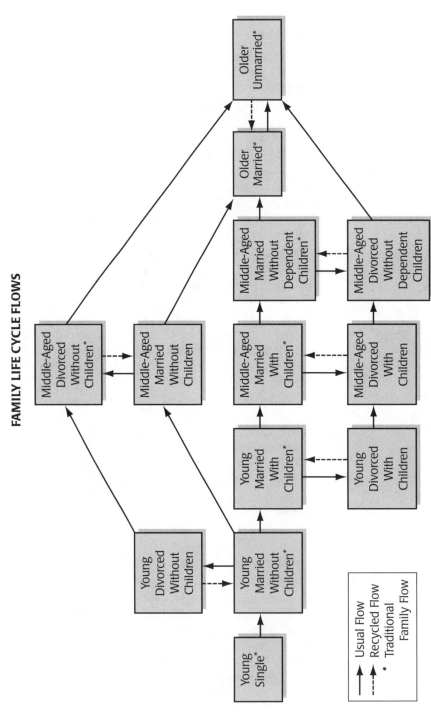

FIGURE 4-5 The Modernized Family Life Cycle

Source: Reprinted from Murphy, P.E. and Staples, W.A., A Modernized Family Life Cycle, *Journal of Consumer Research*, Vol. 6, No. 1 (1979), pp. 12–22 with permission of The University of Chicago Press.

garding selecting the source of care. As the household structure changes, however, and women work outside the home in growing numbers, the traditional patterns of decision making are changing. As the woman's income rises relative to her spouse, her influence in decision making increases. For example, women have been found to now influence 80% of all new car purchases.[28] Regarding health care, the number of women in the work force has also affected the health care decision-making situation. In the past, the man often chose the health plan, since he was working outside the home in a setting that offered insurance. That is no longer the case. Increasingly, both spouses may be offered health plan options at their respective work sites.

There are also two other decision-making patterns that emerge in families. One involves *syncratic decisions* in which the husband and wife participate jointly. The other form includes *autonomous decisions*, those decisions of lesser importance that the husband or the wife decide independently.

Social Class

A second sociocultural influence on consumer behavior is social class. **Social class** has been defined as relatively stable and homogeneous divisions in society in which individuals, families, or groups share relatively similar interests, values, lifestyles, and behaviors. A combination of factors determine whether an individual belongs to one social class vs. another. Income, education level, source of net worth, and type of housing are but a few of these factors. EXHIBIT 4-7 shows one such topology of social class.

This listing summarizes the characteristics of seven social classes in the United States. Although there are many differences within social classes, there is far greater variation between social classes in terms of behaviors and lifestyles. The percentages represented for each social class are approximations of their distribution in society. To marketers, the issue of social class is valuable in that it shows that more than income relates to a consumer's lifestyle or behavior. People of lower social class tend to shop closer to home. In terms of the consumer behavior model described initially, lower social class members engage less often in external search of information prior to purchase.

Reference Group

Social class is significant to marketers in that other members of a social class often serve as a consumer's reference group. A **reference group** is one that influences an individual's thoughts or behaviors.[29] There are three forms of a reference group.[30,31] The reference group to which one belongs is considered the *membership reference group*. The reference group to which one does not wish to belong is considered the *dissociative reference group*. Finally, the reference group to which one aspires to belong is referred to as the *aspirational reference group*. From a promotional strategy perspective, it's important to understand the differing types of reference groups. Showing images of dissociative reference groups to a target market would destroy the value of a promotional campaign.

Exhibit 4-7	Social Class Distinctions

Upper Americans

Upper-Upper (0.3%)—The "capital S society" world of inherited wealth, aristocratic names

Lower-Upper (1.2%)—The newer social elite, drawn from current professional, corporate leadership

Upper-Middle (12.5%)—The rest of college graduate managers and professionals; lifestyle centers on private clubs, causes, and the arts

Middle Americans

Middle Class (32%)—Average pay white-collar workers and their blue-collar friends; live on the "better side of town," try to "do the proper things"

Working Class (38%)—Average pay blue-collar workers; lead "working class life style" whatever the income, school background, and job

Lower Americans

A lower group of working people but not the lowest (9%)—Working, not on welfare; living standard is just above poverty; behavior judged "crude," "trashy"

Real Lower-Lower (7%)—On welfare, visibly poverty-stricken, usually out of work (or have "the dirtiest jobs"); "bums," "common criminals"

Source: Reprinted from Coleman, R.P., The Continuing Significance of Social Class, *Journal of Consumer Research*, Vol. 10, No. 3 (1983), pp. 265–280 with permission of The University of Chicago Press.

Reference group influence is most significant when use of the product or service is visible to the group.[32] Products such as designer clothing, cars, or brands of sneakers such as Nike or Reebok are greatly affected by the reference group. Reference group influence also tends to be higher the less necessary a product is. The more commitment a person feels to belonging to a particular group, the greater the influence of that group. The more relevant the particular purchase or behavior is to the functioning of the group, the more pressure or influence is exerted by the reference group. The stronger the reference group influence is, the less confidence the individual has in his decision. The example of choosing a health care plan highlights what is often a difficult issue for many consumers. In this case, coworkers also involved in the same decision making may play a major role in influencing the ultimate plan selection.[33]

Culture

Culture, as defined in an earlier chapter, refers to the values, attitudes, and ideas that are transmitted from one generation to another within a group of homogeneous individuals. These values, such as achievement or success, might well influence decision making. American society places a strong value of success in work. Many products and advertisements are directed at ways of demonstrating the fulfillment of this cultural value.

In the United States there has been a growing recognition of subcultures and their different purchasing behaviors, values, and attitudes that affect their decision making. As marketers become more skilled in the management of databases, they will be able to target particular subcultures more effectively through use of micromarketing strategies. Ads, products, and communication strategies can all be tailored to reflect different subcultural norms.

Hispanic Subculture

One of the fastest growing subcultures in the United States is among Hispanics, people of Latin American origin. Predominant in states in the northeast, southeast, and far west regions of the United States, Hispanics will represent significant proportions of the population in many major metropolitan areas. In 2005, Hispanics became the largest ethnic minority in the United States. One out of every three Hispanics, however, has no health insurance. As an ethnic group, Hispanics are 65% Mexican American, 11% Puerto Rican, 8% Cuban, and 16% Central and South American and from other Spanish-speaking countries. In dealing with the health care system, Hispanics often find they are subjected to a health system with limited knowledge of the Hispanic culture and language. Hispanic physicians number about 4% of the physician work force in the United States.[34] Many distinct media have been established to target this group. It is essential to recognize the differences in certain subcultures. For example, within some segments of the Hispanic population, gynecological examinations are considered only for the promiscuous.[35]

Marketers have found some interesting buying pattern consistencies among Hispanics.

1. Hispanics tend to be quality and brand conscious.
2. Hispanics' buying preferences are strongly influenced by friends and family.
3. Hispanics consider advertising a credible information source.
4. Hispanics prefer buying American-made products.[36]

■ African-American Subculture

Presently 13% of the population in the United States is African American.[37] The income levels of this group on average have been below the average for Caucasians and Hispanics (as was shown in Figure 3–3). Another factor that this group has had to overcome has been historic problems of racism and segregation and their impact on the education of successive generations. Marketers are increasingly recognizing the growing influence and buying power of this particular subculture as historic boundaries and limitations have been removed. Distinct media vehicles have also been developed on television and in print to target this subculture. Differences in buying patterns are greater within the African-American subculture due to levels of socioeconomic status than between African Americans and whites of similar status. Even though similarities outweigh differences, there are consumption patterns that do differ between African Americans and whites.[38] African Americans spend more for online services, have distinct preferences for shelter and cars, and the typical family is five years younger than whites.[39]

From a health care perspective, there have been multiple issues and challenges to respond better to the African-American health care needs. For example;

- The prevalence of diabetes among African Americans is about 70% higher than among white Americans.
- Infant mortality rates are twice as high for African Americans as for white Americans.
- The 5-year survival rate for cancer among African Americans diagnosed for 1986–1992 was about 44%, compared with 59% for white Americans.[40]

■ Industrial Buyer Behavior

The customer for health care products and plans is changing, as witnessed in the 1990s during the national debate about health care reform. Historically, a health care organization considered its customers to be physicians and patients. With the burgeoning growth of managed care in the United States beginning in the late 1970s, many health care organizations and providers now face a more formidable and complex customer—employers. Employers represent all types of businesses, from a large company that purchases health care for its employees through an occupational medicine program, to an MCO that contracts for inpatient services, to a nursing home that might purchase the services of a physician to monitor the health status of its residents.

In the 1990s, especially small companies, but often even public health plans, banded together to form purchasing coalitions to buy health care coverage for their members at affordable prices. For example, the Cooperative Health Network in Ohio covers 14,000 people and includes four health funds, while the Health Care Cost Containment Cooperative of the Mid-Atlantic Region covers 350,000 people.[41]

In any case, marketing to large corporations, small companies, and other business organizations requires an understanding of organizational buyer behavior and how it differs from the individual consumer behavior described earlier. Understanding these differences fosters the development of a more effective marketing strategy relative to the four Ps of the marketing mix.

Organizational Differences

Organizations differ from consumers in terms of the buying process along several distinct characteristics.

Number of Organizations

Compared to consumers, the industrial, or organizational, market is smaller. While a hospital serves hundreds of thousands of consumers in any given year, that same hospital may deal with only two or three managed health care plans in its respective market.

Demand Variations

A second major aspect of organizational buying is the variation in demand. One aspect of industrial demand, referred to as **derived demand,** is the demand for one product or service (such as the managed health care plan) that is derived from the demand for another service or product (consumer need for health care services). In marketing to organizations, providers need to understand who the organization's customers are.[42] To market effectively to a managed care plan, a medical group should know what services the managed care plan's subscribers expect to receive from a medical group that they would select for care.

Another dimension of industrial demand is the tendency to be price inelastic. Demand is considered price inelastic when price cuts or price hikes have little effect on total level of demand. Since industrial demand is derived demand, there is less opportunity for health care organizations to influence or stimulate primary demand in the industrial market than there is in the consumer market.

If the price of Tylenol drops, it is unlikely that a hospital, for example, would order a significantly larger amount of the product. If the price reduction is short-term, there may be some loading up on inventory, but only to a point, since Tylenol does not account for a significant proportion of the cost of treating a particular patient. Similarly, the price of Tylenol would have to rise substantially before a hospital might decide to shift to another product. In this example, the demand is price inelastic. Among individual consumers, demand would probably be far more elastic. A coupon offering a 50% price reduction on a large bottle of Tylenol would, no doubt, stimulate significant demand. On the other hand, a doubling of the Tylenol's price would likely lead to a dramatic reduction in demand.

Greater Total Sales Volume

Another characteristic of organizational buying is that its total sales volume is greater than that of the consumer market. For example, a consumer purchase of a particular pharmaceutical product represents the sale of one unit sold in the retail market. That sale on the industrial side represents multiple sales from the purchase of raw materials and other goods to support the production of the product.

Geographical Concentration

Industrial markets are often characterized by greater geographical concentration than consumer markets. In the Cincinnati metropolitan area, for example, Cigna Companies, a national insurance company headquartered in Bloomfield, Connecticut, can market to a half-dozen hospitals within a five-to-ten-mile radius of the downtown area. Many consumers in the Cincinnati metropolitan area, however, actually reside beyond the state of Ohio in neighboring Kentucky.

Professional Buying

Organizations differ from consumers in that their buying function is usually a structured, formal decision-making process. Many large companies, for example, have purchasing departments that institutionalize the buying process. Other businesses or organizations have a contract negotiation department to deal with the "buying" of health care services from providers or facilities.

Often in these settings, individual providers are judged by defined, well-established buying criteria. To a large degree, these buying characteristics are similar to the evaluative criteria used by consumers in the alternative evaluation stage of the decision process.

Buying Center

The major difference between the industrial vs. consumer market is the **buying center,** a group of people involved in the decision to purchase a product or service. The buying center allows for many perspectives and broad expertise to be brought to bear on the purchase. For a company selecting a health care plan, the buying center might include the firm's medical director, financial officer, human resources director, union representative, and possibly, the employee assistance representative.

The buying center makes organizational marketing more complex for the organization offering a service. The firm making a presentation to a buying center has to deal with many views and must gauge the relative influence each party has in the buying process. To market effectively to the buying center, four questions must be answered:

1. Which individuals in the buying center are responsible for our particular product or service?
2. What is the relative influence of each member of this group?
3. What are each member's decision criteria?
4. How does each member of the group perceive our firm, our products, and our salespeople?[43]

Negotiation Variations

Industrial buying also differs from consumer buying in terms of two aspects of the negotiation process: frequency and complexity. Organizational purchases are made less frequently than consumer purchases. A consumer buys primary care medical services several times during the year. A managed care plan, however, most likely will negotiate a contract with a medical group annually. Marketing to organizations, then, requires a detailed knowledge of the timing of their purchase cycle.

Organizational buying is also more complex than consumer purchasing—many details of a contract must be negotiated before agreement is reached. A manufacturer, for example, might negotiate with an occupational medicine clinic regarding the services to be performed on site, the handling of workers' compensation claims, and the contract's payment terms.

With the growing emphasis on managed care, health care organizations are now sharing risk with vendors. In risk-sharing arrangements, the supplier will receive greater reward if the buyer meets the objectives. In health care, risk sharing is increasing between suppliers and buyers and between providers and buyers. For example, Group Health of Puget Sound in Seattle, Washington, is a large HMO. In pursuing its goal to control the cost of care, Group Health signed a capitated agreement with Owens and Minor, a large distributor of hospital and physician supplies and equipment. Group Health pays the supplier a set fee per subscriber per month for medical-surgical products. The more products Group Health uses, the less Owens makes. The supplier now tries to ensure proper training and inventory control because both the buyer and supplier now have the same incentive.[44]

Vendor Solicitation

An additional difference between consumer and industrial behavior relates to the solicitation of vendors. When a business organization identifies a need for a product or service, it solicits vendors to submit bids or make presentations for supplying the product or service. When individual customers identify a need, they actively identify solutions to address the need.

Close Buyer–Seller Relationships

With most consumer purchases, the seller rarely develops a significant relationship with the individual. Industrial buying is just the opposite. Since there are fewer customers and the negotiations are often complex, the vendor develops a detailed knowledge of the customer.

The Industrial Buying Process

Similar to consumer behavior, industrial buying can be divided into three basic types of purchasing situations: new task, modified rebuy, and straight rebuy.[45]

New Task Buying

In the new task buying situation, organizations face a new situation in which a purchase is required. In this buying situation, a company gathers information from various vendors who can meet the need. This situation is like an extended problem-solving scenario for the consumer and is often very time-consuming.[46] Employers are often approaching health care as a new task buying problem and so need to collect quantifiable information.

Modified Rebuy

In the modified rebuy situation, the buyer seeks to modify or alter the purchase. Changes can be made to the price or to product specifications. A company might re-open negotiations with an insurance company, asking it to provide a managed care plan in addition to the indemnity product offered to employees. In the modified rebuy scenario, the existing vendor protects against losing the customer.

Straight Rebuy

Straight rebuy involves making repeated purchases of a product that has generated a positive experience and good past evaluations. Straight rebuy decisions are usually programmed purchases that involve little complexity. Basic industrial supplies are often purchased in a straight rebuy mode. A medical group might purchase checks or office supplies through a straight rebuy sequence. Straight rebuys rarely involve buying centers and usually do not require negotiation for the purchase.

The Buying Center

The buying center was identified as a major difference between industrial and consumer buying behavior. As described earlier, there are many participants in the buying center and these participants can assume one of several roles within it.[47]

Users—These are the people who will use the product. They may include an individual such as an employee representative, who provides the user perspective regarding the particular health plan, judging it for convenience and patient responsiveness.

Influencers—Influencers are individuals both inside and outside the organization who affect the final decision. The chief financial officer in a hospital is often a major influencer, regarding the specific financial details of managed care contracts that are signed. A company might hire a benefits consultant to review alternative health insurance products.

Gatekeepers—Gatekeepers are the individuals who control the flow of information into the buying organization. Many pharmaceutical companies must develop strategies for dealing with the physician's gatekeeper, who is often the secretary.

Deciders—This is the person who has the authority to make the final choice between vendors. The management level at which decision authority rests depends on the cost of the purchase or the risk to the organization. In most hospitals, the director of purchasing would be considered the decider for a capital equipment purchase such as a wheelchair. Yet, in the use of infusion pump equipment, the decider would more likely be a clinician involved in the treatment regimen using this specialized equipment.

Buyers—Those responsible for dealing directly with the suppliers are the buyers, often called purchasing agents. Purchasing agents often are solely responsible for managing straight rebuy situations, without consulting with the buying center.

Understanding how the customer behaves is at the core of effective marketing strategy. Consumer decision making involves a series of steps and is affected by a variety of internal and external factors. Industrial buying behavior is a formal process in which the decision-maker role is complicated by the type of purchase and composition of the buying center. As health care rapidly moves to a managed care environment, this aspect of decision making will require greater understanding in order to develop effective marketing strategy.

■ Key Terms

Consumer Decision-Making Process
Evaluative Criteria
Involvement
Routine Decision Making
Brand Loyalty
Complex Decision Making
Limited Decision Making
Motivation
Attitudes

Lifestyle
Learning
Perception
Family Life Cycle
Social Class
Reference Group
Derived Demand
Buying Center

■ Chapter Summary

1. Buyer behavior that results in purchase is a multistage process involving problem recognition, search, evaluation, purchase, and post-purchase evaluation.
2. Post-purchase evaluation is a critical component of buyer behavior. Organizations should assess whether customer expectations are confirmed or disconfirmed by their interactions with the service or use of the product.
3. Consumer decision making depends to a large degree on the amount of consumer involvement in the purchase. The level of involvement is related to the degree of risk and the extent of search behavior.
4. The consumer decision-making process is affected by several influences: motivation, attitudes, lifestyles, learning, and perception.
5. Perception is an important aspect of buyer behavior and must be considered in marketing strategy. Perception affects what people see, understand, and retain.
6. Individual behavior is related to the stage a person is in his or her life cycle. As the composition of the typical family has changed, so have the traditional stages of the life cycle been modified.

7. Within the United States, there are several distinct social classes, each of which reflects norms of behavior, attitudes, and values.

8. Culture is recognized as the transmission of attitudes, values, and norms from one generation to the next. Within the United States there is the growing emergence of several distinct subcultures that influence buying behavior.

9. Organizational buying behavior is characterized by, among other things, the number of companies, demand variations, sales volume, professionalism of the buyer, and geographic concentration.

10. A major defining characteristic of organizational buying behavior is the buying center, which involves many individuals at different levels and positions within the firm.

11. There are three variations of industrial buying: new task, modified rebuy, and straight rebuy.

■ Chapter Problems

1. For several years, Annie Brouck's employer has offered a traditional indemnity plan for health care coverage for herself, her husband Jim, and their children, Tess and Tasha. Recently, the cost of the monthly premium for this insurance coverage increased dramatically. Annie's employer has decided to offer an HMO in addition to this traditional insurance plan. Describe the steps Annie might follow in deciding whether to choose this plan.

2. In recent years, there has been a growing attempt to measure the performance of health care providers. The federal government has published data on how hospitals are compared to acceptable clinical standards with regard to pneumonia. Explain how these data could affect the consumer decision-making process.

3. In terms of decision-making sequences, how would you explain and describe: (a) the 25-year-old, healthy worker who sees the same physician for minor medical needs; (b) the retired individual who calls the state medical society and seeks a second opinion prior to open-heart surgery; and (c) the consumer who sees a new brand of headache remedy on the shelf and decides to try it?

4. On what level of Maslow's Hierarchy of Needs would you place each of the following decisions: (a) buying health insurance, (b) going skiing, (c) following a low-fat diet?

5. Select Care MCO has decided to offer the first managed care product in a small community of 25,000 people in West Virginia. Prepaid health care is a concept that is new to this region. In conducting a consumer survey prior to the introduction of the plan, Select Care finds that attitudes toward MCOs are very negative. Some people believe they will be denied care if they join an MCO, while others feel this form of health care delivery is a socialistic approach to medicine. What options are open to Select Care in trying to change these attitudes?

6. The United States is experiencing a decline of the middle class. What does this trend imply for the future of organizations such as: (a) the U.S. Public Health Service, which operates many inner-city health clinics for the economically disadvantaged, and (b) the Scripps Clinic, a large multi-specialty group practice in southern California? For years, the Scripps Clinic was seen as an exclusive medical provider known not only for treatment but for its research.

7. A medical group has decided to develop an industrial medicine program for employers. This program would help in the treatment of on-the-job injuries, workers' compensation requirements, health education, and toxicology analysis. The group has hired a new salesperson to approach a major furniture manufacturer in the community about the program. In preparing for her first call, the salesperson makes a list of the possible members of the buying center. Prepare the list.

■ Notes

1. A description of this model was developed extensively in J. F. Engel, R. D. Blackwell, and P. W. Miniard, *Consumer Behavior*, 7th ed. (New York: The Dryden Press, 1993).

2. J. F. Engel, R. D. Blackwell, and P. Miniard, *Consumer Behavior*, 7th ed. (New York: The Dryden Press, 1993).

3. For external search approaches, see J. E. Urban, P. Dickson, and W. L. Wilkie, "Buyer Uncertainty and Information Search," *Journal of Consumer Research* 16, no. 2 (1989): 208–215.

4. See S. E. Beatty and S. M. Smith, "External Search Effort: An Investigation Across Several Product Categories," *Journal of Consumer Research* 14, no. 1 (1987): 83–95.

5. Laurie Lee, "Survey Data Provide Strategic Insight into Healthcare Behavior," *COR Healthcare Market Strategist* 4, no. 12 (December 2003): 120–124.

6. Judith H. Hibbard and Jacquelyn J. Jewitt, "Will Quality Report Cards Help Consumers?," *Health Affairs* 16, no. 3: 218–228.

7. J. D. Johnson and H. Meischke, "Cancer Information: Women's Source and Content Preferences," *Journal of Health Care Marketing* 11, no. 1 (1991): 37–44.

8. "Quality Ratings Have Almost No Influence on Consumer Choices of Hospitals, Health Plans, and Physicians," *Harris Interactive Health Care Research* 2, no. 11 (October 11, 2002).

9. A useful discussion of evoked set formation is found in J. E. Brisoux and M. Laroche, "Evoked Set Formation and Composition: An Empirical Investigation under Routinized Response Behavior Situation," in *Advances in Consumer Research* 8, ed. K. B. Monroe (Ann Arbor, MI: Association for Consumer Research, 1981): 357–361.

10. J. A. Howard, *Consumer Behavior in Marketing Strategy* (Englewood Cliffs, NJ: Prentice Hall, 1989): 176–177.

11. M. Fishbein, "An Investigation of the Relationships between Beliefs about an Object and the Attitude Toward That Object," *Human Relations* 16, no. 3 (1963): 233–240.

12. For additional discussion of post-purchase behavior and feelings, see M. C. Gilly and B. D. Gelb, "Post Purchase Consumer Process and the Complaining Consumer," *Journal of Consumer Research* 9, no. 3 (1982): 323–328.

13. L. Festinger, *A Theory of Cognitive Dissonance* (Stanford, CA: Stanford University Press, 1957): 260.

14. C. Costley, "Meta Analysis of Involvement Research," in *Advances in Consumer Research* 15, ed. M. Houston (Provo, UT: Association for Consumer Research, 1988): 554–562.

15. A. H. Maslow, *Motivation and Personality* (New York: Harper, 1954): 80–106.

16. D. Krech, R. S. Crutchfield, and E. L. Ballachey, *Individual and Society* (New York: McGraw-Hill, 1962).

17. R. Lutz, "Changing Brand Attitudes through Modification of Cognitive Structure," *Journal of Consumer Research* 1, no. 4 (1975): 49–59.

18. H. Assael, *Consumer Behavior and Marketing Action*, 3rd ed. (Boston: Kent Publishing, 1990): 275.

19. See J. T. Plummer, "The Concept and Application of Lifestyle Segmentation," *Journal of Marketing* 38, no. 1 (1974): 33–37.

20. For further explanation and detail on VALS, see *The VALS2™ Segmentation System* (Menlo Park, CA: SRI International, 1989).

21. For a review of the consumer perception process and marketing implications, see J. R. Bettman, *An Information Theory of Consumer Choice* (Reading, MA: Addison-Wesley, 1979).

22. J. Taylor, "The Role of Risk in Consumer Behavior," *Journal of Marketing* 38, no. 2 (1974): 54–60.

23. J. C. Mowen, *Consumer Behavior* (New York: Macmillan, 1993).

24. W. D. Wells and G. Gubar, "Life Cycle Concept in Marketing Research," *Journal of Marketing Research* 3, no. 4 (1966): 355–363.

25. J. Wagner and S. Hanna, "The Effectiveness of Family Life Cycle Variables in Consumer Expenditure Research," *Journal of Consumer Research* 10, no. 3 (1983): 281–291.

26. P. E. Murphy and W. A. Staples, "A Modernized Family Life Cycle," *Journal of Consumer Research* 6, no. 1 (1979): 12–22.

27. Ibid., 17.

28. For a discussion of the purchasing roles of husbands and wives, see S. C. Bennett and E. W. Stuart, "In Search of Association Between Personal Values and Household Decision Processes: An Exploratory Analysis," in *AMA Educators Conference Proceedings* (Chicago, IL: American Marketing Association, 1989): 259–264; and E. W. Stuart and S. C. Bennett, "Perception of Marital Roles in Decision Processes: A 1980s Update," in *AMA Educators Conference Proceedings* (Chicago, IL: American Marketing Association, 1988): 77.

29. R. P. Coleman, "The Continuing Significance of Social Class," *Journal of Consumer Research* 10, no. 3 (1983): 183–194.

30. D. Brinberg and L. Plimpton, "Self Monitoring and Product Conspicuousness on Reference Group Influence," in *Advances in Consumer Research* 13, ed. R. Lutz (Provo, UT: Association for Consumer Research, 1986): 297–300.

31. W. O. Bearden and M. J. Etzel, "Reference Group Influence on Product and Brand Choice," *Journal of Consumer Research* 9, no. 2 (1982): 183–194.

32. Bearden and Etzel, "Reference Group Influence," 183–194.

33. Ibid., 188–192.

34. "NHMA Resident Leadership Program," National Hispanic Medical Association, Washington, DC (http://www.nhmamd.org/resident.htm).

35. M. C. Jaklevic, "Programs and Campaigns Reach Out to Members of Ethnic Communities," *Modern Healthcare* 24, no. 1 (1994): 32.

36. "A Little Latin Logic," *Brandweek* (July 20, 1998): 12.

37. "Marketing to Hispanics," *Advertising Age* (August 24, 1998): S1–S27.

38. Statistical Abstract of the United States 2004–2005, U.S. Census Bureau, 15.

39. Eric N. Berkowitz, Roger Kerin, Steven Hartley, and William Rudelius, *Marketing* (Boston: Irwin/McGraw Hill, 2000): 169.

40. H. P. McAdoo, ed. *Black Families* (Newbury Park, CA: Sage Publications, 1988).

41. BlackHealthCare.com, http://www.blackhealthcare.com/.

42. "Health Care Purchasing Coalitions," *Collective Bargaining Reporter* (American Federation Employees, 2000), no. 2, http://www.afscme.org/wrkplace/cbr200_2.htm.

43. W. S. Bishop, J. L. Graham, and M. H. Jones, "Volatility of Derived Demand in Industrial Markets and Its Management Implications," *Journal of Marketing* 50, no. 1 (Fall 1984): 95–103.

44. T. Bonoma, "Major Sales: Who Really Does the Buying?" *Harvard Business Review* 60, no. 3 (1982): 111–119.

45. L. Scott, "Hospitals Feel Vendors' Cost Cuts," *Modern Healthcare* 24, no. 46 (1994): 62.

46. Ibid.

47. P. J. Robinson, C. W. Farris, and Y. Wind, *Industrial Buying and Creative Marketing* (Newton, MA: Allyn & Bacon, 1967).

48. F. Webster, Jr., and Y. Wind, *Organizational Buying Behavior* (Englewood Cliffs, NJ: Prentice Hall, 1972).

Marketing Research

After reading this chapter you should be able to:

- Understand the nature of the marketing research process
- Know the difference between primary and secondary data
- Recognize the range of alternative sampling methodologies
- Understand the value of alternative data collection methodologies
- Appreciate the necessity of a marketing information system

■ The Marketing Research Process

Marketing research is a multistep process that involves the systematic gathering of consumer information or data that will help an organization identify specific issues of concern to consumers. Organizations use these data to design marketing strategies that will address consumer needs. Conducting marketing research involves a five-stage process, which is displayed in FIGURE 5-1. Following these steps will ensure that the data finally collected will help in managerial decision making. The five steps to marketing research include: (1) problem recognition, (2) identification of research objectives, (3) research design, (4) data collection, and (5) analysis and evaluation of results.

■ Problem Recognition

The first stage of the marketing research process, problem recognition, involves the definition of the problem. In order to collect the appropriate information to answer an organization's question, a clear definition of what should be researched is important. Clearly specified, problem definition leads to better articulation of the research objectives.

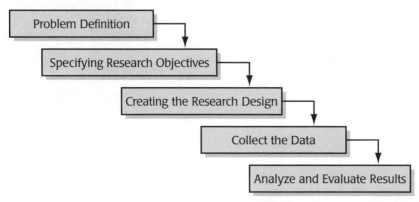

FIGURE 5-1 The Key Steps to Marketing Research

A managed care organization (MCO), for example, might find that acceptance of its plan among corporate health benefit officers is less than expected. Now, the problem might be defined as one of understanding the competitive position of this plan when compared to competing MCOs. A second way to define this problem might be to understand health benefit officers' attitudes toward prepaid health care plans. Or, a third definition of the problem might be to assess the image of this particular MCO among corporate health benefit officers. In each instance, the type of information and possibly the methodology used to collect the data might vary.

Because the problem recognition stage is critical to the resultant research process, all important members of the organization should be included in this phase of the research. Involvement of both management and clinical personnel is essential to obtain an accurate assessment of the problem definition.

Identification of Research Objectives

Determining the research objectives is the second stage of the market research process. Research objectives can take one of four forms. One common research objective is exploratory, when an organization needs to determine the cause of the problem. For example, an MCO might conduct exploratory research to determine what is causing membership attrition. A second common research objective is descriptive. These marketing research efforts attempt to identify new issues or markets. For example, a study might be conducted to describe the needs of referral physicians in dealing with a physician relations department at an academic medical center. A third common objective of marketing research is to test hypotheses. A marketing director at a hospital, for example, might want to determine what impact doubling the advertising budget for a women's mammography screening program will have on demand for appointments. A final research objective is predictive, in which an organization tries to forecast demand for a service. A study might be conducted to predict the demand for an occupational medicine program in which routine lab work is performed at the company site.

It is important to recognize that the individuals involved in problem definition and in the subsequent stage of specifying the research objectives are often different from those individuals who actually conduct the research. Those involved in the first two stages of the research are the people affected by the issue. Implementation of the actual research process is usually done by marketing research staff or by outside organizations skilled in the methodology of market research.

Research Design

After the research objectives have been specified, it is necessary to create the research design. This step is of critical importance. The research design is the plan for the entire study. This plan will specify the data needed, and the methods that will be used to collect them and to analyze and interpret the results. The data needs could consist of either primary data or secondary data.

Primary Data

Primary data are information collected to address a specific research question. There are many alternative methods that are used to acquire primary data. These methods consist of qualitative and quantitative data-gathering forms. Qualitative information is information that is not quantified. Quantitative data consist of empirical information. To collect either form of data, companies can either observe individuals or ask individuals questions. There are many alternative methods that must be decided upon in conducting marketing research. A number of these will be discussed later in this chapter.

The major advantage of primary data is that the information is collected for the particular problem or issue under investigation, which usually means that the data are current. Another major advantage is that primary data collection allows the organization to maintain confidentiality about the problem and the resulting information collected. Primary data, however, have some disadvantages. The collection of primary data can entail significant cost and can require an extended period of time to accomplish.

Secondary Data

Secondary data are data that were collected previously for another purpose.[1] These data could be collected either within the organization or by outside agencies. A hospital might collect patient information for admissions and then use this information to help develop a profile of who is using the facility. While not originally collected for other purposes, admissions information can be a useful source of secondary data to address other questions that the organization might have.

Useful secondary data are collected by the federal and state governments, as well as by many commercial organizations. EXHIBIT 5-1 lists various types of secondary data. The *Statistical Abstract of the United States* publishes information such as fertility rates, births, and marital status on various segments of the population. Much of these data, for example, might be incorporated into the planning for a women's health

Exhibit 5-1   Selected Secondary Data

Statistical Abstract of the United States

U.S. Bureau of Census, Department of Commerce
Washington, DC 20230

This guide provides a general overview of statistics collected by the federal government and other public and private organizations. Some of the topics covered include geography and environment, labor force, communications, population, employment and earnings, business enterprises, vital statistics, transportation, energy, manufacturers, foreign commerce and aid, standard metro area statistics, and more.

Social Indicators
Government Printing Office, Washington, DC 20402

Triennial. Charts and tables on population; the family; housing; social security and welfare; health and nutrition; public safety; education and training; "work," income, wealth, and expenses; culture, leisure, and the use of time; social mobility, and participation. International data are provided for comparison. Extensive technical notes accompany each section. Includes references for further reading and a subject index.

Standard & Poor's Industry Surveys
Standard & Poor Corp., New York

Separate pamphlets for 33 industries, updated quarterly and annually. This is a valuable source for basic data on 33 industries, with financial comparisons of the leading companies in each industry. For each industry there is a "Basic Analysis" (about 40 pages) revised annually, and a short "Current Analysis" (about 8 pages) published 3 times per year. Received with this is a 4-page monthly on "Trends and Projections," which includes tables of economic and industry indicators, and a monthly "Earnings Supplement," giving concise, up-to-date revenue, income, and profitability data on over 100 leading companies in 33 major industries.

Standard Rate & Data Service
Skokie, Illinois

SRDS publications (11 for the United States and 8 to cover foreign countries) give data on advertising rates, specifications, and circulation for individual magazines, newspapers, and other media.

The U.S. services are for business publications (monthly); community publications (semiannual); consumer magazines and farm publications (monthly); co-op source directory (semiannual); direct mail lists (quarterly); newspapers (monthly) and newspaper circulation analysis; print media production (quarterly); spot radio (monthly); spot radio small markets (semiannual); spot television (monthly). The international editions include all media in one volume and are in the language of the country. There are monthlies for Canada, Britain; bimonthlies for Italy and West Germany; quarterlies for France and Mexico; semiannuals for Austria and Switzerland. Three of the monthlies—the ones for newspapers, spot radio, and for spot television—

(continues)

contain useful market estimates. At the beginning of each state's sections are estimates by county, city and MSA, for population, households, consumer spendable income (by income categories), total and per household retail sales, retail sales for 7 store groups, passenger car registration, farm population, and gross farm income. "Market Data Summary" at the front show rankings of these various statistics and areas of dominant influence; also population by age and sex.

Handbook of Labor Statistics (annual)
   U.S. Bureau of Labor Statistics

   The best one-volume source for U.S. labor statistics covering, for 10 and sometimes 20 years, essentially the same statistics as can be found currently in the *Monthly Labor Review*. For complete historical data see its *Handbook of Labor Statistics*, 1975: *Reference Edition*, issued as *BLS Bulletin 1865*.

   The Bureau of Labor Statistics publishes many other statistical bulletins on specific topics. For a subject list of Department of Labor Publications see *Publications of the U.S. Department of Labor: Subject Listing*.

Statistics of Income (annual)
   U.S. Internal Revenue Service

   This series is actually published as several separate annuals, the most important of which are (1) *Corporation Income Tax Returns*, which covers balance sheet and income statement statistics for corporations, and includes statistics for corporations, and includes statistics by major industry, and by size of total assets; (2) annual statistics on *Partnership Returns* and *Sold Proprietorship Returns*; (3) *Individual Income Tax Returns*. These are usually published first as short preliminary reports and then as detailed final reports. Unfortunately, the statistics are often quite old.

program. Baylor Health Care System in Dallas uses Medstat's State Data Analyst database (www.medstat.com/) to forecast future demand for its budgeting and strategic planning purposes.[2]

There are many commercial firms that provide valuable secondary data sources, including one such as Urban Decision Systems, Inc., which offers a useful way to examine a variety of census data.[3] This company can provide both a historical and a forecasted census analysis to a hospital that is considering opening a clinic in a particular location. This analysis can be done on a variety of parameters, including a one-mile and two-mile radius around the intended location. Table 5-1 provides a sample analysis of a proposed clinic site. As the data in this table indicate, a significant decline in the number of households with an income level between $40,000 and $49,000 (from 13.6% in 1989 to 9.3% in 1994) was projected at this proposed clinic site. Yet, a significant increase was projected in the $60,000–$74,999 income group. This shift

Table 5-1	Establishing a Satellite Clinic: Sample Census Data

INCOME: 1980-89-94   URBAN DECISION SYSTEMS. INC.
MINNEAPOLIS, MN: LYNDALE AV & 53RD ST   10/26/89
1.0 MILE RING

	1980 Census		1989 Est.		1994 Proj.	
POPULATION	21,646		19,991		19,175	
In Group Quarters	304		346		359	
PER CAPITA INCOME	$10,570		$19,360		$24,078	
AGGREGATE INCOME ($Mil)	228.8		387.0		461.7	
HOUSEHOLDS	8214	%	8364	%	8358	%
By Income						
Less than $ 5,000	416	5.1	141	1.7	89	1.1
$ 5,000–$ 9,999	869	10.6	577	6.9	449	5.4
$10,000–$14,999	943	11.5	703	8.4	756	9.0
$15,000–$19,999	941	11.5	633	7.6	514	6.2
$20,000–$24,999	923	11.2	602	7.2	524	6.3
$25,000–$29,999	1084	13.2	545	6.5	515	6.2
$30,000–$34,999	919	11.2	537	6.4	447	5.3
$35,000–$39,999	602	7.3	478	5.7	451	5.4
$40,000–$49,999	696	8.5	1136	13.6	778	9.3
$50,000–$59,999	385	4.7	1012	12.1	930	11.1
$60,000–$74,999	235	2.9	866	10.4	1194	14.3
$75,000–$99,999	127	1.5	643	7.7	866	10.4
$100,000 +	74	0.9	492	5.9	845	10.1
Median Household Income	$25,085		$39,652		$45,583	
Average Household Income	$27,600		$46,275		$55,238	
FAMILIES	5867	%	5522	%	5246	%
By Income						
Less than $ 5,000	79	1.3	24	0.4	15	0.3
$ 5,000–$ 9,999	386	6.6	135	2.5	81	1.5
$10,000–$14,999	497	8.5	246	4.5	192	3.7
$15,000–$19,999	615	10.5	295	5.3	197	3.8
$20,000–$24,999	706	12.0	276	5.0	240	4.6
$25,000–$29,999	922	15.7	312	5.6	215	4.1
$30,000–$34,999	803	13.7	348	6.3	242	4.6
$35,000–$39,999	512	8.7	328	5.9	276	5.3
$40,000–$49,999	591	10.1	919	16.6	517	9.8
$50,000–$59,000	354	6.0	868	15.7	749	14.3
$60,000–$74,999	216	3.7	735	13.3	1016	19.4
$75,000–$99,999	117	2.0	579	10.5	726	13.8
$100,000+	68	1.2	457	8.3	781	14.9
Median Family Income	$28,536		$48,665		$58,669	
Average Family Income	$31,549		$55,433		$67,994	

Source: Steven G. Hillestad and Eric N. Berkowitz, *Health Care Marketing Plans: From Strategy to Action*, 1991: Jones and Bartlett Publishers, Sudbury, MA. www.jbpub.com. Reprinted with permission.

in income might suggest the need to develop a clinic that provides services tailored to an upscale consumer.

In health care a growing amount of syndicated secondary market research is becoming available. **Syndicated marketing research** is commercial secondary data that regularly provides information on a particular question or problem area. These data provide benchmark information to hospital managers. The major limitation to syndicated information is that these same data can be purchased by competitors in the identical market.

There are several syndicated marketing research databases available. National Research Corporation *Healthcare Market Guide* is based on an annual survey of 140,000 households in the top 100 markets in the United States. It can provide trend data for a three-year time period covering hospitals and health plans. National, state, and regional summaries are also part of the report (www.nationalresearch.com/hcmg.aspx).

The *Healthcare Market Guide* provides a review of several syndicated secondary research bases available to health care marketers.

1. The *Primary Health Care Decision Maker Profile* provides information on customers, including their demographics, economic status, and level of usage of alternative services.
2. The *Quality Image Profile* includes information on which hospitals within the market are perceived as the industry leaders in overall quality and in a variety of factors, such as best physicians, best nurses, and most personalized care. A sample of this report is presented in Table 5-2. A total of 1203 households are included in these data. As can be seen in Table 5-2, 37% think the Texas Medical Center facilities are best for overall quality. Sixty percent, however, of those households that do not have a personal physician think this same facility is the best. The problem for the Texas Medical Center is that this market segment (no physician) is small: It represents only 72 households of the total sample of 1203 households.
3. The *Hospital Product Line Preference Report* indicates the preferences of consumers for a variety of medical and health care services ranging from cancer treatment and heart care to physical therapy and geriatric care.
4. The *Physician Relationships Report* makes it possible to identify which households in each of the top 100 markets have physicians in both primary care and certain specialty areas. Furthermore, the likelihood that their patients will switch care is also examined.

In the pharmaceutical industry one of the most comprehensive secondary data sources is provided by NDC Health Information Services (www.ndchealth.com). One of their databases, NDC Patient Trends, tracks how many new patients have started a particular therapy in the past 12 months, switched to another therapy, what conditions

Table 5-2 | The NCR Health Care Market Guide: Quality

QUALITY PROFILE—HOUSTON,TX
HOSPITAL/FACILITY RECOMMENDED OR GO TO FOR: BEST OVERALL QUALITY

	Total area house holds	NRC Fusion Super Groups									Service Utilization			Physician Association		
		Single achievers	Starting a family	Full house	Baby boom families	Single again	Couple cluster	Golden years	Old & alone	Less fortunate	No usage	Light usage (1–4)	Heavy usage (5+)	No Phys	Primary Phys Only	Both Prtm/ Spec Phys
TOTAL AREA HOUSEHOLDS (000)	1203 100.0 100.0	179 14.9 100.0	217 18.0 100.0	128 10.6 100.0	162 13.5 100.0	124 10.3 100.0	113 9.4 100.0	112 9.3 100.0	59 4.9 100.0	110 9.1 100.0	331 27.5 100.0	601 50.0 100.0	271 22.5 100.0	72 6.0 100.0	893 74.2 100.0	228 19.0 100.0
DON'T KNOW/ NO IMAGE PERCEPTION HOUSEHOLDS	779 100.0 64.8	117 15.0 65.4	138 17.7 63.6	68 8.7 53.1	104 13.4 64.2	82 10.5 66.1	71 9.1 62.8	75 9.6 67.0	41 5.3 69.5	84 10.8 76.4	284 36.5 85.8	386 49.6 64.2	110 14.1 40.6	62 8.0 86.1	590 75.7 66.1	121 15.5 53.1
HOUSEHOLDS WITH IMAGE PERCEPTION	424 100.0 35.2	62 14.6 34.6	79 18.6 36.4	61 14.4 47.7	58 13.7 35.8	41 9.7 33.1	42 9.9 37.2	37 8.7 33.0	18 4.2 30.5	26 6.1 23.6	47 11.1 14.2	215 50.7 35.8	162 38.2 59.8	10 2.4 13.9	303 71.5 33.9	107 25.2 46.9

Table 5-2   Continued

QUALITY PROFILE—HOUSTON,TX
PRIMARY DECISION MAKER HOSPITAL IMAGERY FOR: BEST OVERALL QUALITY

	Total area house holds	NRC Fusion Super Groups									Service Utilization			Physician Association		
		Single achievers	Starting a family	Full house	Baby boom families	Single again	Couple cluster	Golden years	Old & alone	Less fortunate	No usage	Light usage (1–4)	Heavy usage (5+)	No Phys	Primary Phys Only	Both Prim/Spec Phys
TOTAL TEXAS MEDICAL CENTER FACILITIES	158	28	32	22	23	17	14	13	4	4	10	83	65	6	116	35
	100.0	17.7	20.3	13.9	14.6	10.8	8.9	8.2	2.5	2.5	6.3	52.5	41.1	3.8	73.4	22.2
	37.3	45.2	40.5	36.1	39.7	41.5	33.3	35.1	22.2	15.4	21.3	38.6	40.1	60.0	38.3	32.7
ST.LUKE'S EPISCOPAL HOSPITAL	54	7	5	7	14	7	7	2	3	1	5	28	21	1	36	16
	100.0	13.0	9.3	13.0	25.9	13.0	13.0	3.7	5.6	1.9	9.3	51.9	38.9	1.9	66.7	29.6
	12.7	11.3	6.3	11.5	24.1	17.1	16.7	5.4	16.7	3.8	10.6	13.0	13.0	10.0	11.9	15.0
HERMANN HOSPITAL	38	6	7	5	3	2	4	5	1	3	1	18	16	5	24	7
	100.0	16.7	19.4	13.9	8.3	5.6	11.1	13.9	2.8	8.3	2.8	50.0	44.4	13.9	66.7	19.4
	8.5	9.7	8.9	8.2	5.2	4.9	9.5	13.5	5.6	11.5	2.1	8.4	9.9	50.0	7.9	6.5
UNIVERSITY OF TEXAS: ANDERSON HOSPITAL	25	3	3	3	3	6	1	5		1	1	12	12		19	6
	100.0	12.0	12.0	12.0	12.0	24.0	4.0	20.0		4.0	4.0	48.0	48.0		76.0	24.0
	5.9	4.8	3.8	4.9	5.2	14.6	2.4	13.5		3.8	2.1	5.6	7.4		6.3	5.6
TEXAS MEDICAL CENTER	24	10	9	1	1	1	1	1			2	16	6		19	4
	100.0	41.7	37.5	4.2	4.2	4.2	4.2	4.2			8.3	68.7	25.0		79.2	16.7
	5.7	16.1	11.4	1.6	1.7	2.4	2.4	2.7			4.3	7.4	3.7		6.3	3.7

Source: Reprinted from *The NRC Healthcare Market Guide II* with permission of the National Research Corporation, © 1989.

Source: Steven G. Hillestad and Eric N. Berkowitz, *Health Care Marketing Plans: From Strategy to Action*, 1991: Jones and Bartlett Publishers, Sudbury, MA. www.jbpub.com. Reprinted with permission.

patients suffer when staying on a particular therapy, and a host of related issues. The company also offers NDC Pharmaceutical Audit Suite, which provides weekly audits of retail and mail audit of pharmaceutical sales. And there is another secondary database called NDC ADOPT RX, which provides intelligence on early adopter physicians. The importance of identifying early adopters is discussed in the new product process in Chapter 8.

Online Databases

The advent of computer technology has greatly eased the search of secondary data sources. There are some 5000 online databases available to anyone with a computer and modem. *Disclosure Database* (go to http://library.dialog.com/bluesheets and enter the bluesheet number 0101) is one online source that provides data on more than 12,000 publicly traded companies. *County and City Data Book* (http://www .census.gov/statab/www/ccdb.html) provides online information on social and economic statistics from the U.S. Census Bureau and 15 other federal agencies.

These are some of the commercial services available. Each one demonstrates that, for many organizations, the research plan might include purchase of secondary data as opposed to the collection of primary research information. The amount of online medical information and digital journals available is making access to information increasingly easy with sources such as Lexis Nexis® (www.lexisnexis.com), which provides online business, legal, and public record information.

With many of the secondary data sources just discussed, there are several advantages. Many available secondary data are relatively inexpensive to collect. This suggests that, regardless of the issues being investigated, it is helpful to begin with a search of existing noncommercial secondary data sources. An additional advantage is that, unlike primary data collection efforts, secondary data can usually be acquired in a timely manner. Also, secondary data can often be more objective, since they are typically collected by a third party.

In utilizing any secondary data, but most particularly with online sources, there are four criteria on which it must be judged:

a. Relevant—Do the secondary data fit the project needs or question being considered?
b. Accurate—Are the secondary data reliably collected and reported?
c. Current—Is the information up-to-date enough for the decision being made?
d. Impartial—Are the data objectively collected and reported?[4]

EXHIBIT 5-2 shows some useful on-line sources for health care marketing purposes:

Data Collection

There are a variety of research methods that can be employed to collect primary data. These many methods can be classified into: (1) observational, (2) experimental, and (3) survey research.

Exhibit 5-2 Useful Online Marketing Sources

- www.cyberatlas.com—Internet trends and statistics with a section devoted to health care
- www.pewinternet.org—ongoing research on consumers' health care issues and internet use
- www.jmir.org—Journal of Medical Internet Research; articles on Internet-related communication and health care
- www.harrisinteractive.com/news/newsletters_healthcare.asp—Harris poll sites on health care
- www.solucient.com/—Solucient studies on health care issues
- www.healthleaders.com—news on health care management issues
- www.healthfinder.gov—federal government site offering daily headlines
- www.clickz.com/stats—information about Internet and its users from consumers to e-commerce
- www.iab.net—statistics about advertising on the net
- www.jupiterresearch.com—monitors WEB traffic and ranks most popular sites
- www.demographics.com—reports on demographic trends in the United States
- www.arbitron.com—provides local market and radio audience advertising expenditure information
- www.compuserve.com—provides access to databases of business and consumer demographics, government reports plus articles from newspapers, newsletters, and research reports

Observational Research

Using the **observational research** method, consumers are either observed by another individual or through a mechanical device such as a camera. The most well-known commercial observational method may well be the A. C. Nielsen Company's recording of people's television viewing habits. A mechanical device is attached to the television set, which then records when the television is on and the station that is being viewed. The information is sent, via telephone lines, to the Nielsen Company each evening. From these data, television show ratings are then produced.

The limitation of this information is that it requires viewers to press a button whenever they watch television. It is questionable whether this process is always followed. Eventually, A. C. Nielsen plans to have a system that does not require the viewer to activate the system when watching a television show.

Observational data have also been gathered with hidden cameras in supermarkets. These cameras will track the eye movements of individuals as they scan a supermarket shelf. These eye-tracking studies can then facilitate package design.

Occasionally, organizations will use trained individuals to observe patterns of behavior. For example, a hospital might place a trained observer in its waiting area to observe the admitting process. Observers might track individual patients from their initial encounter in admitting up to their examination in the emergency room. The Campbell Health System in Weatherford, Texas, uses mystery shoppers who report details of the patient and visitor experience of their service encounters.[5] This approach is a basic form of observational research. Observational data are useful in observing what people do; however, they cannot address why people behave in certain ways.

Experimental Research

A second form of data collection is an **experiment**, where factors are manipulated to determine a causal relationship. Experiments are common in fields such as psychology in which specific variables can be measured and controlled to assess the impact of one factor on another. Marketing experiments are often conducted in academic settings. The advantage of experimental research is that it can measure the actual effects of one variable, such as the effect that the size of an advertisement has on message retention. The major limitation to this method is whether the results can be generalized in the real world. As a result of this concern of real-world transferability, experimental research has had less relevance in health care marketing.[6]

Because of experimental limitations, a more common form of experimental research in marketing is the **quasi-experimental design**, in which the data gathering is set up similar to a laboratory experiment, although lacking in control over all variables.

A common example of a quasi-experimental design is a test market. A hospital designs a study to test two alternative media strategies regarding calls to a physician referral line. Two cities are found that have similar characteristics—size of the population, number of competing hospitals, specialty physician population, and telephone ownership. In the first city, the referral line is promoted through a campaign of billboards and limited newspaper advertising. In the second city, television might be the primary communication vehicle with a similar level of advertising support. Responses to the referral line are then assessed across the two cities. While modeled after an experimental design, this in-the-field test cannot control for every variable. There may be other factors, such as a competitor's response in a particular market, which could affect the tests differentially. Yet, in spite of this lack of controls, this quasi-experimental design may present a truer measure of an issue than a pure laboratory experiment.

Survey Research

A third common method for acquiring primary data is through **survey research**. Survey research can be obtained through one of four common forms: (1) telephone interviews, (2) personal interviews, (3) focus groups, and (4) mail surveys. Table 5-3 lists some of the trade-offs to consider in the use of the four survey research methods discussed in the following pages.

Telephone Interviews

Telephone interviews are a quick way to acquire information. Using multiple interviewers in a telephone interview bank, data can be acquired within a short time frame.

Approach Criteria	Personal Interview	Telephone Survey	Mail Survey	Focus Groups
Economy	Most expensive.	Avoids interviewer travel, relatively expensive. Trained interviewers needed.	Potentially lowest costs (if response rate sufficient).	Relatively expensive.
Interviewer bias	High likelihood of bias. Trust. Appearance.	Less than personal interviewer. No face-to-face contact. Suspicion of phone call.	Interviewer bias eliminated. Anonymity provided.	Need trained moderator.
Flexibility	Most flexible method. Responses can be probed. Assistance can be provided in completing forms. Observations can be made.	Cannot make observations. Probing possible to a degree.	Least flexible method.	Very flexible.
Sampling and respondent cooperation	Most complete sample possible, with sufficient call back strategy.	Limited to people with telephone. No answers. Refusals are common.	Mailing list problem. Nonresponse a major problem.	Need close selection.

Table 5-3   **Alternative Marketing Research Methodologies**

Source: Steven G. Hillestad and Eric N. Berkowitz, *Health Care Marketing Plans: From Strategy to Action*, 2004: Jones and Bartlett Publishers, Sudbury, MA. www.jbpub.com. Reprinted with permission.

When the questionnaire is short, trained interviewers can usually be successful in obtaining a high completion rate from respondents. Telephone interviewing also allows for the targeting of responses. Using qualifying questions, a telephone interviewer can target the profile of respondent desired.

The speed advantage of telephone data gathering has been demonstrated at the Cleveland Clinic. In late May 1987, a surgical resident was reported to have acquired immune deficiency syndrome. Publicity was heightened by several news stories. The resident's death occurred five days after the newspaper stories first appeared. The clinic used overnight telephone polling services to get next-morning market assessment of any public concerns or issues to which the clinic had to respond.[7] Computer technology has greatly improved the telephone interviewing process. At many commercial marketing research firms, the phone survey is done by computer. Questions can be randomly reordered on the computer display screen, eliminating potential interviewer bias. Data can be directly entered as the questions are asked to increase the speed of analysis. This direct transmission can also help eliminate the possibilities for errors and missing data. Technology has also helped in the development of computer programs that make calls to unlisted numbers through such procedures as random digit dialing. In this method, calls are made to a randomly drawn sequence of numbers within a particular exchange area. In recent years the use of Wide Area Telephone Systems has helped reduce the cost of telephone surveys conducted over broad geographic areas.

Most readers of this text can speak to the limitations of telephone surveys. Many consumers find them intrusive. It is easy for the respondent to terminate the interview by disconnecting. Telephone surveys are also limited regarding the type of questions that respondents can be asked. Many individuals hesitate to answer confidential questions when they are unsure of the caller's identity. Health care organizations can minimize this problem by sending out a pre-survey letter to inform consumers of the incoming call. The notification can often increase the survey's response rate.

Personal Interviews

A second way to survey individuals is through personal interviews. Personal interviews can take two forms: One method consists of one-to-one interviewing between interviewer and respondent; the second form is the group method referred to as "focus groups" (see below).

An individual interview is a valuable way to collect data when the respondent must be probed regarding his or her answers. Complicated questions or questions that do not lend themselves to simple dichotomous responses often require personal interviews. This method also has the highest completion rate since the interviewer has the opportunity to develop some rapport with the respondent. Personal interviews are the preferred method when the survey requires the presentation of visual cues or a product demonstration.

Personal interviews have some limitations, with cost being a major factor. Personal interviews require trained interviewers. And, there are often costs related to the interviewer's travel time. The potential for bias is great as the respondents often have concerns about how they appear or what they say to the researcher. A trained interviewer, however, can often effectively minimize the amount of social desirability. Sensitive questions, such as those regarding health issues, can be difficult.

Focus Groups

Another method of conducting survey research is the focus group, a version of the personal interview conducted with a group of consumers simultaneously. **Focus groups** are interviews typically conducted with eight to ten people and a trained moderator following an interview guide. Focus groups have become a more common, useful approach for acquiring health care information.[8] Focus groups are often used in two aspects of the research process. First, focus groups can be conducted to develop hypotheses. For example, if a manufacturer of hypodermic needles that have long been the preferred brand among nurses finds that sales to hospitals have declined in recent years, this manufacturer might not understand why sales have dropped. To determine some of the possible reasons for such a decline in sales, the company might conduct focus groups and then investigate these reasons in a larger study. A second common use of focus groups is to gain insight into the results of quantitative studies. An MCO might conduct a study to determine the image of competing plans in their market among households with young children. The study might report that 40% of the respondents do not think this particular MCO is good for young families. Focus groups might then be conducted among people with young children to try to gain insight into why this perception is held.

The typical arrangement for a focus group consists of a group of people who are recruited to discuss a particular topic. EXHIBIT 5-3 shows a portion of the focus group guide that was used in a study to examine physicians' and women's attitudes toward breast cancer screening. The focus group moderator is a trained professional who uses

Exhibit 5-3 Sample Focus Group Questions

1. Today, it seems that we can rarely pick up a magazine or read a newspaper without hearing about cancer and what might cause it. Are there any forms of cancer that you think women should be particularly concerned about? Are you doing anything to check for this potential health problem?

    PROBE: What do you see as the real risks of a women getting breast cancer?

    PROBE: Do you think there is some age when getting breast cancer is most likely? Do you think there is some age when getting breast cancer is no longer very likely?

2. Based on what you've read or people whom you've talked to, what types of tests do you think can be done to check a woman for breast cancer?

3. When women are in their childbearing years, they often feel that their gynecologist or obstetrician is responsible for looking after women's problems such as breast, uterine, or cervical cancer. Do you think so? How does this change as the woman gets older?

4. Now I'd like to focus our discussion in the little time left to the problem of breast cancer, specifically. Most of us tend to rely on our physician to inform us of the health care tests we need, and when we need them. When it comes to the area of breast cancer, what does your doctor say to you, or suggest to you?

5. There are many alternative methods that have been suggested for the detection of breast cancer. Specifically, some experts have suggested self-exams, thermography (give description), ultrasound (give description) and mammography (give description). Based on what you've heard, read, or experienced, what do you think about each of these different testing methods?

    Note: Proceed through list individually. First, let me get your reactions to self-exams . . .

    Probe: Probe on effectiveness, fear, frequency with which test should be conducted.

this guide to generate discussion among the group's members. As can be seen in reading these questions, the focus group guide provides an expansive question to the participants to generate discussion. The moderator is there to facilitate the flow of discussion among participants. Focus groups are often used early in the research process when the researcher is not sure of the correct or exact questions to ask in a survey. An analysis of the focus group response can reveal issues that the researcher should explore quantitatively to determine how extensive they are in the general population.

Data from focus groups consist of transcripts of the discussions and often videotapes. At Texas Children's Hospital in Houston, focus groups of patients' concerns are shown to department managers.[9] The analysis of the focus group consists of looking for major themes or issues that emerged in the discussion. Typically, a company will conduct several focus groups using the same question guide. In this way, the analysis can examine consistent themes that emerge from the multiple groups. Research has demonstrated that when focus group themes are consistent across multiple groups, a larger-scale survey tends to validate these themes.

The major benefit to a focus group is the synergy that often occurs from a group discussion. Also, there are many questions that cannot be fully explored in a more formal survey. Focus groups are often used to examine the reasons why a particular behavior or response occurred in a population. A limitation of focus groups is that they, by design, consist of a limited number of participants. There is no statistical exactness or estimation that can be applied to a focus group since the data are qualitative in origin. As with any method in which an individual is involved in collecting the data, there is always the potential for bias, especially with a moderator who is not well trained.

Mail Surveys

Mail surveys are the fourth common form of survey research. Mail surveys have the advantage of being a relatively inexpensive way to collect data. Typically, costs involve the reproduction of the survey and postage to send and return it. A major advantage of mail surveys is that they provide anonymity to the respondent. Mail is also an inexpensive, efficient way to contact individuals who are dispersed over a large geographical area. In health care, mail surveys have often been used to collect patient satisfaction data. Another advantage to mail surveys is the elimination of interviewer bias.

While mail surveys have these distinct advantages, there are several major disadvantages. The major limitation pertains to response rate and who returns the form. SunHealth Alliance, a hospital consulting firm in Charlotte, North Carolina, surveyed 85% of its hospitals and got only a 13% response rate to its mail surveys (and an 85% response rate to its telephone surveys). While there are several strategies that can be used to improve response rates, as indicated in EXHIBIT 5-4, no real controls can be enforced to ensure that the person targeted for the survey did, in fact, complete the survey. There is also the concern that the people who complied and returned the survey may, in fact, be different from those who did not respond. While mail surveys provide the advantage of eliminating interviewer bias, they do not allow for any probing of respondents. Completion rates are affected by question format. Too many open-ended questions requiring respondents to explain their answers in great depth often result in lower return rates.

Designing a Sample

When conducting a study, a basic issue to determine is who should be surveyed. Most marketing research involves a **sample**, which is a collection of data from only a portion of a target population. A **census** is when data are collected from all members of the target population. The sampling process involves six steps.

Step One

Initially, it is essential to define the population. The *population* is the description of all people or elements of interest to researchers and from which a sample will be selected. For example, an academic medical center might define the population as "all pediatricians in the state who referred to a tertiary care facility within the past two-year period."

Step Two

The second step is to specify the *sampling frame*, which is the means of representing the sample population. The sampling frame may be a telephone directory or the medical society mailing list. A perfect sampling frame is one in which every element of the population is represented only once.

Step Three

The third step involves specifying the sampling unit. The *sampling unit* contains the elements of the population to be sampled. For example, if a survey was going to include clinical directors of comprehensive cancer programs, and there was no such directory, the sampling unit might have to be hospitals. The sampling unit is also partially dependent upon the overall design of the project. If, for example, the survey is to be conducted by telephone, the sampling unit will necessarily be telephone numbers. A mail survey requires a sampling unit of addresses.

Step Four

Selection of the sampling method is the fourth step. The *sampling method* is the way the sampling units are to be selected. Any sampling method is dependent on five choices:

1. probability vs. nonprobability
2. single unit vs. cluster of units
3. stratified vs. unstratified
4. equal unit vs. unequal probability
5. single stage vs. multistage

When combined, these five choices provide a possibility of 32 different sampling schemes.

Probability vs. Nonprobability Sampling

A *probability sampling* is one in which the sampling units are selected by chance—for each unit, there is a known chance of being selected. The advantage of a probability sample is that an objective measure of the sample's reliability can be made. An additional advantage is that probability sampling often does not require much detailed information about the population to be surveyed.

A major disadvantage to probability sampling is that a listing of the universe population, or at least a good estimate, is needed. In most research, one may not want to take a probability sample. For example, in an exploratory study, one might want to sample just the successful MCO salespeople to determine what they are doing to win accounts, rather than sampling all MCO salespeople.

There are two basic forms of probability sampling. *Simple random sampling* is a process that requires that each unit's chance of being chosen is known and equal. Simple random samples have the advantage of being easy to understand, and the data analysis techniques are simple. The major disadvantage to simple random samples is that they require a list and number of every item in the universe. Additionally, when there are large variations in the data, it's possible to gather highly misleading samples. Table 5-4 shows some data for household expenditures on medical care during the past year. Two simple random samples could lead to dramatic differences in the inferences drawn regarding health care expenditures, as shown in the lower half of the figure.

Systematic sampling is similar to the simple random sampling process. This approach involves picking a random starting point, and then taking every "Kth" unit in the frame. If, for example, a hospital wanted a sample of 500 patients from a total universe of 100,000, the "Kth" unit would be 200, and then every 200th unit in the frame would be included in the sample.

The advantage of systematic sampling is that, unlike simple random sampling, a designated number does not need to be assigned to every item in the universe. In fact, this approach does not even require a list if units are being sampled over time such as

Table 5-4	Variations in Simple Random Samples		
Household	Medicine Expenditure	Household	Medicine Expenditure
1	$ 60	9	$ 900
2	2700	10	1400
3	500	11	1100
4	1200	12	3000
5	180	13	4500
6	800	14	650
7	4200	15	1300
8	120	16	900
	Total = $23,510		Average/Household = $1469.38
			Standard Deviation = $1344

Sample A		Sample B	
Household	Expenditure	Household	Expenditure
1	$ 50	7	$4200
14	650	12	3000
9	900	15	1300
5	180	2	2700
8	120	10	1400
	Total Expenditure = $1900		Total Expenditure = $12,600
	Average/Household = $ 380		Average/Household = $2520
	Estimate of total		Estimate of total
Universe =	$6112	Universe =	$40,320

is common to patient satisfaction surveys (e.g., the hospital in the above example surveying every 200th patient). There is some difficulty with this approach, however, when trying to measure sampling error. A well-designed probability sample often does not require large numbers to estimate the results confidently. Table 5-5 shows the sample sizes needed in order for the researcher to be 95% and 90% confident in the results for defined populations. It is important to realize that as the population becomes more finely specified, the size of the sample increases relative to each characteristic.

A *nonprobability sample* is one in which the chance selection procedures are not used. Nonprobability samples have the advantage of offering better selection of respondents. This factor is particularly true in exploratory research. The major disadvantage, as with all nonprobability samples, is that no mathematical calculation of sampling error is possible. Selection is often based on the judgment of the researcher, which could limit the ability to generalize the results. There are several variations of a nonprobability sample.

Table 5-5	Sizes of Samples to Be Confident of Accuracy	
Population	Sample Size That Will Provide 95% Confidence Level	Sample Size That Will Provide 90% Confidence Level
Infinity	384	271
100,000	384	271
50,000	381	269
10,000	370	263
5,000	357	257
3,000	341	248
2,000	322	238
1,000	278	213
500	217	176
100	80	73

Note: Error margin held constant at +/−5 percent points

Source: "Finding Out How People Feel about Local Schools," (Columbia, MD: National Committee for Citizens Education, 1984), 36.

A convenience sample is a nonprobability sample where the only criterion for inclusion is the convenience of the unit to the researcher. The advantage of this approach is obvious—it is fast and uncomplicated. The major problem of this method is that the sampling error cannot be determined.

Purposive samples are a nonprobability approach in which units are selected from the universe population on the basis of some form of "expert" judgment. The problems with this method are similar to convenience samples. There is also no way to measure the expertise of the judge in reducing sampling errors.

Of all the nonprobability samples, quota samples involve the most systematic approach to obtaining a representative sample. In a quota sample, the characteristics believed to relate to a representative sample of the population are identified. Then, the proportion of the universe population having the characteristic of interest is estimated. The sample is then allocated among those cells. For example, if it was estimated that women were responsible for the selection of the primary care provider in 80% of all families, then 80% of households included in the quota sample would contain females.

The quota sample is the most attractive of all nonprobability sampling approaches in trying to control reliability. This method also requires the researcher to focus on relevant population subgroups and minimizes the possibility of unusual samples. Its major disadvantage is that it is hard to use more than a limited number of control characteristics on which to develop a quota sample.

In deciding between probability or nonprobability samples, researchers must consider what kind of error tolerance is needed in the results. Highly accurate estimates of the population values would require a probability sample. A related concern is whether nonsampling errors are likely to be large. If the population is relatively homogeneous on the variables of interest, a nonprobability sample might be sufficient.

Single Unit vs. Cluster Sampling

Single unit vs. cluster sampling is the second variation to sampling methods. In *single unit sampling*, each sampling unit is selected individually. In *cluster sampling*, units are selected in groups. For example, if the unit to be sampled is a household, single unit sampling would require that each household be selected separately. One form of cluster sampling would be to change the sampling unit to city blocks. Then, every household on the particular block selected would be included in the sample.

With cluster sampling, the population to be sampled is divided into mutually exclusive and exhaustive subsets. A random sample of these subsets is then selected. A *one-stage cluster sample* is one in which all the population elements in the selected subsets are included in the sample. If, however, a sample of elements is selected from within each subset, this is referred to as a *two-stage cluster sample*. Since a sample of subgroups is chosen with a cluster sample, it is desirable that each subgroup be a small-scale model of the population. In cluster sampling, the subgroups formed should be as heterogeneous as possible.

The choice between single unit and cluster sampling is an economic issue between cost and value. Cluster sampling usually costs less per sampling unit than does single unit sampling; yet for similar sample sizes, the sampling error will be greater with a cluster sample than with a single unit sample. This greater sampling error occurs because there is less variability within a cluster than for a population as a whole. Since single unit sampling uses the population as a whole, this method of sampling reduces sampling error.

Stratified vs. Unstratified Sampling

This is a third sampling variation. A *stratified sample* is a probability sample that involves dividing the population into mutually exclusive and exhaustive subsets and randomly sampling elements from each group. In an unstratified sample, the population is not divided into subsets. This approach is similar to cluster sampling in that both divide the population into mutually exclusive and exhaustive subsets. The difference is that, with stratified sampling, a sample of elements is chosen from each subgroup, while with cluster sampling, a sample of the subgroups are selected. In stratified sampling, each element of the population must be divided into only one subset.

A stratified sample is a common approach in health care research. Consider an MCO that wants to survey member satisfaction. If surveys are administered at the clinic site, it is likely that heavy users of the MCO might be oversampled relative to the total membership, since heavy users are receiving more care. To protect against this oversampling, the MCO might divide its members' strata based upon the amount of their utilization. User groups might be divided into heavy, medium, light, and non-clinic users. Members from each group would be sampled based on the proportion of the membership base that each group represents. If the MCO wants to survey users' satisfaction, the sample proportions would be drawn to represent the heavy users as a proportion of their use relative to the other strata. The strata are drawn so that each individual group is as homogeneous as possible. This type of sample is referred to as a proportionate stratified sample.

Not all stratified samples are proportionate. When some strata have greater variability, more units might be sampled. For example, to determine the average income of physicians across specialties, it might be necessary to disproportionately sample within a specialty, such as neurosurgery, in which the range is broader than a specialty, such as pediatrics, where the income range is narrower.

Equal Unit Probability vs. Unequal Unit Probability

This is the fourth method for selecting sampling units. The only instance in which there is equal unit probability of selection in the sample is when there is no difference in variance among the strata.

Single Stage vs. Multistage Sampling

The final consideration when choosing a sampling method pertains to the number of stages in the sampling process. The researcher must choose between *single stage* or *multistage sampling*. If a perfect sampling frame exists that lists each unit of the population from which the sample is to be drawn, then only a single stage sampling process is needed. Without a perfect sampling frame, a multistage process is often required. Another advantage to multistage sampling is that it often provides a better estimate of the population variance.

Step Five

The fifth step in the sampling process is determination of the sample size. Table 5-5, discussed earlier, shows the required sample sizes for certain populations. Yet more detailed sampling size determinations are possible with the use of sampling theory.

Step Six

The sixth step is to specify the sampling plan, which involves specifying how to implement the sampling choices made in the previous five steps.

Questionnaire Design

Questionnaires must be designed to collect survey information. There are several elements that must be considered. Foremost in designing any survey instrument is the requirement for clarity of meaning to the terms that are used. All well-designed survey instruments utilize a pretest in which the survey is administered to a small group of people similar to those who will ultimately participate in the survey. Difficulties with questionnaire design, its wording, and its completeness can all be revealed in a pretest. If the survey requires major revision, this revision can be followed with an additional pretest. EXHIBIT 5-5 lists the six questions that should be asked about each word in a good survey question.

In addition to pretesting, there are other factors to consider when designing questionnaires. Questions should be written as simply as possible. They should use terms and language with which the audience is familiar. Abbreviations should be avoided.

Exhibit 5-5 Good Survey Research: Questioning Each Word

1. Does it mean what we intend?
2. Does it have any other meaning?
3. If so, does the content make the intended meaning clear?
4. Does the word have more than one pronunciation?
5. Is there any word of similar pronunciation that might be confused?
6. Is a single word or phrase suggested?

Sending a survey to consumers in which they are asked to indicate their interest or need in referrals to a physiatrist may be meaningless, since a technical specialty designation may be unknown or confusing to the potential respondents.

A second caveat in writing any survey question is to ensure that a certain state of affairs is not presupposed. For example, the following question assumes the patient has contacted the nurse practitioner:

Did you find the nurse practitioner to be helpful?
___ Yes   ___ No

In writing any question, one must ensure that the respondent is capable of giving an accurate answer. The wording of the question must be clear to communicate whether one is seeking a factual answer or an opinion. Some individuals will not respond if they believe a factual answer is required and they are unsure of the correct answer.

Question of fact:
How long did you wait before seeing a physician? _____

Question of opinion?
How long do you think you waited before seeing a physician? _____

With factual questions it is important to remember that memories diminish rapidly with time.

Another concern in questionnaire design is to make sure that only one piece of information is asked for at one time. The following question will yield confusion for the respondents and unclear results for the researcher.

Were the billing office and receptionist courteous?
___ Yes   ___ No

Finally, extreme caution should be taken when using adjectives, adverbs, or vaguely defined words. Words such as "several," "most," and "usually" can all have different meanings to different people. For a manager, these definitions complicate actionable results.

Exhibit 5-6   Patient Satisfaction Survey

1. Do you think our level of tertiary care is sufficient in nephrology?

    _____ yes _____ no

2. Did the telephone receptionist answer your call promptly?

    _____ yes _____ no

3. Rate us on each of the following dimensions:

	Good	Very Good	Outstanding
Caring attitude	1	2	3
Physician's knowledge	1	2	3
Hours of scheduling	1	2	3
Prescription service	1	2	3

4. Is our facility clean and easy to use? _____ yes _____ no

5. What is your age?

    _____ under 20   _____ 46 to 55

    _____ 21 to 30   _____ 56 to 70

    _____ 31 to 45   _____ over 70

6. How many children do you have?

    _____ One child

    _____ Two to four

    _____ More than four

EXHIBIT 5-6 shows a sample patient satisfaction questionnaire that contains many of the questionnaire design problems discussed in this section. Review this survey and critique these items according to the caveats expressed.

Question Formats

There are various question formats that can be used in any survey instrument. Consider the example of a multispecialty clinic that would like to examine the expansion of office hours to include evening appointments. The clinic survey questions could be presented in one of several ways:

1. *Open-ended questions* ask individuals to respond based on their own words. These can take the completely unstructured approach:

   What is your opinion of appointment hours?

   An alternative would provide more direct response mechanisms.

2. *Multichotomous questions* are those that present the respondent with a fixed alternative. These questions can be phrased in a dichotomous way in which there are two choices presented (Yes or No):

Would you prefer evening hours by appointment?   ___ Yes   ___ No

They can also be phrased through the application of a scale or options list such as the following examples:

(a) Likert scale: Indicates the degree of agreement or disagreement.
I think evening hours would be more convenient for me.

(Circle the choice that reflects your view)

(b) Semantic differential scale: Uses bipolar adjectives.

Evening hours by appointment are: Convenient __ __ __ __ __ __ Inconvenient

(c) Intention to buy or use scale: Assesses purchase intention beyond attitude.

If evening hours by appointment were offered, I would:

Definitely Use   Probably Not Use
Probably Use   Definitely Not Use
Not Sure

Analysis and Evaluation of Research

The last stage of the market research process involves the analysis and evaluation of the research results. This analysis might be either qualitative (as in the case of focus groups) or quantitative (using survey methodologies that provide empirical information). In either case, a skilled, unbiased person should conduct the analysis. The quantitative sophistication of marketing analysis has advanced with the use of *multivariate statistical analysis*, which considers the impact of multiple variables on a dependent variable. For example, regression analysis is a multivariate statistical technique that has one dependent variable, such as level of monthly smoking activity, and multiple independent variables, such as age of smoker, gender of smoker, amount of alcohol consumed weekly. The regression analysis can determine how much each variable accounts for smoking consumption, as well as how much the effects of the multiple variables together account for the level of smoking consumption.

Even the most sophisticated analysis, however, is useless if the people within the organization cannot understand the results or translate them into managerial actions. For this reason, it is often helpful to have the analyst prepare mock tables that would appear in the final report. Management personnel can examine whether they would see value in a table that might analyze consumer attitude toward a closed panel HMO by gender, or whether a more important table might provide a breakdown of attitude toward a closed panel HMO by type of health insurance of the individuals surveyed.

In this way, the people involved with implementing the changes or dealing with the question being examined can look at what the information might be like. These administrators or managers can then decide whether receiving such data would be helpful. It is essential and important to have data that would lead to a management action.

Yet it is in this last stage of analysis and evaluation of research results that weaknesses in the problem definition are revealed. Too often, in the presentation of market research, a comment is heard, such as: "That's interesting, but what can we do with it?" The cause of such frustrations is not so much that the data analysis was poor, or that the questions that led to the information were incorrect, or even that the method of data collection was inappropriate. Rather it is more likely caused by an improperly defined problem and poorly specified research objectives.

Finally, for most health care organizations, it is essential to recognize that the marketplace is dynamic. Competitors are always changing their strategies, customer attitudes might shift as a function of new health care alternatives being offered to them, physician loyalties might change because of new alliances formed between providers. The dynamic nature of the market necessitates a continual monitoring of the marketplace with ongoing market research. Organizations must also manage and coordinate the flow of this information to the decision makers within the company in an organized fashion. The recognition of this requirement has led to the creation of marketing information systems.

■ Marketing Information Systems

With the onset of more marketing information, individuals are trying to manage the flow of data and information in a more organized fashion. A **marketing information system** (MIS) is "a structured, interacting complex of persons, machines, and procedures designed to generate an orderly flow of pertinent information collected from intra- and extra-firm sources, for use as the bases for decision making in specific responsibility areas of marketing management."[10]

The structure of a hospital's MIS might link admissions data with patient and physician referral information. Online database information and syndicated marketing research information could also be accessed. Key employees would have remote terminal access by modem to the necessary information. Ideally, an effective MIS would be able to construct succinct information reports to the necessary managers on a regular basis.

There are several important ingredients needed to create an organized MIS. Mechanisms must be in place to gather and store the data. Data analysis must be performed, and there must be a way to access the data on a regular or as-needed basis.

The biggest need for an effective MIS is because of the growth in database marketing. **Database marketing** may be defined as "an automated system to identify people—

both customers and prospects—by name, and to use quantifiable information about these people to define the best possible purchasers and prospects for a given offer at a given point in time."[11] The objective of database marketing is to target particular customers more effectively. In implementing a database marketing approach, each patient's record, when entered into the MIS, is assigned a distinct code. In that way, every patient who used the hospital's services can be identified by a database code and targeted mailings could be directed to specific people through these preassigned codes. Building such an MIS for targeted marketing is the strategy of Mid-Michigan Regional Medical Center in Midland. This provider developed a promotional campaign to encourage consumers to complete a free health assessment quiz. Consumers provided information about lifestyle, family status, and clinical status that could be entered into the MIS for future targeted marketing efforts.[12]

A cardiology department, as another example, might decide in conjunction with nutrition and rehabilitative medicine to offer a health education program called "Healthy Heart." Rather than just advertising broadly in the media, the hospital might access those individuals who utilized related services within the past two years, or whose demographic profile might be relevant for this program.

An effective MIS at Hinsdale Hospital in Illinois was described by Maholtra. This hospital used a support system called the Travenol Market Model, which integrated internal hospital and physician records with marketing data and hospitalization rates. Using these data, the hospital identified potential high-growth services and geographic locations.[13]

■ Conclusions

Fewer areas of marketing are being more rapidly affected by technology than marketing research and information systems. In health care, ongoing market research efforts are needed to understand the customer to market the organization effectively.

■ Key Terms

Marketing Research
Primary Data
Secondary Data
Syndicated Marketing Research
Observational Research
Experiment
Quasi-Experimental Design

Survey Research
Focus Groups
Sample
Census
Marketing Information System
Database Marketing

Chapter Summary

1. Marketing research is a process that involves the collection of primary and secondary data, or a combination of both. These data can be either quantitative or qualitative in form.
2. Secondary data can be obtained from the organization itself, from regulatory agencies, and from commercial firms.
3. The collection of primary market research data can be accomplished through observation, experiments, interviews, and surveys.
4. Mail, telephone, and personal interviews vary in terms of flexibility, cost, and respondent cooperation.
5. An increasingly common qualitative data-gathering method in health care is the focus group, used to develop hypotheses or to obtain explanations.
6. In conducting market research, organizations can collect data from all members of the target population—referred to as a census—or they can use a subset of the population—referred to as a sample. Designing a sample begins with a definition of the target population.
7. Any sampling method is dependent on five factors: (1) probability, (2) stratification, (3) equal likelihood of selection, (4) number of stages, and (5) level of the unit.
8. In order to develop any survey instrument appropriately, it is essential to pretest the instrument among a group of people similar to those who will receive the final survey.
9. Marketing information systems are an approach to organizing an array of data for use in strategic marketing decisions.
10. Organizations are developing database marketing efforts that allow them to identify, profile, and reach individual customers.

Chapter Problems

1. A hospital marketing director has several research projects to undertake this quarter. He must try to determine the appropriate sampling methodology in light of each problem. Provide your recommendation on each issue:
    (a) The hospital urology department wants to establish a sexual dysfunction clinic. The department head wants to get an estimate of the number of males ages 35 to 60 in the community suffering some form of sexual dysfunction.
    (b) A primary care medical group is trying to determine whether patients are being greeted and serviced appropriately by the billing and admitting departments.
    (c) An MCO is trying to determine what concerns physicians have in agreeing to become part of its panel of physicians who will treat the managed care plan's subscribers.
2. A health group wants to identify consumers who: (a) once belonged to an MCO, but left the plan; (b) have at least one child; and (c) live in the primary service

area of the town's hospital. Write the questions to target this population and suggest the best method for getting this information.

3. The American Academy of Pediatrics wants to conduct a survey of recently graduated family practitioners to assess why they did not choose pediatrics for their specialization. Provide a definition of the population, suggest a sampling frame, and indicate the appropriate sampling unit.

4. In the previously cited example (Problem 3), suggest the appropriate sampling method in terms of:
   (a) probability vs. nonprobability   (d) equal unit vs. unequal unit
   (b) single unit vs. cluster unit   (e) single stage vs. multistage
   (c) stratified vs. unstratified

5. Listed below are the alternative samples obtained by a health care marketing research firm for its clients. Describe the type of sample each represents.
   (a) Ten people sitting in the waiting room are asked to describe the ambiance of the facility and the attitude of the receptionist.
   (b) The medical school samples alumni regarding an evaluation of their education. Respondents are selected in an amount equal to the same population of specialties from the graduating class.
   (c) The MCO calls every 15th subscriber to assess whether the patient handbook was received, and whether the subscriber has any questions.

6. A nursing home has decided to conduct a short survey to assess whether the family members who are responsible for an elderly resident are satisfied with the care being given. A portion of the survey is listed below.

---

1. How often do you visit your relative?
   ___ Daily   ___ 3 to 4 times a week   ___ 2 to 3 times a week
   ___ Less than once a week

2. Please rate each aspect of care:

	Excellent	Very good	Good
Nursing quality	1	2	3
Room cleanliness	1	2	3

3. Do you like our newsletters and phone call updates?
   ___ Yes   ___ No

4. Why do you think we are the best nursing home in the area?
   _____

5. Please tell us your age:
   ___ Under 25   ___ 35 to 50   ___ Over 65
   ___ 26 to 35   ___ 51 to 65

Please critique this survey.

■ Notes

1. For a useful reference to secondary data sources, see L. McDaniels, *Sources of External Marketing Data*, #580–107 (Cambridge, MA: Harvard Business School Press, 1986).

2. Steve Larose, "Hospitals Predict Market Share with the Help of Public Databases," *Data Strategies & Benchmarks* (January 2003): 1, 3–10.

3. This discussion and the following on commercial secondary data are drawn from S. G. Hillestad and E. N. Berkowitz, *Health Care Marketing Plans: From Strategy to Action* (Gaithersburg, MD: Aspen Publishers, Inc., 1991): 65–106.

4. Philip Kotler and Gary Armstrong, *Principles of Marketing*, 11th ed. (Upper Saddle River, NJ: Prentice Hall, 2006): 108.

5. J. B. Millstead, "Satisfying Your Customers: Mystery Shopping in Your Organization," *Healthcare Executive* 13, no. 3 (1999): 66–67.

6. P. Cooper and R. D. Hisrich, "Marketing Research for Health Services: Understanding Applying Various Techniques," *Journal of Health Care Marketing* 7, no. 1 (1987): 54–60.

7. W. R. Gombeski, Jr., J. R. Day, and L. Honacek, "Overnight Assessment of Marketing Crises," *Journal of Health Care Marketing* 11, no. 1 (1991): 51–54.

8. A useful study of the application of focus group research is presented by E. J. Wargo, "Assessing the Potential of an Industrial Medicine Program," *Journal of Health Care Marketing* 7, no. 1 (1987): 79–85.

9. "Texas Children's Hospital Films Focus Groups to Improve Service," *Hospital Patient Relations Report* 8, no. 3 (1993): 1–2.

10. R. H. Brien and J. E. Stafford, "Marketing Information Systems: A New Dimension for Marketing Research," *Journal of Marketing* 32, no. 3 (1968): 19–23.

11. S. K. Jones, *Creative Strategy in Direct Marketing* (Lincolnwood, IL: NTC Publishing, 1991), 5.

12. L. R. Uttich and G. Dobbins, "The Database Difference," *MPR Exchange* 20, no. 3 (1993): 4–5.

13. N. K. Maholtra, "Decision Support Systems for Health Care Marketing Managers," *Journal of Health Care Marketing* 9, no. 2 (1989): 20–28.

Market Segmentation

After reading this chapter you should be able to:

- Understand alternative market segmentation strategies
- Recognize relevant criteria for selecting market segments
- Identify alternative bases for industrial segmentation
- Appreciate the hierarchy of segmentation alternatives

A basic issue facing most organizations and businesses is deciding which customers to attract to buy their product or use their service. Targeting the market is a major aspect of marketing strategy, as discussed earlier in Chapter 2. A company can decide to target everyone, one market segment, or multiple segments with a different marketing mix strategy.

■ Mass Marketing

A mass marketing strategy is an approach in which an organization develops its marketing mix (the four Ps) to appeal to the broadest group, or largest number of people possible. One of the better-known advocates of this approach was Henry Ford, who was quoted as saying, "You can have any color car you want, as long as it is black." This is a mass marketing strategy at its ultimate—one color car for the entire car-buying market. The early Model T produced by Ford also did not come with the familiar array of options available to car buyers today.

The underlying rationale of a mass marketing strategy is that everyone in the market wants the same product—delivered, priced, and promoted the same way. Or, if there are differences within the market, they are not usually significant enough to affect demand, nor do they merit being addressed by the organization with a different marketing mix strategy.

A mass marketing strategy has some distinct advantages. Foremost is the cost. A mass marketing strategy for a manufactured product often eliminates retooling costs and can ensure longer production runs. Similarly, a mass marketing strategy makes sense when it is economically impractical to produce variations in the marketing mix.

The limitations of a mass marketing strategy, however, underscore its limited usefulness. In reality, there are often large differences within a broad consumer market that do affect demand. People have different shopping patterns or work habits, which, for instance, might necessitate different clinic hours for appointments. Differing income levels require differential pricing for certain services or products. A mass marketing strategy can often cause distribution problems. If a product is available at every outlet, no one particular outlet will feel it is worthwhile to push the product. Finally, the major limitation to a mass marketing strategy relates to competitive considerations. A mass marketing strategy that tries to appeal to everyone leaves a company susceptible to having a group, or segment, of its customers won over by another firm that more closely tailors its marketing mix to attract that particular subgroup. It is competition that provides a strong rationale for a market segmentation strategy.

■ Market Segmentation

Market segmentation is the process of grouping into clusters consumers who have similar wants or needs to which an organization can respond by tailoring one or more elements of the marketing mix. While a mass marketing strategy can be described as bending demand to the will of supply, market segmentation has been described as the bending of supply to the will of demand.[1] Consider the modern automobile industry. Henry Ford would not recognize the production and sales of cars today. Consumers can choose from an array of colors, makes, models, and options. Nike has segmented the market for athletic footwear by the type of athletic activity in which the buyer participates. The Nike line consists of running shoes, weightlifting shoes, basketball shoes, racquetball footwear, tennis, golf, hiking, and even walking footwear. This listing does not even provide a full picture of the colors and variations within each athletic footwear category.

While this view describes a *product* change to respond to individual differences, segmentation can be accomplished with any element of the marketing mix. Individuals in a particular market segment would respond in a like way to one or more elements of the marketing mix. Market segmentation strategies usually fall into one of two categories: (1) concentration strategies, or (2) multisegment strategies.

Concentration Strategy

As described previously in Chapter 2, targeting one segment of the market is referred to as a **concentration strategy**. By focusing on just one market segment, a firm is able to tailor its strategy in an attempt to solidify its position in the marketplace. One advantage of a concentration strategy for the smaller firm is that it may allow the business to target a group that may not be attractive to a larger competitor.

The biggest problem with the concentration strategy is what has been referred to as the **majority fallacy**. Organizations, in deciding to concentrate, will sometimes focus on the largest segment of the market in the belief that it represents the greatest revenue and profit potential. Other competitors may also be attracted to this particular segment for the exact same reasons. As a result of its large size and attractiveness to competitors, the largest segment becomes competitively the most intense, and hence, the least profitable one to target.

An organization that follows a concentration strategy must be able to defend its choice of market segment. The company has no other segments upon which to spread its risk if it is unsuccessful. Another limitation to this strategy is that a firm can develop a reputation that identifies it with just one segment of the market, making it difficult to expand its business to serve other segments. For years, Timex has been known as the manufacturer of reliable, inexpensive watches. It might be very difficult, however, for Timex to market a premium-priced watch. So too, in health care, Kaiser Permanente may have been seen as an organization that concentrated on one segment of the market by targeting the affordable health care segment.

Niche Strategy

A variation of the concentration strategy is referred to as the niche strategy. A **niche** is a very small, specialized market segment with a highly defined set of needs. A **niche strategy** targets this narrow segment with specialized products or services. For example, a clinic could be established to target only wealthy clientele, the trend with boutique medicine clinics. A niche within this group might include just senior members of governments or royalty. This niche might have highly specialized needs in terms of travel arrangements, dietary requirements, security precautions, and even accommodations. In 1994, several faculty groups from the Harvard Medical School tried targeting wealthy patients in Europe and the Middle East. With the support of tax incentives from the Irish government, a hospital was established in Ireland to woo patients from these regions. Surgery was to be provided by some of the world's best clinicians. Yet, advanced medical skills and technologies in Europe and the Middle East made it difficult to attract this upscale niche. These wealthy consumers did not feel a need to seek quality care outside their own countries.[2]

Multisegment Strategy

In a multisegment strategy, an organization can pursue several market segments with varying mixes. One approach a company can use is **product differentiation**, a strategy of altering one or more marketing mix elements to respond to various wants and needs of different groups. There are several versions of this strategy. In one version of product differentiation, a company can take the same product, and through different advertising campaigns or pricing, position it differently to two different groups.[3] The KIA automobile might be positioned as an economical car for a young married couple starting out, or as a fun car for the college-aged buyer. A second strategy of product differentiation might involve taking two products and marketing them to two different segments. Kaiser Foundation Health Plan of California can offer its traditional closed-panel health maintenance organization (HMO) model in markets familiar with that type of health plan. In other markets, Kaiser might develop a point-of-service plan that allows members to use an out-of-plan physician for an additional co-payment or higher deductible.

Selecting Market Segments

Any company that follows a segmentation strategy must identify which market segments to target. Segments should be selected according to the following criteria.

1. A good market segment should be *identifiable*, that is, easily profiled. The more distinctly a segment can be defined, the more efficiently a company can tailor the marketing mix.
2. *Accessibility* is a second criterion. Can the market segment be reached through distribution or promotion efforts? Do these consumers shop in a particular store, or can they be targeted through a specialized magazine or newspaper? It is easy to target physicians as a group through an array of publications like the *American Medical News* or *The New England Journal of Medicine*. There is no easy promotional medium, however, to access some physician groups, such as the segment of physicians who refer to academic medical centers for tertiary care problems.
3. A third important criterion for selecting a market segment is whether its members are *inclined*, or likely, to buy the product or service. It may be easy to target a market segment of high-income consumers who live within a particular ZIP code. If this market segment is not inclined to purchase the service, it is useless to target the marketing mix to them.
4. A fourth concern is whether members of the market segment are *able* to buy the product or service. This criterion speaks to the economic resources of the market. A medical group might develop a prepaid health plan that is very customer-oriented—appointments are never double-scheduled; physicians stay with patients for as long as needed to answer questions, so that the average appointment interval is one hour; and house calls are made upon request. The cost of the plan, however, might be 10 times that of a competing HMO. While the product is desirable, no one can afford to enroll.
5. A fifth criterion for selecting a market segment is that it should be *profitable* to serve.
6. A group's *desirability* is another criterion by which to judge whom to target. There may be some segments that you do not want to serve because they would

be counter to your image or inconsistent with the needs or values of other groups who use your services.

7. A seventh criterion that is relevant when an organization appeals to multiple segments is *consistency*. Are the market segments consistent with each other? Attracting diverse market segments is often difficult because one group may buy or use a product that another group finds irrelevant to its own needs.

8. The final criterion is the *availability* of a market segment. Competitors may already be serving the particular targeted segment, making it hard to shift customers' loyalties.

■ Bases for Segmentation

There are a variety of ways in which a market can be segmented. These can be described as sociodemographic, geographic, psychographic, usage, and cohort segmentation.

Sociodemographic Segmentation

There are many common social and demographic variables used for market segmentation. Some of the variables that are especially pertinent to health care marketing include age, gender, and ethnicity.

Age

In health care marketing, age segmentation has particular relevancy. A medical group practice might develop a specific communication strategy geared to the needs of its patients' age group. An internist might publish a brochure in a larger type size. Patients needing to make outside phone calls can use telephones with volume controls. Specialized forms could be developed to help patients remember when to take medications. The group practice might even designate one employee as the senior citizen assistance representative who, for example, could help in the filing of insurance forms. Aultman Hospital in Canton, Ohio has developed its Prime Time Seniors Program, which has a wide range of services geared to consumers who are age 50 and older. Having over 70,000 members, the program's segmented consumers get assistance filling out forms, discounts at area merchants, free parking, and invitations to educational, social, and travel programs (www.aultman.com/contentindex.asp?ID=115).

Age segmentation exists in terms of product. Geriatric medicine is a clinical program geared to the elderly. Based on the environmental analysis presented in Chapter 3, members of older age groups respond well to marketing programs targeted for their market segment. Baystate Medical Center, a large tertiary hospital in Springfield, Massachusetts, has developed a senior class program that offers tours, lectures, screenings, and other free services. Eighteen thousand senior citizens are members. In 1993, the hospital generated $25 million in gross revenues from this market segment.[4]

Gender

Gender segmentation strategies have been apparent in health care for several years. Studies consistently have found that after age 14, women see physicians 25% more often than men, and women also have a 15% higher hospitalization rate than men.[5-8] Since the mid-1980s, a service of growing popularity in many hospitals has been women's health programs. Research has shown that women in their 30s and 40s are the key health care decision makers for four generations: their own, their children, their parents, and their grandparents.[9] In a recent survey by Solucient, individuals were asked if they made the decisions regarding physicians and hospitals for their families. Of survey respondents who answered "yes," 75% were female. In a corresponding question that asked whether the spouse makes the health care decisions, between 75 and 80% of those who answered "yes" were males.[10] Women's health services segment the market based on gender in an attempt to package a bundle of clinical services that are important to women and are provided in a convenient fashion. One of the more controversial programs in recent years that has been targeted to overweight women has been bariatric surgery programs. The average operative age for people is slightly over 39 years old, and between 1998 and 2001, 86% of the patients for this service were women.[11]

Ethnicity

In recent years, greater attention has been paid to cultural and ethnic diversity as a variable to consider in market segmentation. In the United States, the growing presence and importance of the Hispanic market has led many marketers to tailor their marketing strategies to reach this group.[12] Kaiser Permanente in California is responding to the growing Hispanic market in the state. In television advertisements, Kaiser highlights that Hispanics can request Spanish-speaking physicians, that call centers are available with Spanish-speaking operators and nurses, and that translation services are available in all clinics.[13] Many large metropolitan areas have specialized Spanish-language television shows. St. Francis Hospital, in San Francisco, California, has for many years employed a team of Asian translators to assist in dealing with this patient constituency. The hospital promotes these services through specialized Asian media in the Bay Area. FHP Health Care, a national HMO company based in Fountain Valley, California, has contracted with medical groups who serve Vietnamese and Chinese segments of the population.

In 1993, recognition of cultural and ethnic diversity led the American Medical Association to prepare a monograph on "cultural competence" for physicians. The five key components are:

1. Awareness and acceptance of how cultural differences can affect the delivery of health care
2. Ability to recognize how one's own culture affects behavior and attitudes
3. Awareness that misunderstandings and misinterpretations can occur when a provider from one culture interacts with a patient from a different culture

4. Enough knowledge of each patient's culture to anticipate barriers, plus an awareness that cultures are too complex to understand fully
5. Ability to adapt and refine one's skills to provide culturally competent care[14]

There is a journal within the field of nursing entitled the *Journal of Transcultural Nursing*, which is an online publication highlighting research on the issues of cultural diversity that can affect care. Several of the findings within this journal have important implications to marketers in the delivery of health care services (http://tcn.sagepub .com/current.dtl). Other common sociodemographic variables often used in segmentation strategies include occupation (creating tailored health education programs to particular occupational groups based on the incidence of problems suffered), family status, and education.[15]

Income Segmentation

In recent years in health care there has been a growing tendency to segment the market by income. This strategy is most visible with the rise of "boutique" medical practices. These practices have typically targeted the upper income consumer who also has insurance coverage. In the "boutique" practice, the physician limits the number of patients he or she will see. Patients are given a significant amount of time for an office visit and the physicians are almost always "on call." The fees for being a patient in one of these practices can vary. For example at MDVIP in Boca Raton, the physician manages 600 patients, and each one is charged an annual retainer of $1500 (http:// www.mdvip.com/). In Seattle, a similar boutique practice limits the number of patients to 100 per physician. Patients are charged $10,000 per year (www.md2.com/md2 .html).[16] Tufts New England Medical Center is one of the first academic-based organizations to offer boutique care for patients willing to spend $1800 per year; for this additional fee they will get a private waiting area as well as longer appointments. This approach was taken to help generate increased revenue for the medical center.[17]

Geographic Segmentation

A second major way to segment the market is geographically. Many U.S. manufacturers have found that consumers in different regions of the country have unique preferences for certain food products. Spicier foods, for example, are popular in the Southwest,[18] and Japanese-made automobiles have had stronger appeals to consumers on both coasts compared to those in the midwestern parts of the United States.

In health care, geographic segmentation is rarely national; far more often it is regional or local. The major geographic distinctions relevant to health care are urban vs. rural or urban vs. suburban. An urban academic medical center, for example, may pursue a geographic segmentation strategy in attracting patients. In the primary and secondary service areas of the academic medical center, the center may find that it receives few referrals from community physicians. Most of these physicians may admit to their own local hospitals and refer patients to specialists on the staffs of these facilities. There may also be a concern among local community physicians that their patients, once referred to the academic medical center, might become loyal patients of the medical center.

Following a geographic segmentation strategy, then, the academic medical center might open primary care satellites staffed by its own primary care physicians within its primary service area. Outside the primary and secondary service areas, the medical center may find a stronger referral flow. Physicians in the outlying areas are less concerned about patients going to the academic medical center for routine care, since the medical center is 50 or 100 miles away. In these outlying communities, the academic medical center does not set up primary care satellites. Rather, it establishes a physician relations department to assist with patient referrals from these physicians and to reinforce and encourage their referral pattern. Or, the clinic might set up a range of satellites across a wide geographic area to capture referrals as well as primary care patients as was done by the Scott and White Clinic. The main clinic is based in Temple, Texas; however, it has specialty clinics and surgery centers throughout the region as shown in FIGURE 6-1 (www.sw.org).

For most health care marketing, geographic segmentation allows organizations located in markets with rather heterogeneous factors to tailor a marketing mix on the basis of location.

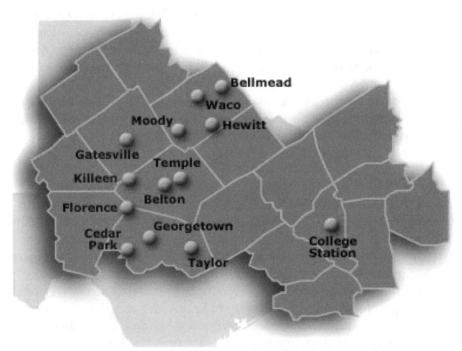

FIGURE 6-1 Geographic Segmentation of Scott and White Hospitals and Clinics

Source: © 2005. Scott & White.

Psychographic Segmentation

A third major way to segment the market is psychographically, which refers to lifestyle and social class.

Lifestyles

Segmentation by lifestyle is a common approach to segmenting the market. Individuals are grouped, based on their behavioral characteristics, attitudes, and opinions. To conduct lifestyle segmentation, marketing researchers profile consumers based on their responses to attitude, interest, and opinion (AIO) statements. An example of some responses to health care–related AIO statements was shown in Chapter 4. Such questions, rated on a scale ranging from "strongly agree" to "strongly disagree" help identify a health-conscious consumer's AIOs. A research firm can then match specific demographic characteristics to this profile of a health-conscious consumer in order to more closely profile this market segment.

In Chapter 4, the VALS2™ system of profiling consumers was discussed. This system is a version of psychographic segmentation. The PRIZM system, also described in Chapter 4, is a version of psychographic segmentation that is tied to demographic and geographic segmentation bases. The PRIZM system describes lifestyle profiles of different neighborhoods. A selection of some PRIZM profiles is shown in Table 6-1. Developed by Claritas (www.claritas.com), Prizm has been a useful segmentation approach for satellite location as well as to target contributors to foundations.

A health care version of psychographic segmentation is being used by Stanford University of Palo Alto, California, in conjunction with Consumer Insights, a marketing consulting firm in San Rafael, California. The company uses a 25-question survey and a

Table 6-1	The PRIZM Profiles	% of U.S. Households
Blue Blood Estates: America's wealthiest neighborhoods		1.1
Norm Rae-Ville: Lower middle class mill towns, and industrial suburbs primarily in the South		2.3
Gray Power: Upper middle class retirement communities		2.9
Single City Blues: Downscale, urban, singles' districts		3.3
Towns and Gowns: America's college towns		1.2
Furs & Station Wagons: New money in metropolitan bedroom suburbs		3.2
Heavy Industry: Lower working class districts in the nation's older industrial cities.		2.8

Source: Selected PRIZM profiles from *Clustering of America* by Michael J. Weiss. Copyright © 1988 by Michael J. Weiss. Used by permission.

mathematical algorithm to classify consumers into nine market segments, called Profiles of Attitudes Toward Healthcare. Segments are given names such as "clinic cynics" and "ready users." Stanford University identified psychographic segments in its market area and is reshaping its advertising strategy to respond to these groups.[19]

One marketing care consulting firm, Strategic Directions, Inc. has focused on the 40s and older age group and their psychographic profiles. Based on their psychographic profiles, they have grouped people based on their attitudes toward their use of health products and services, how they use health information, and their degree of health compliance with providers' instructions. And, while Claritas and Vals have generalized descriptors of the populations, Strategic Directions Group, Inc. has developed psychographic profiles such as the "faithful patient," someone who is aware he or she should eat well but who does little to remain healthy; or another psychographic segment as the "resentful complier," which is a group that confirm the importance of taking medication as directed, although they do not believe their doctor listens or cares about them.[20]

Social Class

Social class is included in the Chapter 4 discussion of consumer behavior. It is often used as a basis for psychographic segmentation. Individuals within certain social classes hold similar attitudes and have similar purchasing patterns. Many advertisements are directed to particular social classes in their appeal for products.

Usage Segmentation

Another major category for segmentation is grouping people based on product usage or purchase. Of all the bases for segmentation, usage segmentation may be one of the most valuable. This approach segments the market based on the percentage of a product that consumers buy or a service that they use. Since the ultimate goal of any marketing strategy is to affect a consumer's purchase decision, segmenting based on purchase can relate marketing strategy directly to consumer actions. There are several ways in which this can be done: usage rates, type of usage, brand loyalty, and benefit segmentation.

Usage Rates

One interesting basis for segmentation that is relevant for health care is usage rates. Table 6-2 describes some usage rates for three product categories: colas, beer, and canned hash. Within marketing, a phenomenon called the **heavy half consumer** has been identified, in which a small group of consumers account for a disproportionate amount of a product's sales. Sometimes this is referred to as the 80/20 rule: 80% of a product's sales are accounted for by 20% of the people who purchase the product.

While a heavy half segment does not mean that the group always must purchase 80% of a product's sales, this segment does account for a disproportionate percentage of the sales relative to its size in the total market.

Table 6-2			The Heavy Half Consumer					
COLAS			**BEER**			**CANNED HASH**		
H–22%	H–39%	H–39%	H–67%	H–16%	H–17%	H–68%	H–16%	H–16%
U–0%	U–10%	U–90%	U–0%	U–12%	U–88%	U–0%	U–14%	U–86%

Table 6-2 displays data indicating the existence of a heavy half segment across three product categories: colas, beer, and canned hash. Looking at the far right-hand column, one can see that 39% of consumers buy 90% of all the soft drinks sold. Here is an instance where a small (39%) segment of the market accounts for a disproportionate percent of product consumption. The heavy half segments are more dramatic for beer and canned hash. Seventeen percent of all people account for 88% of all beer consumed, and 16% consume 86% of all the canned hash sold.

A similar case for heavy half segments can be made within health care. Many HMOs, for example, have experienced heavy utilization by a small segment of their subscriber panel. A small percentage of the primary care physicians (PCPs) who refer to a specialty group account for a disproportionate share of all referrals.

Heavy half segmentation has some important marketing implications. Consider the heavy half segment for beer (i.e., the 17% that consumes 88% of all beer sold). The major marketing objective of a beer company is to maintain its loyalty. No changes in the product or service should be made until it is pretested with these heavy half purchasers. For the medium users (the 16% of the market that consumes 12% of all beer sold), a brewer's marketing objective is different. The goal here is to increase purchases in this group. A beer brewery may try to convince these individuals that ordering a fine imported beer—as opposed to ordering a glass of fine Chardonnay—will imply they are sophisticated consumers. A company might use a slogan such as, "Come to think of it, I'll have a Heineken!" Finally, there is the third group of nonusers. Sixty-seven percent of consumers do not buy any beer. With a nonuser group, marketing research is necessary to determine why people do not use a product. Typically, there are two subsegments within this population. Some people do not buy beer because they do not like it. For a beer company, little can be done with this segment. Some people, however, do not purchase beer, but they have never tested it. The key here is to determine a legal (for an alcoholic beverage company) way for this segment to sample beer.

Heavy half segments also exist within health care. A specialist can examine the referral patterns by primary care referrers and will, most likely, find the existence of this phenomenon. Twenty or 30% of all the PCPs may account for a disproportionate share of all the referrals to the specialist. A similar effect has been observed within the Veteran's Administration health care system where a small percentage of the older veterans (World War II and Korean War veterans) account for a disproportionate share of the utilization in the community clinics.

Consider the implications of heavy half segmentation in health care. The strategies and marketing objectives differ in a fee-for-service versus a managed care model. In a fee-for-service setting, the objectives are similar to the beer company. A specialist who has a heavy half segment of PCP referrals wants to maintain the loyalty of that group. No changes will be made regarding how patient referrals are handled unless first checked with the loyal users. The worst strategy would be to change the service in response to a few complaints, only to find that the change is unpopular among the heavy half segment.

With the middle group, marketing strategy must examine ways to increase referrals. Does this mean improving access? Providing better feedback? Expanding the type of specialties represented in the group? In a particular service area, a specialist might find a large number of physicians who do not refer at all to the medical practice. What must be determined is which physicians don't refer because they are satisfied with their present referral source. Some portion of the physicians who do not refer are in this group because they are unfamiliar with the practice or the physicians within the group. This segment is one to which a promotional strategy effort must be directed.

To increase referrals and attract referrals from physicians who presently do not use the Cleveland Clinic Foundation, this organization has established the Cleveland Clinic CompreCare Affiliate program. Open to physicians who are not affiliated with the Cleveland Clinic Foundation, this program has no cost to participating physicians or minimum referral requirements. Among other benefits, the program provides a monthly newsletter, a toll-free telephone line for scheduling appointments, a guarantee regarding information feedback, and continuing medical education courses. The Foundation has tracked referrals from physicians who participate in the CompreCare program and found a 77% increase among those who had not referred prior to the incentive program, and a 34% increase among medium referrers (one to six patients a year). The third group included physicians who had been heavy previous referrers.[21]

This heavy half scenario and related objectives change dramatically in a managed care setting. In a managed care model, the objective is to identify the heavy users of health services and to determine how to reduce their demand. For example, an HMO might profile the heavy users to determine whether there are any consistent usage patterns. This might lead to some intervention or more thorough screening prior to appointment scheduling. It also might require shifting certain deductible requirements to minimize excessive use. The middle users are, for most managed care plans, the individuals who follow standard levels of use and requirements. It is the last group, the nonusers among the subscriber pool, which is the financial lifeblood of the managed care plan. For this segment of the market, the managed care plan must develop retention strategies to ensure that these nonusers see value in the product that they purchased.

For traditional marketers, there are some commercial sources available to help them in profiling heavy half users, along with their media habits. Table 6-3 displays a sample from a media usage database published by Simmons Market Research of

Table 6-3		Usage Data and Profiling Information				

SUNDAY NEWSPAPERS AND SYRUP USER FREQUENCY
NCS/NHCS: SPRING 2005 ADULT 2-YEAR COMBINED UNIFIED (MAY 2003–MAY 2005)

	ELEMENTS	4 TIMES A DAY OR MORE OFTEN	2 OR 3 TIMES A DAY	ONCE A DAY	1 TO 3 TIMES A WEEK	LESS THAN ONCE A WEEK
Total Sample	Sample	52,860	1,646	11,779	4,593	2,595	3,198
	(000)	211,727	5,909	45,383	18,020	10,009	11,921
	Vertical	100%	100%	100%	100%	100%	100%
	Horizontal	100%	2.79%	21%	8.51%	4.73%	5.63%
	Index	100	100	100	100	100	100
	Base	100%	2.79%	21%	8.51%	4.73%	5.63%

SUNDAY NEWSPAPERS: SUNDAY NEWSPAPERS - READ: SUNDAY NEWSPAPERS - READ ANY (NET)

	Sample	39,715	1,247	9,239	3,619	1,900	2,347
	(000)	121,109	3,517	27,650	10,945	5,387	6,474
	Vertical	57%	60%	61%	61%	54%	54%
	Horizontal	100%	2.90%	23%	9.04%	4.45%	5.35%
	Index	100	104	107	106	94	95
	Base	57%	1.66%	13%	5.17%	2.54%	3.06%
Total Sample	Sample	52,860	1,646	11,779	4,593	2,595	3,198
	(000)	211,727	5,909	45,383	18,020	10,009	11,921
	Vertical	100%	100%	100%	100%	100%	100%
	Horizontal	100%	2.79%	21%	8.51%	4.73%	5.63%
	Index	100	100	100	100	100	100
	Base	100%	2.79%	21%	8.51%	4.73%	5.63%

MAGAZINES: MAGAZINES - READ/LOOK INTO LAST 6 MOS: AARP, THE MAGAZINE

	Sample	8,738	241	1,923	775	334	458
	(000)	38,293	977	8,243	3,253	1,727	2,136
	Vertical	18%	17%	18%	18%	17%	18%
	Horizontal	100%	2.55%	22%	8.49%	4.51%	5.58%
	Index	100	91	100	100	95	99
	Base	18%	0.46%	3.89%	1.54%	0.82%	1.01%

MAGAZINES: MAGAZINES - READ/LOOK INTO LAST 6 MOS: ALLURE

	Sample	2,504	102	608	209	151	169
	(000)	10,112	402	2,382	846	599	722
	Vertical	4.78%	6.81%	5.25%	4.70%	5.99%	6.05%
	Horizontal	100%	3.98%	24%	8.37%	5.93%	7.14%
	Index	100	143	110	98	125	127
	Base	4.78%	0.19%	1.13%	0.40%	0.28%	0.34%

MAGAZINES: MAGAZINES - READ/LOOK INTO LAST 6 MOS: THE AMERICAN LEGION

	Sample	1,150	39	224	97	57	79
	(000)	5,397	186	980	369	378	405
	Vertical	2.55%	3.15%	2.16%	2.05%	3.77%	3.39%
	Horizontal	100%	3.44%	18%	6.84%	7.00%	7.49%
	Index	100	123	85	80	148	133
	Base	2.55%	0.09%	0.46%	0.17%	0.18%	0.19%

MAGAZINES: MAGAZINES - READ/LOOK INTO LAST 6 MOS: AMERICAN RIFLEMAN

	Sample	1,302	34	249	113	76	84
	(000)	6,555	128	1,234	572	585	440
	Vertical	3.10%	2.16%	2.72%	3.18%	5.85%	3.69%
	Horizontal	100%	1.95%	19%	8.73%	8.93%	6.71%
	Index	100	70	88	103	189	119
	Base	3.10%	0.06%	0.58%	0.27%	0.28%	0.21%

(continues)

Table 6-3	Usage Data and Profiling Information (continued)

SUNDAY NEWSPAPERS AND SYRUP USER FREQUENCY
NCS/NHCS: SPRING 2005 ADULT 2-YEAR COMBINED UNIFIED (MAY 2003–MAY 2005)

ELEMENTS	4 TIMES A DAY OR MORE OFTEN	2 OR 3 TIMES A DAY	ONCE A DAY	1 TO 3 TIMES A WEEK	LESS THAN ONCE A WEEK
MAGAZINES: MAGAZINES - READ/LOOK INTO LAST 6 MOS: AMERICAN WAY (AMERICAN AIRLINES)					
Sample	1,934	60	431	191	74	88
(000)	6,520	203	1,440	558	312	250
Vertical	3.08%	3.43%	3.17%	3.10%	3.12%	2.10%
Horizontal	100%	3.11%	22%	8.56%	4.78%	3.84%
Index	100	111	103	101	101	68
Base	3.08%	0.10%	0.68%	0.26%	0.15%	0.12%
MAGAZINES: MAGAZINES - READ/LOOK INTO LAST 6 MOS: ARCHITECTURAL DIGEST					
Sample	2,187	76	479	177	100	114
(000)	8,199	285	1,774	548	499	385
Vertical	3.87%	4.83%	3.91%	3.04%	4.98%	3.23%
Horizontal	100%	3.48%	22%	6.68%	6.08%	4.69%
Index	100	125	101	79	129	83
Base	3.87%	0.13%	0.84%	0.26%	0.24%	0.18%
MAGAZINES: MAGAZINES - READ/LOOK INTO LAST 6 MOS: ARTHRITIS TODAY					
Sample	1,370	63	314	106	70	93
(000)	6,105	234	1,572	373	311	402
Vertical	2.88%	3.95%	3.46%	2.07%	3.11%	3.37%
Horizontal	100%	3.83%	26%	6.11%	5.10%	6.58%
Index	100	137	120	72	108	117
Base	2.88%	0.11%	0.74%	0.18%	0.15%	0.19%
MAGAZINES: MAGAZINES - READ/LOOK INTO LAST 6 MOS: THE ATLANTIC MONTHLY					
Sample	847	31	160	66	33	51
(000)	3,117	60	529	214	150	179
Vertical	1.47%	1.02%	1.17%	1.19%	1.50%	1.50%
Horizontal	100%	1.94%	17%	6.85%	4.82%	5.73%
Index	100	69	79	81	102	102
Base	1.47%	0.03%	0.25%	0.10%	0.07%	0.08%
MAGAZINES: MAGAZINES - READ/LOOK INTO LAST 6 MOS: ATTACHE (US AIRWAYS)					
Sample	971	32	231	75	47	41
(000)	4,692	136	1,260	380	240	167
Vertical	2.22%	2.30%	2.78%	2.11%	2.40%	1.40%
Horizontal	100%	2.90%	27%	8.10%	5.12%	3.56%
Index	100	104	125	95	108	63
Base	2.22%	0.06%	0.60%	0.18%	0.11%	0.08%
MAGAZINES: MAGAZINES - READ/LOOK INTO LAST 6 MOS: AUTOMOBILE					
Sample	1,716	66	379	121	98	137
(000)	7,749	186	1,742	529	519	523
Vertical	3.66%	3.14%	3.84%	2.93%	5.19%	4.38%
Horizontal	100%	2.40%	22%	6.82%	6.70%	6.75%
Index	100	86	105	80	142	120
Base	3.66%	0.09%	0.82%	0.25%	0.25%	0.25%
MAGAZINES: MAGAZINES - READ/LOOK INTO LAST 6 MOS: AUTOWEEK					
Sample	1,394	61	287	119	79	102
(000)	6,037	242	1,124	488	344	419
Vertical	2.85%	4.09%	2.48%	2.71%	3.43%	3.52%
Horizontal	100%	4.00%	19%	8.09%	5.69%	6.94%
Index	100	143	87	95	120	123
Base	2.85%	0.11%	0.53%	0.23%	0.16%	0.20%

| Table 6-3 | **continued** |

SUNDAY NEWSPAPERS AND SYRUP USER FREQUENCY
NCS/NHCS: SPRING 2005 ADULT 2-YEAR COMBINED UNIFIED (MAY 2003–MAY 2005)

ELEMENTS		4 TIMES A DAY OR MORE OFTEN	2 OR 3 TIMES A DAY	ONCE A DAY	1 TO 3 TIMES A WEEK	LESS THAN ONCE A WEEK
MAGAZINES: MAGAZINES - READ/LOOK INTO LAST 6 MOS: AMERICAN BABY						
	Sample	2,570	124	669	220	175	189
	(000)	9,587	493	2,421	821	629	536
	Vertical	4.53%	8.34%	5.33%	4.56%	6.28%	4.50%
	Horizontal	100%	5.14%	25%	8.56%	6.56%	5.59%
	Index	100	184	118	101	139	99
	Base	4.53%	0.23%	1.14%	0.39%	0.30%	0.25%
MAGAZINES: MAGAZINES - READ/LOOK INTO LAST 6 MOS: BABY TALK						
	Sample	1,925	89	486	151	133	151
	(000)	7,902	384	1,922	577	626	533
	Vertical	3.73%	6.50%	4.23%	3.20%	6.26%	4.47%
	Horizontal	100%	4.86%	24%	7.30%	7.93%	6.74%
	Index	100	174	113	86	168	120
	Base	3.73%	0.18%	0.91%	0.27%	0.30%	0.25%
MAGAZINES: MAGAZINES - READ/LOOK INTO LAST 6 MOS: BARRON'S						
	Sample	826	33	174	74	32	55
	(000)	3,123	115	663	200	153	277
	Vertical	1.48%	1.95%	1.46%	1.11%	1.53%	2.32%
	Horizontal	100%	3.68%	21%	6.40%	4.89%	8.87%
	Index	100	132	99	75	104	158
	Base	1.48%	0.05%	0.31%	0.09%	0.07%	0.13%
MAGAZINES: MAGAZINES - READ/LOOK INTO LAST 6 MOS: BASSMASTER						
	Sample	773	25	163	64	50	47
	(000)	4,173	46	997	346	309	291
	Vertical	1.97%	0.77%	2.20%	1.92%	3.09%	2.44%
	Horizontal	100%	1.10%	24%	8.30%	7.41%	6.97%
	Index	100	39	111	97	157	124
	Base	1.97%	0.02%	0.47%	0.16%	0.15%	0.14%
MAGAZINES: MAGAZINES - READ/LOOK INTO LAST 6 MOS: HARPER'S BAZAAR						
	Sample	1,852	98	472	145	93	132
	(000)	6,373	275	1,423	371	328	518
	Vertical	3.01%	4.65%	3.14%	2.06%	3.28%	4.35%
	Horizontal	100%	4.31%	22%	5.82%	5.15%	8.13%
	Index	100	154	104	68	109	144
	Base	3.01%	0.13%	0.67%	0.18%	0.16%	0.24%
MAGAZINES: MAGAZINES - READ/LOOK INTO LAST 6 MOS: BETTER HOMES AND GARDENS						
	Sample	11,875	367	3,054	1,193	531	646
	(000)	52,627	1,596	13,349	4,930	2,199	2,819
	Vertical	25%	27%	29%	27%	22%	24%
	Horizontal	100%	3.03%	25%	9.37%	4.18%	5.36%
	Index	100	109	118	110	88	95
	Base	25%	0.75%	6.30%	2.33%	1.04%	1.33%
MAGAZINES: MAGAZINES - READ/LOOK INTO LAST 6 MOS: BICYCLING						
	Sample	770	32	140	65	45	51
	(000)	3,003	133	588	206	135	146
	Vertical	1.42%	2.25%	1.30%	1.14%	1.35%	1.22%
	Horizontal	100%	4.43%	20%	6.86%	4.49%	4.85%
	Index	100	159	91	81	95	86
	Base	1.42%	0.06%	0.28%	0.10%	0.06%	0.07%

(continues)

Table 6-3	Usage Data and Profiling Information (continued)

ELEMENTS		4 TIMES A DAY OR MORE OFTEN	2 OR 3 TIMES A DAY	ONCE A DAY	1 TO 3 TIMES A WEEK	LESS THAN ONCE A WEEK
MAGAZINES: MAGAZINES - READ/LOOK INTO LAST 6 MOS: BLACK ENTERPRISE						
	Sample	902	41	198	53	71	83
	(000)	5,702	240	1,298	240	610	468
	Vertical	2.69%	4.07%	2.86%	1.33%	6.09%	3.92%
	Horizontal	100%	4.22%	23%	4.21%	11%	8.21%
	Index	100	151	106	49	226	146
	Base	2.69%	0.11%	0.61%	0.11%	0.29%	0.22%
MAGAZINES: MAGAZINES - READ/LOOK INTO LAST 6 MOS: BOATING						
	Sample	944	25	194	80	38	59
	(000)	4,081	60	827	343	237	249
	Vertical	1.93%	1.01%	1.82%	1.90%	2.37%	2.09%
	Horizontal	100%	1.47%	20%	8.40%	5.81%	6.11%
	Index	100	53	95	99	123	109
	Base	1.93%	0.03%	0.39%	0.16%	0.11%	0.12%
MAGAZINES: MAGAZINES - READ/LOOK INTO LAST 6 MOS: BON APPETIT						
	Sample	2,455	90	607	201	97	151
	(000)	9,934	343	2,450	801	448	607
	Vertical	4.69%	5.81%	5.40%	4.45%	4.48%	5.09%
	Horizontal	100%	3.46%	25%	8.07%	4.51%	6.11%
	Index	100	124	115	95	95	109
	Base	4.69%	0.16%	1.16%	0.38%	0.21%	0.29%
MAGAZINES: MAGAZINES - READ/LOOK INTO LAST 6 MOS: BRIDE'S						
	Sample	1,830	77	472	155	107	131
	(000)	7,334	254	1,884	637	433	533
	Vertical	3.46%	4.30%	4.15%	3.54%	4.32%	4.47%
	Horizontal	100%	3.47%	26%	8.69%	5.90%	7.27%
	Index	100	124	120	102	125	129
	Base	3.46%	0.12%	0.89%	0.30%	0.20%	0.25%
MAGAZINES: MAGAZINES - READ/LOOK INTO LAST 6 MOS: ARTHUR FROMMER'S BUDGET TRAVEL						
	Sample	853	38	187	72	47	48
	(000)	3,142	135	679	235	213	187
	Vertical	1.48%	2.28%	1.50%	1.31%	2.13%	1.57%
	Horizontal	100%	4.29%	22%	7.49%	6.79%	5.96%
	Index	100	154	101	88	144	106
	Base	1.48%	0.06%	0.32%	0.11%	0.10%	0.09%
MAGAZINES: MAGAZINES - READ/LOOK INTO LAST 6 MOS: BUSINESS WEEK						
	Sample	2,613	87	559	237	97	140
	(000)	10,939	409	2,142	958	451	608
	Vertical	5.17%	6.92%	4.72%	5.32%	4.51%	5.10%
	Horizontal	100%	3.74%	20%	8.76%	4.12%	5.55%
	Index	100	134	91	103	87	99
	Base	5.17%	0.19%	1.01%	0.45%	0.21%	0.29%

Magazines read in the last 6 months, by cough syrup frequency

Chicago, Illinois. This source provides an overview of heavy half users for a wide variety of product categories. These sample pages show the magazines read according to frequency of the use of cough syrup. Simmons also provides a breakdown of their media habits.

Type of Usage

A second segmentation based on type of usage, or how the product is used.[22] Orange juice manufacturers can develop different marketing mix strategies geared to different types of usage segments. Orange juice can be used as a breakfast drink, a mixer for alcoholic beverages, or as an alternative to other beverages. The marketing mix strategies will be tailored specifically for each of these segments. For the breakfast drink market, the product needs to be distributed in grocery stores; advertisements should show it being used in the morning; and the pricing should compare to other morning drinks, such as grapefruit juice. For the alcoholic beverage mix segment, the distribution strategy must shift to liquor stores. The alternative beverage segment might require a packaging change. For instance, orange juice can be packaged in single-serving cans or juice boxes for children's lunches. Vending machine distribution also becomes a major element of this marketing mix strategy.

A recent drug in health care that has seen different usage segments appear has been Botox. One distinct segment is for injections in cosmetic surgery. A second usage segment is in the treatment of migraines, the results of which came about accidentally.[23] And, a third usage segment is for underarm sweating.

Brand Loyalty

A third usage segment categorizes consumers by their level of brand loyalty or the degree to which they purchase or use the same brand of product or service. Some consumers who repeatedly use the same multispecialty group practice for all their medical care can be described as *hard core loyal*. Some consumers might occasionally use the medical group for some services and use practitioners outside the group for different clinical needs. These individuals might be termed *split loyalists*. A third group, defined as *switchers*, tries different facilities for care. Profiling these segments helps a medical group develop a better understanding of who belongs to a respective target market. This profiling can assist in developing strategies for increasing the loyalties of the *split loyalty* segment. For example, McStravic has suggested targeting loyal hospital users with newsletters, birthday cards, health tips, and update reports to reinforce positive impressions.[24]

Benefit Segmentation

A final basis for usage segmentation is **benefit segmentation**, the grouping of people based on the benefits sought from the product.[25] To implement this approach, an organization must understand what benefit customers are seeking from the product purchase, and then must analyze the existing brands available on the market. This process

Table 6-4	Benefit Segmentation of the Toothpaste Market		
Benefits/ingredients	Fluoride	Abrasive	Flavoring
Decay prevention	Crest		
Cosmetic		Ultra Brite	
Taste			AIM

can help to identify benefit segments not presently being served. Table 6-4 displays a benefit segmentation approach for the toothpaste market. Three major benefit segments are identified. One segment prefers decay prevention in their toothpaste, a second wants to improve their cosmetic appearance, while the third group prefers taste. To appeal to each of these segments, there are distinct product ingredients. A fluoride will provide for decay prevention, an abrasive improves the whitening of teeth for cosmetic value, and adding flavoring targets the taste-benefit segment. As Table 6-4 shows, some major brands have been positioned for each benefit segment. Crest is best known for its decay prevention properties. Ultra Brite has long touted what it will do to brighten a person's smile, and AIM is positioned for taste. An interesting addition to the competition among toothpaste brands has been the appearance of Mentadent by Lever Brothers, an international consumer products company in New York. Mentadent touts its decay prevention *and* tooth whitening properties. The product package shows two separate streams of toothpaste on a person's brush. Clearly, Lever Brothers is trying to appeal to two benefit segments, the decay prevention and cosmetic segments.

A similar benefit segmentation approach has been proposed for the preventive health care market. John and Miaoulis, two academic health care marketing researchers, conducted an exploratory study with 175 consumers. While conducting in-depth interviews, the researchers identified six segments, shown in Table 6-5. This representation suggests important implications for vitamin marketers in targeting the hypochondriac segment where brand preference rather than product utility is the key, since this is a proactive group of purchasers. The self-sufficient segment may be a potential target market for health clubs, if these organizations position themselves correctly. When seen as a means to avoid using the medical system, health clubs could attract the self-sufficient market segment.[26]

Cohort Segmentation

One of the newest ways to segment the market with possibly the greatest strategic implications for health care organizations is referred to as **cohort segmentation**. Historically, in traditional industries customers were viewed from a generational perspective. A generation is viewed as 20 to 22 years of time. Thus, when we discussed patients or consumers, we often talked of them as the "over 65" year-old consumer or the "under 17" year-old patient. In viewing patients or customers from a cohort perspective, it is different.

Table 6-5	Preventive Health Care Benefit Segments		
Name of Segment	Health Seekers	Followers	Band-Aiders
Benefits sought	Long, life, continued good health.	Want someone else to be concerned about their health, looking for guidance.	Recognition for being hard workers and rarely sick.
Category beliefs	Preventive medical services are the key to a longer and healthier life.	Not sure whether preventive services can deliver what they offer, best to follow the crowd.	Preventive care is for other people who get sick a lot. When your time is up, it's up!
Health services sought	Very broad range of services; nutritional counseling, exercise programs, hypertension tests, dental, etc.	Generally the annual physical, await symptoms before seeking medical services.	Primary treatment oriented; seek only essential preventive services, e.g., vaccinations.
Degree of participation	High, very active, continuous.	Sporadic.	Minimal.
Occasions of use	Corresponds to particular health needs at various life stages.	Depends on the degree of persuasiveness of the preventive service.	Following work-inhibiting symptoms, accidents, etc.
Personality/lifestyle	Rational, open-minded, appreciates "savings" from preventive services. Plan ahead, body conscious.	Other-directed, highly impressionable by "knowledgeable others."	Family-oriented, set in ways; not impressed by wonders of science.

(continues)

Table 6-5	continued		
Name of Segment	Do Not Bug Me	Hypochondriacs	Self-Sufficient
Benefits sought	Relief from everyday pressures and tensions. Looking for ways to cope with problems.	Tremendous need for recognition, want people to notice them and to assure them that they are okay.	Self-reliance. Home remedies do the job.
Category beliefs	Needs to smoke, eat, etc. to deal with tension. It is just too tough to quit.	Do not wait—see the doctor right away. Must get all possible medical attention to make sure everything is okay.	I can take care of myself. Don't trust doctors and hospitals.
Health services sought	Annual physical.	Any and all.	Home remedies and over-the-counter drugs.
Degree of participation	Seldom.	Excessive.	Nonparticipation in institutional medicine.
Occasions of use	To keep employer and/or family off his/her back.	Symptom-of-the-day club members.	Only have remedies.
Personality/lifestyle	Easygoing, gregarious on the outside; atrocious and very nervous on the inside.	Dependent and lacking self-confidence. Seeks attention from others.	Independent, previous bad experiences with doctors.

Source: From John, J., and Miaoulis, G., A Model for Understanding Benefit Segmentation in Preventive Health Care from *Health Care Management Review*, Vol. 17, No. 2, pp. 24–25, 1992.

A cohort is a group of people bound together in history by a set of events. These events can be major technological upheavals, wars, sociological upheavals, or political dislocations. These major events form and shape attitudes. And, these attitudes stay with people even as they age. It is this attitude shaping aspect of cohorts that stay with them that makes cohort segmentation so unique.[27] So, for example, while many people in health care make assumptions that the elderly patient acts a certain way, the cohort perspective suggests that can only be true about that particular cohort. When the next cohorts move into that age group, they will bring with them a different set of attitudes and values. The health care organization must respond accordingly by changing strategies and tactics for each cohort.

To understand how companies are responding today, look at the advertisements for Cadillac and the design of the Cadillac automobile today. Historically seen as a conservative automobile, General Motors recognizes that the over 50-year-old segment is today's cohort of Boomers. Their attitudes and values are different from the over-50 segment of 20 years ago. Boomers are more individualistic, reared in the 1960s. Cadillac has redesigned its cars to sport sharper lines and stiffer suspensions. Their ads feature background music of Janis Joplin harkening back to the days of Haight Asbury. The Cadillac of today is less the conservative car of the 1960s and 1970s.

In the United States today several major cohort groups have been identified:

- Depression—This cohort was born between 1912 and 1921 and was defined by the great depression. Financial security rules their thinking. Paying their bills was a central concern, be it to the hospital or the physician.
- World War II—Born between 1922 to 1927, this group came of age during World War II. For many of these individuals, the highest status ever achieved was during the war. These individuals were and are great patients, because what they learned was to accept authority. Their defining experience was to accept an authority. This value system stayed with them for their entire life, first as young soldiers, now as aging patients.
- Post-War—This cohort was born between 1928 and 1945 and came of age between 1946 and 1963 during the Eisenhower era. It was a period of time that promoted conformity. People who came of age in this era have a great trust in institutions and authority.
- Boomers I and II—The Boomers are really subsegmented as two groups. The leading edge Boomers were born between 1946 and 1954. They were the first to experience television as a pervasive influence on culture. Indulgent of self, leading edge Boomers question everything. Trailing Boomers are far more cynical. When they came of age (1973–1983), the country was in a major economic recession, President Nixon was being impeached, and faith in institutions was gone. Trailing Boomers are far more cynical.
- Generation X—Born between 1966 and 1977, Generation X represents slightly more than 21% of the population. This group is often referred to as "latchkey kids"

whose parents both worked so they went home and let themselves in after school. They are also the product of families with the highest divorce rates. Politically, Generation X is a politically conservative cohort.

- **N-Gen**—Often referred to as Generation Y, born between 1978 and 1985, they represent 29 million younger adults. The crystallizing events for this cohort were the Internet and terrorism. Many individuals who study cohorts say this group holds values similar to the World War II group. They are positive, idealistic, and stress team play.
- **Millenials**—Born between 1986 and 2000, this group consistently rates their parents as their most admired role models. They trust their grandparents, followed then by their parents. This group is always connected 24/7. The message they have received is achieve now, be inclusive, and serve your community. To this cohort computers are not technology; they have never known a life without computers. The Internet is better than television. In fact television viewing has declined during their lifetime. Multitasking is a way of life.

The implications of these cohorts for health care marketing are shown in Table 6-6. Each cohort has a different set of values that defines them. As a result, when interacting with a medical provider or organization, these cohorts will have a different set of expectations, and to communicate with these cohorts effectively will also require a different approach. As can be seen in Table 6-6, the pre-Boomers (depression and World War II) will wait for the physician or service provider. Yet, the Boomer I lives on the concept of billable

Table 6-6	Cohort Patient Expectations				
	Pre-boomer	Boomer I	Boomer II	Gen x'er	N-Gens/ Millenials
Service/ promptness	Will wait for good bedside manner	Get me out fast	Get me out fast	Get me out fast	Now
MD personality	Marcus Welby	Academic	ER	Not important	Not important
Staff	Friendly	Professional	Efficient	Quick	Quick
Office environment	Cheerful	Professional	Where's a video	No opinion	No opinion
Quality care means	Optimism	Clear explanations	Latest technology	Latest technology	Web-based links
Reaction to prognosis	Accepting	Second opinion	Second opinion	Third opinion	Check sites
Approach to promote	Analog	Detailed communication	Detailed communication	Interact with message	Real time

Source: Adapted from Marilyn Moats Kennedy, "Managing Change: Understanding the Demographics of the Evolving Workplace."

hours. Moreover, the N-Gens and Millenials have grown up on the Internet with a "now speed" mentality. Waiting for their computer to boot up is too long. That same "serve me now" value orientation will stay with them even as they age—that is the perspective of cohort segmentation. Consider too the issue of office staff or physician personality. While so important to the pre-Boomer cohort, it is of little concern or importance to later cohorts who have grown up making transactions over the Internet. And, when a medical organization considers its promotional strategy, the same approach must be taken into account. While the newspaper and magazines were the media that dominated the Depression through Post-War cohorts, the highest educational level exists among Boomers. They prefer to see very detailed information. Gen Xers and later cohorts prefer to interact with the information. Check out the Web sites for Nike where you can customize your own shoe: (www.nikeid.com) or Volkswagen where you can take a 360 degree tour of their cars: (www.vw.com and search for a virtual tour)—these cohorts do not want a static message from the medical organization.

■ Segmenting Business Markets

Because health care represents a significant size of a company's cost structure, health care organizations will continue directing their marketing strategies and products to employers and business organizations of all sizes. Segmenting industrial markets requires different perspectives than those used in segmenting consumer markets. Four broad classifications might be considered for business markets: demographics, operating variables, purchasing approaches, and usage requirements.

Demographics

Business demographics consist of variables such as size of the company (in terms of revenue or number of employees), industry type, and customer location.

Size of Company

Size of company is a particularly relevant variable for health care organization segmentation. For example, small companies have different price sensitivities, and clinical needs for occupational medicine contracts from large companies. A small company might also require the assistance of a third-party administrator in the analysis of alternative health care plans, or stop-loss insurance as it considers health coverage options for its employees. Group Health of Puget Sound has several plan options based on the size of the company. There is an option for a small group of 2 employees to larger companies with more than 50 (www.ghc.org).

Industry Type

Industry type is a valuable segmentation variable. The federal government provides a classification scheme referred to as the **Standard Industrial Classification (SIC) Code.**

The SIC system groups organizations based on their major business activity or the major service or product that firms provide. The SIC system provides a way for health care organizations to identify the SIC codes of the businesses it is trying to target, and possibly to identify or group them according to similar product or clinical needs. While the SIC codes are a useful way to access data collected on company segments, there are some limitations to their usefulness. First, the government assigns each company only one particular SIC designation. For large companies that engage in several business areas, the diversity that exists within the company will be lost by this classification method. Second, the codes are not available for every industry within every geographical area. The federal government will not reveal data when two or fewer organizations exist with a particular classification code within a specific geographic area.

Customer Location

Customer location is a third useful segmentation scheme. A hospital may provide off-site services, such as laboratory or minor emergency care, in locations where its major business customers are located.

Operating Variables

A second manner in which companies might be segmented is by operating variables, which include company technology, product use, and customer capabilities.

Technology

The technology that a company utilizes in its own business often heavily affects its own particular buying needs. For example, a company that is a sophisticated technical service business might employ a large number of highly educated consumers. Its work force's medical needs might involve more psychosocial elements compared to medical interventions required by a firm engaged in the manufacture of steel fire escapes. This latter firm would have a work force that engages in a significant amount of heavy lifting. This work force may have a lower formal educational level. And, since prior research in health care has shown that health status is correlated to educational level, employees of the steel plant with lower educational levels might require more health education seminars, such as smoking cessation clinics or dietary intervention, to improve their health status and physical fitness.

Product Use

A second operating variable on which segmentation can be based is product use. Companies that use a similar product or service generally have other characteristics in common. For example, a health insurance company might target companies that offer to their employees the same product or indemnity plan from the insurance company's competitor. This analysis provides insight into which factors result or contribute to the buying decision. Identifying a segment of customers who purchase particular health care products or services from a weaker competitor can also provide a target group from which to generate additional revenue.

Customer Capabilities

Analyzing the distinct capabilities or position of companies can result in defined market segments. For example, small companies might have no in-house medical director to assist in analyzing medical plans. Such companies represent a segment receptive to contract management strategies to assist in plan selection. Other companies might not have an in-house physician to assist in job-related injuries. A medical group could provide onsite clinical assistance.

Purchasing Approaches

A third way to segment business markets is to classify companies by the way they make their purchasing decisions.

Purchasing Procedures

Companies differ in terms of the procedures they employ in dealing with sellers. The customer's purchasing process should be a defining consideration in setting up the marketing strategy to target the prospective company. Some businesses approach the health care buying decision through contracts, others mix that approach with a traditional insurance approach. In segmenting by the way companies make purchases, a health care provider might have to develop a range of possible responses, as shown in Table 6-7. A contractually dominant buyer might be a preferred provider organization, while a noncontractual buyer is the traditional corporate purchaser. The health care buying market is moving increasingly toward a contractually dominant setting. If buyers selectively purchase, or carve out, coverage of certain clinical areas, strategic business units would have to be established to compete for service-specific contracts.[28]

Purchasing Criteria

Most companies have some purchasing criteria by which they evaluate vendor bids. Some firms have explicit criteria that are published and made available to prospective sellers, while other companies have more subjective criteria. These purchasing criteria are similar to the benefit segmentation described with consumers. Some firms might emphasize the plan's cost as their primary criterion, while others consider employee satisfaction relative to the plan's cost. Within purchasing criteria, some employers have established health care performance criteria by which to judge alternative health plans. Now with Health Plan Employer Data and Information Set report cards, some plans such as Aetna are making these very easy to access on their Web sites. Data provided by Aetna cover not only member satisfaction by state but also issues on prevention, appropriate use of medications, timely follow-up, and annual screening. (Follow links to "Service and Tools," then "Quality Report Cards" on www.aetna.com.)

Table 6-7	Purchase Procedure Segmentation		
	Market Structure		
	Bundled Dominant	Mixed	Discrete Dominant
Noncontractual dominant	Develop broad service and general marketing capabilities.	Offer a midrange of services, but focus on certain specialties. Target marketing efforts to general population and specific target groups.	Offer a narrow range of specialty services. Target marketing efforts. Strongly coordinate market-ing and production functions
Contractual arrangement mixed	Develop broad service capability. Target marketing effforts to general population, em-ployers, third parties, and enrollees.	Offer a midrange of services, but focus on certain specialties. Target marketing efforts to general population, target groups, employers, third parties, employees, patients, potential patients, and enrollees.	Offer a narrow range of specialty services. Target marketing efforts to patients and potential patients, employers, and third parties. Strongly coordinate marketing and production functions.
Contractual dominant	Develop broad service capability. Target marketing efforts primarily to employers, third parties, and enrollees.	Offer a midrange of services, but focus on certain specialties. Target market efforts primarily to employers, third parties, patients, potential patients, and enrollees.	Offer a narrow range of specialty services. Target marketing primarily to patients, potential patients, and third parties. Set up strategic business units.

Source: William N. Zelman and Curtis P. McLaughlin, Product Lines in a Complex Marketplace: Matching Organizational Strategy to Buyer Behavior from *Health Care Management Review,* Vol. 17, No. 2, pp. 24–25, 1992.

This information can be made available to subscribers, as well as to prospective customer businesses to show that the provider is assessing its own performance and can demonstrate it to the buyer. Segmenting the market by purchasing criteria allows for a more tailored marketing mix strategy.

In health care, purchasing criteria of growing importance are the service charac-teristics demanded by the buyer. Company needs vary regarding how they expect or desire their particular account (and those of their employees) to be serviced by a health care organization.

Usage Requirements

Similar to consumers, companies can also be segmented, based on usage factors, which can include variables such as the volume of purchase, frequency of purchase, or the application. For the most part, these are similar to previously described consumer usage variables. Again, it is crucial to consider that organizations, just like consumers, also can represent a heavy half segment. The same issues and marketing objectives are also relevant in industrial segmentation strategies.

■ The Heuristics of Segmentation

Described within this chapter were several possible methods for segmenting the market, whether targeting individuals or companies. Health care marketers should decide what is the most helpful way to segment, as well as determine, how these alternative methods relate to each other. Health care marketers need to recognize that, by segmenting, provider organizations are trying to produce a differential response from the market segment as opposed to the mass market. In other words, if segmenting the market and tailoring the marketing mix to particular consumers has no effect on purchase consumption, then there is no value to segmenting. To know that there are large hospitals and small hospitals relative to bed size is to describe segments demographically. However, if this demographic segmentation scheme cannot be related to a purchase difference, then it is purely descriptive and irrelevant to marketing strategy. If, however, larger hospitals have different purchasing criteria, and separate purchasing managers, and chief executive officers (CEOs) who frequently read a particular trade publication more often than CEOs from small hospitals, then marketing segmentation strategy can affect usage and purchases.

FIGURE 6-2 presents a hierarchy of the various segmentation schemes discussed within this chapter. The best level of market segmentation is represented on the far right-hand side of this figure—actual purchase. It is actual purchase that the marketer wants to affect. As one moves from right to left, each successive segmentation approach is less accurate in terms of predicting how the market segment behaves. From a marketing strategy perspective, it is best to know the consumer at each point on this hierarchy.

For example, it would be valuable to describe the market segments according to their choice of an indemnity plan and a managed care option. It would also help the marketer to know their product preferences regarding health care coverage and their brand preferences. In terms of product design and positioning, knowing the product

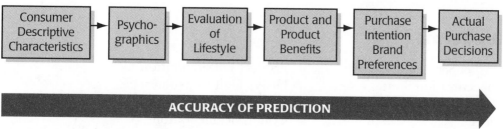

FIGURE 6-2 Segmentation Heuristic

benefits would be invaluable. To develop effective promotional material, as well as possible product features, lifestyle factors would be useful input. Demographics provide the final descriptive characteristics of the market.

Consider working from right to left within the figure. Only knowing the gender or age range of the market segments would be of limited help in designing an attractive managed care organization (MCO) package of services. Some inferences could certainly be made for certain age groups. If, in addition to demographics, a company also had lifestyle and psychographic profiles of customers, it could design a better program. For example, the MCO might decide to offer health club benefits.

If there is a tangible rating of product benefits, then the intended product can be designed to resemble more closely the desired product. Brand name preferences can assist in knowing whether the product can be sold under the medical group's name or whether it should assume a different branding strategy. How likely the consumer is to purchase the described product is the next best way to predict behavior, but actual purchase is the best.

These heuristics also provide the rationale for increasing company use of purchase history to define market segments. In many supermarkets today, customers are provided with their own identity code on a card, which they may present upon checking out. Consumers receive incentives, such as automatic discounts, if the card is displayed. This also allows for purchase histories to be recorded. The data can be sold to companies to analyze market segments. Customers can be grouped based on who purchased a product during a special promotion. Similar profiling characteristics can be identified to tailor future marketing mix strategies.

■ Conclusions

Market segmentation is a common approach used by traditional businesses. Yet, for many years, the health care industry operated close to the dictum of Henry Ford, "You can have health care any way you want, providing it is the one way we deliver it." Segmentation strategies have taken hold, with the realization that the more tailored the marketing strategy is to subgroups within the population, the greater the resulting sales and customers.

■ Key Terms

Market Segmentation	Product Differentiation
Concentration Strategy	Heavy Half Consumer
Majority Fallacy	Benefit Segmentation
Niche	Cohort Segmentation
Niche Strategy	Standard Industrial Classification (SIC) Code

■ Chapter Summary

1. In a mass marketing strategy, the marketing mix is designed to appeal to the broadest market, while in a market segmentation approach, the marketing mix is designed to appeal to subgroups of consumers.

2. In following a concentration strategy of targeting only one segment, an organization should not focus only on the largest segment, because competitive intensity can render this segment the least profitable.

3. In selecting from multiple market segments, there are several criteria to consider: Segments should be identifiable, accessible, inclined to buy, able to buy, profitable, desirable, consistent, and available.

4. Markets can be segmented sociodemographically, geographically, and psychographically by usage, and recently by cohorts.

5. In usage segmentation, it is important to identify the heavy half consumer who purchases a disproportionate share of a product, or who accounts for a disproportionate amount of a service's volume.

6. The important aspect of cohort segmentation is to realize that cohorts' attitudes and value systems stay with them even as they age. Thus a health care organization must develop a strategy to respond to the market and not expect that the boomers of today will respond like the World War II consumers when they are in that age group.

7. Business markets can also be segmented by several criteria. The federal government has developed the SIC coding system, which is a common basis for industrial segmentation.

8. As corporations play an increasingly important role in health care purchases, health care organizations may need to segment them by purchase procedures or purchase criteria.

9. There is a heuristic method to segmentation approaches that moves from purely descriptive measures, such as demographics, to actual purchase, such as usage.

10. The ultimate purpose of segmentation is to tailor an organization's marketing mix with the intent of positively affecting consumer behavior. If segmentation does not differentially affect this response, there is little value to segmenting the market on that particular criterion.

■ Chapter Problems

1. Assume that a multispecialty medical group has decided to segment the market in the community by income level. The group has decided to target a small niche of middle-aged, white-collar professionals who are married, with both spouses working outside the home. How might this medical group tailor its marketing mix to appeal to this segment?

2. A women's health clinic has recognized the need to segment its market. Identify three bases by which this clinic might segment the female market, and identify the manner in which the "product" component of the marketing mix would change in light of the segmentation base used.

3. Examine the benefit segmentation scheme shown in Table 6-5. In what ways might an MCO new to a community try to capture the "follower" segment? How would this strategy differ in trying to attract the "health seekers"?

4. A neurology group practice recently analyzed its level of patient referrals and referral sources. This analysis showed that 60% of all referrals came from 35% of all the physicians who referred to the group. The remaining referrals came from the other 65% of the referral physicians. In examining this referral pattern, it was also revealed that 20% of all the primary care physicians in the group's primary service area had never sent a patient to the group for diagnosis or treatment. As the practice manager of the group, you have been asked by the physicians to develop a marketing strategy to deal with this information.

5. Bethesda Hospital has recently developed an integrated health care system—the hospital and its physicians have formed a new organization, which also is affiliated with a large insurance company. This new structure, called a physician-hospital organization (PHO), offers a prepaid health care plan and competes against other managed care companies. The marketing director of the PHO is planning to approach the employers in the community to encourage them to offer the new health care plan to their employees. Suggest three alternative ways this customer base for the PHO could be segmented, and indicate how each base of segmentation would result in a change in the marketing mix.

6. A new group of primary care physicians have decided to locate in a suburb of Washington, D.C. Having had some primary market research conducted of the area, the research firm characterized the community as comprised of primarily Boomers, Gen Xers, and a significant number of N-Gen white collar workers, all employed by high tech and consulting firms who work in the outer belt that surrounds Washington, D.C. What are the implications of this market profile in terms of how:
   a. the office setting might be configured?
   b. the office scheduling and hours might be constructed?
   c. a plan might be developed to make the market aware of this new group opening its practice?

■ Notes

1. W. R. Smith, "Product Differentiation and Market Segmentation as Alternative Marketing Strategies," *Journal of Marketing* 21, no. 1 (1956): 3–8.

2. L. Ingrassia, "U.S. Overconfidence Leaves This Hospital in Critical Condition," *The Wall Street Journal* (20 December 1994), A1,A9.

3. P. R. Dickson and J. L. Ginter, "Market Segmentation, Product Differentiation, and Marketing Strategy," *Journal of Marketing* 51, no. 2 (1987): 1–10.

4. R. Weiss, "Market Response Systems: A Community Interface," *Health Progress* 75, no. 61 (1994): 68–69.

5. Klea D. Bertakis, R. Azari, L. J. Helms, E. J. Callahan, and J. A. Robbins, "Gender Differences in the Utilization of Health Care Services," *Journal of Family Practice* 49, no. 2 (February 2000): 147–152.

6. P. D. Cleary, D. Mechanic, and J. R. Greenley, "Sex Differences in Medical Care Utilization: An Empirical Investigation," *Journal of Health and Social Behavior* 23 (1982): 106–119.

7. C. A. Mustard, P. Kaufart, A. Korzyrsky, and T. Mayer, "Sex Differences in the Use of Health Care Services," *The New England Journal of Medicine* 338 (1998): 1678–1683.

8. "The Health Industry Finally Asks: What Do Women Want?" *Business Week*, no. 2961 (August 25, 1986): 81.

9. J. S. Ghent, "Childbirth Education: A Natural Approach To Assessing Healthcare Clients," *Healthcare Marketing Report* 12, no. 5 (1994): 14–15.

10. "Understanding the Female Consumer: Healthcare Needs, Impact on Utilization, and Decision-Making Role in Household," A Report from Solucient (www.solucient.com/docs/Womens111403.pdf).

11. Edward E. Mason, Kathleen E. Renquist, Bridget Zimmerman, Wei Zhang, and IBSR Data Contributors, "Trends in Bariatric Surgery, 1998–2001," Presentation, The University of Iowa (http://aboutplastic.surgery.uiowa.edu/ibsr/trends03_files/frame.htm).

12. J. de Cordoba, "More Firms Court Hispanic Consumers, But Find Them a Tough Market To Target," *The Wall Street Journal* (February 18, 1988), 25.

13. Judy Silber, "Kaiser Connects with Latinos," *Contra Costa Times* (March 7, 2004) (www.contracostatimes.com/mld/cctimes/business/8128450.htm).

14. W. Hearn, "Cultural Competence," *American Medical News* 36, no. 40 (1993): 13–15.

15. See, for example, W. Power, "How Not To Break a Leg: 'Arts Medicine' Helps Performers Stay Healthy on the Job," *The Wall Street Journal* (June 5, 1986), 29.

16. Vic Simon, Physician Compensation report (October 2003) (http://aishealth.com).

17. Liz Kowalczyk, "'Boutique' Care Coming to Tufts' Wealthy Patients," *Boston Globe* 264, no. 42 (August 11, 2003), 1, A4.

18. L. Carpenter, "How To Market to Regions," *American Demographics* 9, no. 11 (1987): 11–15.

19. D. Knight, "Psychographics Delivers More Than Targeted Ad Pitches," *Healthcare Marketing Report* 11, no. 11 (1993): 6–8.

20. Carol M. Morgan and Doran J. Levy, "Applying Psychographic Segmentation to Healthcare Marketing and Planning," *COR Healthcare Market Strategist* 4, no. 6 (June 2003): 1, 10–13.

21. "Incentive Programs Can Be Used To Boost Business," *Physician's Marketing and Management* 61, no. 1 (1993): 6–8.

22. R. K. Srivistava, "Usage Situational Influences on Perceptions of Product Markets: Theoretical and Empirical Issues," in *Advances in Consumer Research*, Vol. 8, ed. K. Monroe (Ann Arbor, MI: ACR, 1981), 106–111.

23. Jack A. Klapper, "Botox and Migraine," *American Council for Headache Education* 12, no. 1 (Spring 2001), (http://www.achenet.org).

24. R. McStravic, "Loyalty of Hospital Patients," *Health Care Management Review* 12, no. 2 (Spring 1987): 23–30.

25. R. J. Haley, "Benefit Segmentation: A Decision Oriented Research Tool," *Journal of Marketing* 27, no. 3 (1963): 30–35.

26. J. John and G. Miaoulis, "A Model for Understanding Benefit Segmentation in Preventive Health Care," *Health Care Management Review* 17, no. 2 (Spring 1992): 21–32.

27. There are several sources on cohorts. Some examples are: Rick and Kathy Hicks *Boomers, Xers, and Other Strangers: Understanding the Generational Differences That Divide Us* (Wheaton, IL: Tyndale Publisher, 1999); Claire Raines and Jim Hunt, *The Xers and the Boomers: From Adversaries to Allies—A Diplomat's Guide* (Berkeley, CA: Crisp Publications, 2000); Geoffrey E. Meredith, Charles D. Schewe, and Janice Karlovich, *Defining Markets, Defining Moments* (New York: Hungry Minds, 2002); J. Walker Smith and Ann Clurman, *Rocking the Ages; The Yankelovich Report on Generational Marketing* (New York: Harper Business, 1997); Richard D. Thau and Jay S. Heflin, *Generations Apart: Xers, Boomers, and the Elderly* (Amherst, NY: Prometheus Books, 1997).

28. W. N. Zelamn and C. P. McLaughlin, "Product Lines in a Complex Marketplace: Matching Organizational Strategy to Buyer Behavior," *Health Care Management Review* 15, no. 2 (Spring 1990): 9–14.

Developing Customer Loyalty

In any business whether it be a product or a service, gaining customer loyalty is a primary concern. It has been increasingly documented that the costs of gaining a new customer are five times that of keeping a loyal customer and that the retention of customers can lead to significant increases in profitability.

■ Relationship Marketing

Relationship marketing can be defined as an organization's attempt to develop a long-term, cost-effective link with a customer for the benefit of both the customer and the organization.[1] The foundation of relationship marketing is to develop a strategy that shifts the organization's thinking from the individual transaction, such as getting the patient to come to the clinic, to a relationship focus of longer term loyalty—thus defining the organization as the regular health care provider. In recent years within marketing, thinking is shifting from focusing on the individual transaction (the sale, the referral, the patient visit) to the establishment of a longer term relationship, a loyal customer, patient, referral physician. Table 7-1 shows the shift in focus from a transactional view to a relationship orientation. The relationship marketing orientation changes the health care providers' efforts in several ways.

Table 7-1	The Relationship Marketing Focus	
Criterion	Transactional	Relationship
Goal	Single encounter	Ongoing provider
Customer contact	Episodic	Continuous
Organizational focus	Service elements	Customer value
Customer responsiveness	Little effort	Organizational goal
Quality concern	Focus of clinical staff	Focus of entire staff
Time perspective	Short term	Long term

Source: Adapted from Adrian Payne, Martin Christopher, Helen Peck, and Moira Clark, *Relationship Marketing for Competitive Advantage* (Butterworth-Heinemann, 1995).

Foremost is the goal of the organization. Rather than a strategy of continuing to increase share or track the number of new charts each month, a common group practice perspective, relationship marketing implies a target of being the provider of choice. For a multispecialty organization, it would be more to become the sole source provider for the family unit. The shift, however, to relationship marketing also signals some other changes in terms of the marketing efforts of the organization as well as internal changes in terms of employee focus and quality. A system must be developed in which continuous contact is made with the customer, patient, physician, or company.

In no area of marketing do health care organizations suffer more, or show the need for improvement, than in this aspect of relationship marketing. In a transactional perspective, the health care provider has episodic contact. When the patient arrives at the facility, care is delivered. Any post encounter follow-up is either negative, in the form of a bill, or initiated by the patient in terms of a call for additional medical need. In relationship marketing, the organization maintains regular, ongoing contact with the patient. Newsletters, e-mails, and health care updates are all part of this relationship marketing model. A primary care group, for example, might develop a listing of patients who are skiers or runners. This is built on the premise, of course, that the health care provider uses marketing research and integrates it into a database of its customers. The group might then e-mail health tips to this group of patients/customers prior to ski season on how to prepare for the upcoming activity.

Here too in health care, the role of the Internet may loom large. As of September 2003, between 5 and 10% of hospital sites had set up personalized e-mail engines to help patients reenter the site a second time. Advocate Health Care in Chicago offers online access to personal medical records.[2] Its Web site "My Advocate" personal portal is seen in EXHIBIT 7-1.

The organizational focus dimension is a shift in thinking about what the customer is buying, not what the organization is providing. To a large degree, this aspect of relationship marketing goes to the core of the marketing concept that was discussed in

Exhibit 7-1   Advocate WEB Portal

Welcome to [MyAdvocate]   We're your doctors. We're your hospitals. We're your Advocate.

AdvocateHealth Care

first time visitors
Start Here!

Return to Advocate Health Care
by clicking the logo at any time.

You're about to enter the area of our site dedicated entirely
to you and your health. Our Registration Wizard will help you
create your personal health pages...We're your doctors.
We're your hospitals. We're your Advocate.!

registered users
Log in Here!

to create your
my health pages
click here!
about privacy

Welcome back. Please enter your user
name and password:

Username:

Password:

log in

Forgot your password?

Take a **Tour!**

• Store your "personal health profile"
• Save a printable "my doctors list"
• Personalize "my health calendar"

to begin the
MyAdvocate
Tour
click here!

Source: www.advocatehealth.com Customer Potential Management Corporation, Copyright 1999.

Chapter 1. But it is this element that is the difficult challenge to implementing relationship marketing into health care. In a transactional focus, the people within the company focus on the product that they are producing or the service that is being delivered. A good product or well-delivered service is one that meets the standards of the producer or the provider. In a relationship-marketing context, the focus shifts more to what the customer defines as value from the encounter. It is more than just seeing a physician, but the value might be in terms of a clear explanation, timely access to the physician, a one-stop system where prescriptions can also be obtained. Greater definition of value is provided later in this chapter.

Customer responsiveness speaks to the organization's ability to respond to the customer's needs. American Healthways has a contract with Blue Cross Blue Shield of Minnesota to identify high risk members and recruit them to participate in their risk reduction and disease management program. The contract is on a risk/reward basis between the vendor and the health plan, although it is free to members who join.[3] In a transactional organization, this is often a major basis for defining employee positions.

In a customer responsive organization, the employee is empowered to meet customer needs. Karl Albrecht has described the seven sins of customer service as apathy, the brush-off, coldness, condescension, robotics, the rulebook, and the run-around.[4] In a transaction-focused organization, the individual often responds according to "the rules" or in an almost robotic response. In the waiting room of many emergency departments, while there is no doubt the pace is hectic and the volume can at times be intense, the person at the desk often faces one customer after another with a "Take a seat" response.

In no area is a relationship marketing perspective more significant than in that of quality. Few health care provider organizations would not respond to the fact that quality is essential. Yet to a large degree the quality committees that are formed have a clinical focus and participation. In a relationship marketing organization, quality extends beyond the clinical side of the service delivery to the entire range of what is sought and experienced by the customer. It is these components that drive the relationship marketing effort. In this way, the transactional, situation-to-situation encounter of the patient or customer is replaced with a longer-term effort to retain individual customers—be they a physician, company, or individual.

■ Satisfaction or Loyalty?

Over the past two decades in health care, there has been growing recognition among health care organizations that the customer should be satisfied. And, in fact, there is a wide range of commercial providers that have stepped into this realization with "satisfaction measuring" programs. These efforts often have as their basis some benchmarking of the organization relative to others. To a large degree, the efforts in health care mirror what has been found in other industries. For example, the Juran Institute found in one study that in excess of 90% of top managers from 200 of the United States' largest companies agree with the statement that "Maximizing customer satisfaction will maximize profitability and market share."[5] And, while these satisfaction measures used by health care organizations have some useful relative perspective, there is a dilemma that exists around satisfaction. In the study conducted by the Juran Institute, less than 2% of the 200 respondents were able to measure a bottom line increase in profitability from a documented increase in satisfaction.[6]

Satisfaction itself is not sufficient. It has been found in several instances that a customer can be satisfied. However, not only is there no noticeable corresponding gain in profitability, but there might even be a loss of that same customer. A study by the Forum Corporation reported that up to 40% of the people who claimed to be satisfied, switched suppliers.[7] In the *Harvard Business Review*, 65 to 85% of the customers who reported being satisfied or very satisfied still chose another supplier.[8] While it is obvious that dissatisfied customers will certainly switch, it has been found that even satisfied customers will switch providers or suppliers.[9] Thus satisfaction is not the end state that marketers must work to achieve.

■ The Customer Loyalty Pyramid

From a marketing perspective, a goal must be not only to attract customers but also to develop loyalty. FIGURE 7-1 describes what may be referred to as the **Customer Loyalty Pyramid,** which is a progression of customer psychological movement from awareness to loyalty. As can be seen in this figure, the ultimate is customer loyalty. The achievement of this goal, however, requires attention to several earlier levels of organization/customer interaction. The first three levels of awareness, interest, and evaluation are all components of the promotional strategy of an organization. While these issues are described in more detail in Chapter 12, the first three levels involve making the customer aware of the service offering and generating some positive feelings to the organization. First time purchase is represented by trial. If the first encounter with the health care provider is positive and the service meets the customer's expectations, satisfaction occurs. Satisfaction can result then in repeat purchase. Successive repeat purchase or use of the health care organization results in loyalty, the ultimate objective.

It is important to recognize that many times trial can be achieved. The patient comes into the walk-in clinic, having seen the advertisements on billboards on the highway. Yet often the first time buyer never returns. A common reason is that the customer experiences early problems that sour the relationship. Often there is no communication mechanism established with the decision maker. It is just as easy to return to the competition.[10]

Loyalty is more than satisfaction. In the 1980s Cadillac and AT&T were two companies that both had high satisfaction scores but were still losing market share.[11] Loyalty represents two key components: customer retention and the share of customer

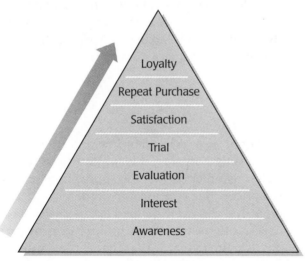

FIGURE 7-1 The Customer Pyramid

Source: Adapted with the permission of The Free Press, a division of Simon & Schuster Adult Publishing Group, from *Delivering Quality Service: Balancing Customer Perceptions and Expectations* by Valerie A. Zeithaml, A. Parasuraman, Leonard L. Berry. Copyright © 1990 by The Free Press. All rights reserved.

purchases. A multispecialty group can have high customer loyalty if the person uses the range of services needed in the group. A family practitioner group might consider itself as having achieved high loyalty if both a husband and a wife use the group. A loyal customer, then, is one who makes frequent and repeat purchases. He or she purchases or uses the organization across the range of service lines and has immunity from the pull of competition.[12] It is this isolation from a competing organization's pull that is the benefit of a loyal customer and the goal of relationship marketing.

The value of a loyal customer is multiple. A major benefit is the reduction in acquisition costs. It has often been said that it costs five times more to acquire a new customer than to keep an existing one. The loyal customer delivers a greater "lifetime value" in terms of profit. Per customer revenue growth has also been cited as greater for the loyal customer. Loyal customers are also more profitable to serve, because both the customer and the employee know how to interact. A patient who understands the scheduling process or how the billing department works or whom to contact with a problem or particular need will be more efficient to service than a customer less familiar with the organization. Loyal customers are advocates. These are people who provide referrals of others to the organization. The word-of-mouth value of a patient has been well recognized in health care. Finally, it has been said that the loyal customer will pay a premium price to stay with the provider.[13]

There is another great advantage to loyal customers that is of particular value in service businesses like health care. Loyal customers have a broader zone of tolerance or are more willing to give an organization a break if there is a problem. Consider the loyal patient. Because he or she has more experience with the physician's office or the health care organization, when there is a problem on a particular day, the loyal patient might be more likely to say "It is not usually like this." It is the patient who is not loyal who is less forgiving and more likely to switch. It is being able to have this zone of tolerance that makes creating loyal patients or customers important.

■ Creating Customer Value

For any organization, health care, or traditional business, a major aspect of marketing efforts is to create customer value. In focusing on value, it is important to recognize a few major factors. Foremost is that the customer defines the appropriate service quality and price level, thereby defining the price/value relationship of the service. The difficult challenge in a competitive market is that the value defined by the customer is relative to competitive offerings. Therefore, as is often lamented by health care providers that a customer's expectations continually rise, the reality is that that is the nature of a dynamic and competitive market.[14] What may be a source of a differential advantage at one point in time is no longer true because other providers offer a similar service. In the 1980s some hospitals established some unique value in obstetrics with labor, delivery, and recovery rooms that were attractively decorated. In today's market, it is only the lack of such a unit that might be a point of difference, but a negative one at that.

To a large degree, an equation can be developed for health care service value. It can be defined by the following equation:

$$\text{Value} = \text{Clinical quality provided} + \text{Process quality} - (\text{Price} + \text{Service Acquisition Cost})[15]$$

It is these four variables, then, that define the value provided by a health care organization. The first variable, clinical quality provided, is obvious. This variable is the result of the technology and expertise represented with the health care organization. The third variable, Price, is also obvious. This is the out-of-pocket cost to access that clinical quality. It is the remaining two variables that need some additional explanation.

Process quality represents the ease with which a customer can access the clinical quality. Can a patient set up an appointment easily or does it require multiple callbacks or endless minutes on hold? Does a primary care referring physician have to call back to get information about a patient, or does the specialty organization have a system in place in which the feedback is provided in a timely, meaningful manner? Service process quality has been said to consist of several dimensions as shown in EXHIBIT 7-2. While most of these dimensions may seem obvious, one of them, authority, at first glance may raise questions regarding a health care organization. At first glance, one might say that of all service providers, health care entities surely deliver on the authority dimension. After all, do not physicians and nurses and others walk around in uniforms, with the symbol of medicine, the stethoscope around their necks? Diplomas and other Board certifications are prominently displayed on the walls of most offices. Yet, authority in terms of service process quality is eliciting confidence in the delivery process. Again, to see where many health care organizations fail, one needs only to sit in the waiting room of any medical facility. Count how often in the course of a day, a patient approaches the admitting desk and is handed a clipboard with instructions to complete the form. The patient often replies that he or she completed this same form only yesterday or last week. The response is often, "Yes, that may be

Exhibit 7-2   Service Process Quality Dimensions

- Dependability—Did the provider do what was promised?
- Responsiveness—Was service provided in a timely manner?
- Authority—Did the provider elicit a feeling of confidence during delivery process?
- Empathy—Was the provider able to take the customer's point of view?
- Tangible evidence—Was evidence left that service was performed?

true, but we can't locate your record right now." Or, how often in an encounter between a physician and the patient does the physician inquire whether the patient followed up with a blood test? When the patient responds positively, the physician quickly scans through the medical record to only respond "The lab results are not back yet" and then proceeds with the visit. In either instance the authority or confidence in the service provider is severely limited.

The importance of the service process quality has been seen directly in health care. Several studies have shown that up to 80% of all medical malpractice suits have nothing to do with the actual clinical quality of the medicine or care delivered. A major explanation for the lawsuits is that the patient or the loved ones were angered by the way in which the service was delivered, independent of whether the care was injurious.[16]

The fourth variable, **service acquisition cost**, refers to how much effort the customer has to use in order to access the service value. There are multiple dimensions to this last variable. These dimensions are most easily seen if one considers a health care organization that has a contract to provide occupational health to a company. The effort cost would include factors such as the cost of contracting, and the setup costs that the customer must bear in having this occupational medicine program. Another factor is the system dislocation costs. For example, the more changes the company must make in terms of its own human resource function, the less value there would be in the occupational medicine program being delivered. The final two aspects of the service acquisition cost are the operating and maintenance costs and the monitoring costs. This last factor refers to whether the provider organization will provide ongoing monitoring of the contract outcomes, or whether the organization must develop its own monitoring system to assess whether it is getting what was promised.

From a health care provider perspective, one might then turn back to this equation and the question of where the organization turns in order to create customer value. The value equation suggests four possible places to turn increase value. For most health care organizations the first variable is of prime concern. And, in fact, one might argue that whenever possible the organization will try to provide better clinical care. The reality of this variable, however, is that the health care provider does not control it. Assuming the quality of care being delivered is high, the only way to significantly enhance quality (to a noticeably higher level) is with some new technological breakthrough. The group then goes out and leases or buys the new equipment, or possibly the surgeon may go off and learn a new, better invasive procedure that has been developed. Or, there is some significant pharmacological breakthrough for which scripts can now be written, such as recent advances in the treatment of mental illness or sexual dysfunction in males.

Similarly, looking at the equation, one can turn to the cost side. An obvious way to improve the value proposition to the customer is to lower the out-of-pocket price that must be paid. Here too, however, most health care organizations would hesitate to turn to this variable since it obviously would lead to margin reduction in an industry with not very attractive margins.

The result of this analysis suggests that there are two places to which an organization can most likely turn to increase customer value: process quality or service acquisition costs. These two variables relate directly to service delivery aspects.

Conducting a Gap Analysis

In order to deliver value to the customer and be able to measure that value to drive for loyalty, satisfaction measures are not sufficient. Rather, a more refined approach to develop value has been referred to as a **Gap Analysis**.[17] These researchers identified five possible gaps that can occur in service delivery and are shown in FIGURE 7-2.

The first gap often exists between expectations of service quality and management perceptions of those expectations. For example, a patient may expect that the privacy of his or her medical records is of utmost concern. The administrator of the health care facility may also have that same expectation. Yet patients may have concerns that their records are not confidential when they see them slotted in a bin for anyone in the office to view or watch a young clerk take them back to the physician for review.

The second gap that often occurs in service delivery is between management perceptions of customer expectations and service quality specifications. This might be termed the "walks the talk" gap. That is, it is one thing for management to realize that customers have an expectation that when they call the clinic, the phone will be answered in less than 10 rings. It is another management level, however, to set standards into place as to what defines good service.

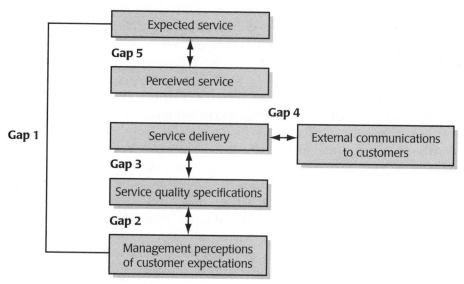

FIGURE 7-2 The Sources of Service Gaps

Source: Adapted with the permission of The Free Press, a Division of Simon & Schuster Adult Publishing Group, from *Delivering Quality Service: Balancing Customer Perceptions and Expectations* by Valerie A. Zeithaml, A. Parasuraman, Leonard L. Berry. Copyright © 1990 by The Free Press. All rights reserved.

The third gap is that which often exists between service quality specifications and the service delivery. This gap is related to resources. These resources are often related to either infrastructure support or personnel. In health care, the service quality specifications suggest that the medical record should be available to the physician when facing a patient encounter. The expectation is also that the record should be up-to-date within some reasonable time frame (48 to 72 hours). The reality, in many health care organizations, is that the medical record system and staff are overwhelmed, and computerization of these records that might result in eliminating this gap is seen as an expense item requiring equipment and personnel. Related to this gap is the issue of personnel.

A service business is by definition one that is based on people rather than products. To a large extent, this gap exists when there is an insufficient, poorly trained, or poorly motivated person involved in the service delivery system. For service workers recent findings by Gallup polls suggest great cause for concern. Gallup reported that 55% of the workers in its database have no enthusiasm for their work. Of greater concern is the finding that one in five workers is so unenthused and negative that he or she poisons the workplace. Gallup refers to these workers as the "not engaged."[18] In a service business, these individuals contribute greatly to the Gap 3 issue.

In health care services, the nonclinical individuals who interact with the customer can be seen as the boundary tier. These people fulfill two critical roles in terms of impression managers and gatekeepers. As impression managers, the employee must recognize that he or she is the organization to the customer/patient. As gatekeepers of information, employees play a key role in terms of the implementation of service delivery standards. It is interesting to note that when boundary employees work for companies in which they report generally positive work attitudes, the customers they serve report high satisfaction levels. Interestingly, when boundary employees report delivering high quality service, customers report the same. Yet when employees report delivering poor service, customers also report the same.[19] The average front line service employee receives $2.80 worth of training per year. Ritz Carlton and Federal Express employees, in contrast, receive on average 40 hours of training prior to having direct contact with the customer.

The fourth gap is a promotional gap. In this instance it is between the actual service delivery and the promise that was made to the marketplace. In health care, this gap has been seen repeatedly in hospitals that have established "fast track" programs within the emergency department. These programs when rolled out are often supported by a media campaign of billboards and radio ads promoting this new quick access in the local hospital emergency department for minor injuries. The reality, however, is that the only fast part of these "fast track" programs is, rather than waiting in the emergency department waiting room, the patients' information is taken and they are moved quickly to an examination room, where they then wait.

Promotion raises customer expectations and educates customers as to what their expectations should be. The relationship between Gap 4 then and Gap 5 is direct. Having seen the promotion, the customer has a perception of what the service should be or will be. When the experience is different from what was promised, the customer then has a changed expectation relative to his or her perception. It is the gap here that often leads to the person not returning and becoming a loyal customer.

Measuring Service Performance

Recognizing the potential for gaps and the important role of customer expectations, the measuring of service performance, then, must meet three criteria. Foremost, the measurement tool must be managerially useful. Secondly, it must recognize the role of customer expectations, and finally, it must direct action to the most relevant areas. In this regard, the first step in developing a measurement tool is to conduct a **customer contact audit**.

Gordon Sasser and Daryl Wyckoff, who teach production management at the Harvard Business School, originally developed the customer contact audit. They used this tool to assess the service delivery process for the Hertz Corporation. In conducting a customer contact audit, the organization flow charts every step in the delivery of the service. These steps are not only the ones that the customer sees, but also those that must be completed in order for the service to occur. FIGURE 7-3 shows the flowchart of the car rental process. In this figure the shaded boxes illustrate the places where the customer directly interacts with Hertz in the rental of a car. The other boxes represent activities that must be performed to ensure a successful service encounter, such as performing scheduled maintenance to ensure that the car runs, but they are facets of the service delivery process that are unseen by the customer. From a service perspective, Hertz must excel at each shaded box point and measure customer expectations at each point of contact. In some service literature, these points of contact are referred to as "Moments of Truth."

A similar approach has been described as **medical service blueprints**, whereby the operational processes of a patient or other external customer's interactions with a clinic or hospital's program or department are mapped. The blueprint or contact audit will reveal where there are bottlenecks in the process, reveal new opportunities for efficiency, and highlight potential opportunities to excel in customer service delivery. FIGURE 7-4 shows the customer contact audit approach for a primary care visit. Each starred box designates where the customer directly interacts with the service deliverer.

In order to measure service performance then, the organization must remember that customer expectations are a key factor in the ultimate level of performance. To build loyalty, health care organizations must ultimately exceed expectations.[20] It is also valuable to consider how important each one of these customer contact points is in terms of the overall satisfaction with the service. Therefore, at each "Moment of Truth," one must ask two questions:

1. How important was "X" in terms of your overall satisfaction with the health center?
2. How well did we meet your expectations in "X"?

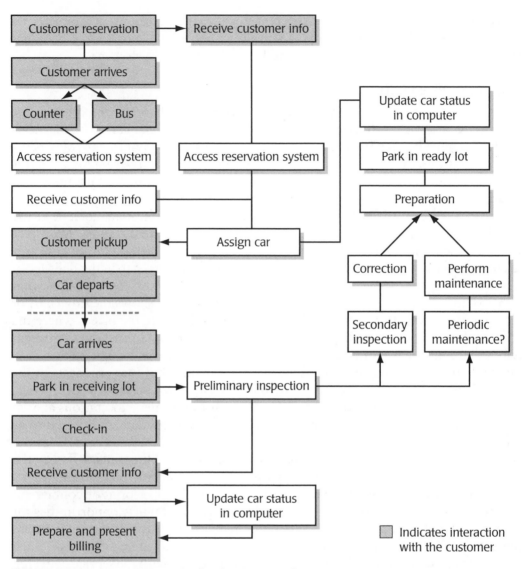

FIGURE 7-3 Customer Contact Audit: The Car Rental Process

Source: Reprinted from *Marketing* by E. N. Berkowitz, R. Kerin, S. Hartley, and C. W. Rudelius, and R. D. Irwin, 1994. Reprinted by permission of the McGraw-Hill Companies.

The first question may be scaled 1 to 5 or 1 to 7 from very important to very unimportant. The second question should be on a scale of "Much better than expected," "Better than expected," "As I expected," "Worse than expected," and "Much worse than expected." This measurement tool will then allow each customer contact point

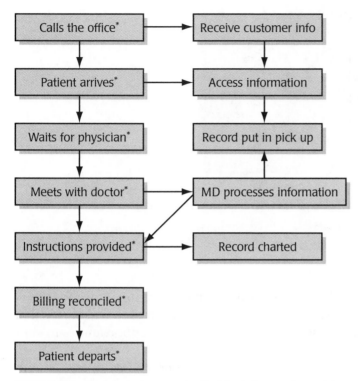

FIGURE 7-4 Customer Contact Audit: The Primary Care Visit

to be put in a matrix similar to what is shown in FIGURE 7-5. This matrix was first introduced in Chapter 4 in Buyer Behavior. However, it is critical to recognize the centrality of this concept to building loyalty.

The upper right-hand quadrant represents the leverage opportunities for an organization. These are the contact points that are very important to the customer, and the organization far exceeds customer expectations. For the managed care organization, then, these are the points that should be highlighted in the newsletter. "Ninety five percent of our subscribers say access to pediatric appointments of sick children is very important, and we far exceeded their expectations on access."

The lower left-hand corner is the status quo box. This quadrant and the lower right quadrant represent the weaknesses with the traditional satisfaction surveys that are often used by health care organizations. The traditional measures do not consider expectations, nor are they really designed for managerial usefulness in targeting the key "Moments of Truth." Any contact point in the lower left box implies that the organization is not meeting expectations, but it is unimportant to the customer. Given the limited financial resources facing most health care organizations, and the limited time of managers and personnel, the level of service delivery here is not a salient concern to the customer.

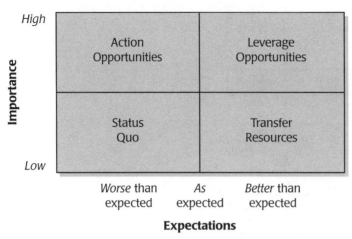

FIGURE 7-5 Directions for Management Change

The lower right quadrant also highlights a problem with existing measures of service delivery. Any contact point here far exceeds expectations, but they are in areas that are not very important to the customer. These points represent opportunities to shift resources.

It is the upper left quadrant, the action opportunities, where a health care administrator needs to focus attention. Contact points here are very important, yet are not meeting customer expectations. However, before any operational change is made within the contact point, additional research is necessary. First, it must be determined whether the reason for the contact point ending here is a *real* problem, or a *perceptual* problem. A real problem is one in which the service delivery was actually not good. For example, consider the emergency department of most hospitals. Wait time is something that is often rated of high importance by the patient. Let us assume that in a particular quarter, the results show wait time to be an "Action Opportunity." The director of the emergency department first needs to assess what the demand was in the emergency department during the measurement period relative to staffing (internal secondary data as discussed in Chapter 5). This analysis reveals that during the measurement period the staffing level was normal, but there were actually three separate incidents when there were major trauma cases transferred to the facility. In three different weeks during the quarter, wait times were truly horrible. What managerial action is taken here? None. It is the nature of running an emergency department. Sometimes a crisis occurs and response must be taken. The crisis can't be predicted or staffed for appropriately in anticipation.

Similarly, an analysis of internal data might reveal a different cause of this "Action Opportunity." During the reporting period two of the emergency department physicians who are in the National Guard were called for deployment. A *locum tenems* agency was hired, yet the replacement physicians did not work as efficiently. Service access suffered. As director of the emergency department, the only action might be to find another backup source for the next such occurrence.

The marketing challenge presents itself when it not a real problem, but rather a perceptual problem. Analyzing the data, the director realizes demand was normal and staffing was normal. Now, the issue is one of managing customer expectations. In situations when demand is above staffing levels, the person's expectations must be brought in line with reality upon checking into the emergency department. An action opportunity here represents a process change. Often, upon going to the emergency department, the patient provides information, and the receptionist or admitting clerk says, "Take a seat." The Walt Disney Company in the running of their theme parks has determined that unexplained waits seem longer than explained waits. Take note the next time you are standing in line at the Magic Kingdom for the little signs that indicate how long you are from getting to ride on Space Mountain. This same approach must be taken in this contact point. The person at admitting must help shape customer expectations. "Usually, the wait is 45 minutes because we take people in order of seriousness. While I am sure that you are uncomfortable and we want to treat you promptly, we have had a major trauma case just brought in to the hospital. The wait time will be at least an hour and thirty minutes. Here is a coupon for a cup of coffee and pie on us in the cafeteria. We will page you there when we have taken care of this medical emergency." This is a very different service delivery experience than "Take a seat."

Developing a Customer Recovery System

A customer **recovery system** is an organized system that anticipates service delivery failures or problems. A defined script indicates how each service person at each level of service delivery will provide a proactive response. A recovery system anticipates that problems will occur in terms of delays with seeing patients or in terms of scheduling and the like. But, recovery is important as the data shows in EXHIBIT 7-3 whereby 68% of the people leave because of benign neglect. At the University of Wisconsin Hospitals and Clinics, a customer recovery system has been implemented. When a patient complains about a wait or some other problem, the person at the desk is empowered to

Exhibit 7-3	Why Customers Leave

- 14% leave because complaints were not handled
- 9% leave because of the competition
- 9% leave because of relocation
- 68% leave for no special reason—benign neglect

Source: From *Customer Loyalty, New and Revised Edition*, by Jill Griffin, 1995. Used with permission of John Wiley & Sons, Inc.

offer some remuneration to ease the problem, such as free parking, or a coupon for a video rental if the family is staying in Madison for treatment. Often, just the recognition of the problem by the health care organization employee is enough of a balm to soothe the dissatisfied patient.

For recovery systems to be effective, however, there are some critical components for successful implementation. These are:

- Focused recovery training must be conducted with all employees.
- Recovery standards must exist.
- The organization must be "easy to complain to."
- Frontline employees must see themselves as part of the system.
- Employees need to believe they are part of a quality-conscious organization.

Ultimately, from a marketing perspective, when there is an opportunity to recover a customer, it should be viewed as an opportunity to create a loyal customer.

■ Conclusions

Developing customer loyalty is the real challenge for health care organizations. While hospitals have been mandated by accreditation reviews to measure satisfaction and many health care organizations have measured this construct, satisfaction alone will not result in loyalty. The key to loyalty is to create a visible value for the customer and to recognize that in a service-driven business such as health care problems will occur. It is the anticipation of those problems and their likelihood of occurrence that leads to opportunities to demonstrate excellent customer service with a recovery system.

■ Key Terms

Relationship Marketing   Gap Analysis
Customer Loyalty Pyramid   Customer Contact Audit
Process Quality   Medical Service Blueprints
Service Acquisition Cost   Recovery System

■ Chapter Summary

1. Relationship marketing is a shift from a transactional perspective to the development of longer term loyalty.
2. In a transactional focus, the perspective is more on what the organization is selling; in a relationship marketing focus, it is more on what the customer values.
3. Satisfaction is not a sufficient goal for customer behavior; rather, the focus must be loyalty.

4. The customer loyalty pyramid has multiple stages: awareness, interest, evaluation, trial, repeat, satisfaction, and ultimately loyalty.

5. The lower levels of the customer pyramid (awareness, interest, evaluation) are referred to as the promotional levels of the pyramid.

6. Loyal customers have multiple benefits in terms of reduced acquisition costs, longer term per revenue growth, more profitable to serve, able to refer others, and more willing to pay a price premium.

7. Loyal patients have a broader zone of tolerance or are more willing to forgive an organization's service lapses.

8. Customer value equation has four variables: clinical quality, service process quality less out of pocket cost less effort expended.

9. Conducting a Gap Analysis can help identify the opportunities for the delivery of customer value.

10. A customer contact audit or medical service blueprint is a flowchart of each step in delivering the service to the patient and shows where the patient interacts with the service deliverer. This approach can highlight opportunities for establishing a differential advantage.

11. Measuring satisfaction is a function of expectations and the importance of each point of contact.

12. A customer recovery system is defined script that anticipates how to react when a problem arises in service delivery.

■ Chapter Problems

1. Most medical specialty groups historically have relied on primary care physician practices for referrals. At a recent society meeting, the senior partner returned with a renewed perspective in terms of looking at the customer base of referrers. "We need to develop relationships with these practices rather than view them as individual transactions when they send us a patient." How might this perspective shift the strategy of the group?

2. For many years health care organizations, as well as traditional businesses, have often struggled in frustration that high scores in satisfaction do not necessarily lead to higher levels of profitability or sales. Explain why this inconsistency tends to exist.

3. Whenever most medical groups can improve clinical quality, they will move in that direction. The ultimate result would be an improvement in the value they deliver to the patient. If clinical value cannot be achieved, however, where else could a health care organization turn to achieve greater value to a customer?

4. Newsletters are important and can tie into the customer satisfaction program of a health care organization. Explain the integration of this strategy in a total marketing program for a health care organization.

■ Notes

1. David Shani and Sujana Chalasani, "Exploiting Niches Using Relationship Marketing," *Journal of Consumer Marketing* (Summer 1992): 33–42.

2. Thomas J. Wall, "Online CRM: On to the Next Level," *Medicine on the Net*, July 2003, pp. 1–5, hcpro.com/services/corhealth/index.cfm.

3. Scott MacStravic, "Cultivating Patient Relationships," *Marketing Health Services* 23, no. 1 (Spring 2003): 24–29.

4. Karl Albrecht, *Delivering Customer Value: It's Everybody's Job* (Portland, OR: Productivity Press, 1995).

5. Chris Fay, "You Can't Get No Satisfaction: Perhaps You Should Stop Trying." White paper, Juran Institute (Wilton, CT: n.d.)

6. Ibid.

7. David I. Strum, and Alain Thiry, "Building Customer Loyalty," *Training and Development Journal,* (April 1991), Vol. 35, pp. 35–36.

8. Frederick F. Reichheld, "Loyalty Based Management," *Harvard Business Review,* (March–April 1993), vol. 71, No. 2, pp. 64–73.

9. Banwari Mittal and Walfried M. Lassar, "Why Do Customers Switch? The Dynamics of Satisfaction versus Loyalty," *The Journal of Services Marketing* 12, no. 3 (1998): 177–194.

10. Jill Griffin, *Customer Loyalty: How to Earn It, How to Keep It* (San Francisco: Jossey-Bass, 1995).

11. R. Eric Reidenbach and Gordon W. McClung, "Managing Stakeholder Loyalty," *Marketing Health Services* (Spring 1999): 21–29.

12. Strum and Thiry, op cit.

13. Frederick F. Reichheld, *The Loyalty Effect* (Cambridge: Harvard Business Review Press, 1996), 40–49.

14. Naumann, 1995.

15. James L. Heskett, W. Earl Sasser, Jr., and Leonard A. Schelesinger, *The Service Profit Chain* (New York: The Free Press, 1997).

16. *The Service Profit Chain*, 41.

17. The concept was developed and articulated by Valerie A. Zeithaml, A. Parasuraman, and Leonard L. Berry, *Delivering Quality Service* (New York: Free Press, 1990).

18. *USA Today*, May 10, 2001, 2a.

19. Benjamin Schneider and David E. Bowen, *Winning the Service Game* (Cambridge, MA: Harvard Business School Press, 1995).

20. Fred Lee, "Stop Measuring Patient Satisfaction," *Marketing Health Services* 23, no. 2 (Summer 2003): 33–37.

The Marketing Mix

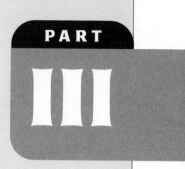

Product Strategy

After reading this chapter, you should be able to:

- Learn the range of product and service variations
- Understand the issues of product line formation
- Identify the strategy considerations over the product life cycle
- Know the strategic implications of alternative branding strategies

■ The Meaning of Products and Services

Ultimately for any business, the focus of marketing revolves around the products and services to meet customer needs. Health care business lines involve a range of products and services. The primary distinction between products and services is their degree of tangibility, or the extent to which they can be examined, touched, or experienced before purchase. Products can be divided into two groups: nondurable goods and durable goods. A **nondurable good** is an item that can be consumed in some defined period of time. Examples of nondurable goods include chewing tobacco, food products, and topical dressings for wounds. A **durable good** is a product that lasts over an extended period of time. Items such as automobiles, computerized tomography (CT) scanners, and computers can all be classified as durable items. A wide range of health care activities involves **services**, which are defined as intangible activities or processes offered to customers to solve problems, and for which the organization is often reimbursed. Open heart surgery, a comprehensive cancer program, and a geriatric medicine clinic are examples of common health care services.

The differences between such items reflect important considerations in any marketing action. Nondurable products are often heavily advertised because consumers frequently purchase such products. Many pharmaceuticals, such as Rogaine®, are heavily advertised directly to the consumer. Retail store displays play a major role in direct marketing to the consumer. For durable products, personal sales often play a major role. General Electric (GE), for example, has an extensive sales force that calls upon hospitals selling the latest GE scanning devices. Durable products usually cost more than nondurable items and are often far more complicated to use. For these products, personal sales are essential to help answer customer questions and to explain the intricacies of the product.

The marketing of services is often more challenging because of their unique elements, given that they are not tangible. Services differ from products on five components, which can be referred to as the five Is.

The Five Is of Services

Service marketing is a challenging and often difficult aspect of marketing. The five characteristics of services that any health care marketer should recognize include: intangibility, inconsistency, inseparability, inventory, and interaction.

Intangibility

Services are intangible in that they cannot be felt, touched, or heard before they are encountered. Cardiac surgery, for example, is intangible. Prior to undergoing such a procedure, a patient cannot see the surgery or examine it as can be done with the purchase of a computer. A major challenge in the marketing of intangible services is to show the tangible benefits from their use.[1] An advertisement for an occupational medicine program, for example, might show a productive worker back on the job; or the hospital birthing center advertisement shows a mother with a contented baby. Because services are intangible, consumer interactions with the processes and the individuals who deliver the service are often the bases by which consumers evaluate the actual service itself.

Inconsistency

Health services are delivered by people—the nurse practitioner, the physician, or the admitting clerk in the group practice. In this regard, service marketing is more difficult than product marketing. In the manufacture of a product, exact standards can be developed by which the production line assembles a car, telephone, or other product within some defined tolerance levels. Deviations in the tolerance can lead to a simple adjustment in the production machines. People-delivered services have inherent variability. The delivery of the service changes with the individual who delivers the service. For example, two surgeons may have noticeably different levels of proficiency at performing a particular procedure. While they perform the same clinical procedure, no one would argue that they are delivering the same service. Similarly, on any given day, the admitting clerks at the hospital may deliver their services differently as a function of their own motivation, morale, or attitude.

For service marketers, the objective in reducing inconsistency is to achieve as much standardization as possible. In McDonald's restaurants, for example, service workers all wear the same uniform to minimize inconsistency. The key, however, to any attempt at reducing inconsistency in people-delivered services is through training.

Inseparability

Services cannot be separated from the individuals who deliver them. The classic example of this characteristic in health care settings is known as the "bedside manner" of the physician. The link between the issues of inseparability and inconsistency underscores the complexity of health care service marketing.

Inventory

Often in the discussion of services, the issue of inventory is ignored. Inventory is a concept that is common to product businesses. In the analysis of costs associated with product businesses, a major concern is the cost of carrying any inventory. Yet services, too, have inventory. Whenever an employee who delivers the service is not being utilized, but is still being paid, an inventory exists. A hospital emergency room physician who is paid on a contract represents an inventory cost that the hospital carries. As long as the emergency room is not being utilized and the physician has down time, the cost of that inventory is large.

Service businesses can manage the cost of inventory by either managing the service deliverer or by shifting the demand. One strategy for managing the delivery of a service is to employ part-time workers who work at peak time periods. Nurses are frequently paid premium wages for working certain shifts or working overtime to cover unusually busy periods of activity.

Managing the demand for a service is more difficult. It involves shifting demand to nonpeak hours to level out the costs of personnel and overhead. Movie theaters, for example, offer discounted admissions during the afternoon, or matinee, shows. Management's goal is to attract customers throughout the day to defray the costs of building maintenance and the movie rental fees. In health care, accomplishing this strategy requires an understanding of the ebb and flow of customers through the business.

Interaction with Customers

Because services involve processes, an important consideration in marketing a service is the quality of the interaction between the customer and the service provider. As was discussed in Chapter 7, the **customer contact audit** or medical practice blueprinting is one approach that highlights the encounters between a customer and the service offering.[2–4]

■ Classification of Products and Services

Products and services vary in two key ways: in terms of durability and tangibility, as we have just discussed. These variations clearly determine the types of marketing strategy developed for each category. Products and services can also be classified on other levels, in terms of who buys them and how they are delivered.

At the most macro level, products can be classified by the type of users who buy them. **Consumer goods** are products purchased by the ultimate consumer. **Industrial products** are products purchased for use in the manufacture of other products, which will, at some point, be purchased by the ultimate consumer. Both consumer and industrial products have several variations, which are discussed in this chapter. Services can be classified by how they are delivered: primarily by individuals or by machines.

Classifying Consumer Products

A major way to classify consumer products is by the amount of effort and manner of search the consumer uses in purchasing the product.[5] Using this classification scheme, consumer goods fall into three categories: (1) convenience goods, (2) shopping goods, and (3) specialty items. **Convenience goods** are products that the consumer purchases frequently and require little deliberation or search prior to purchase. Cold remedies, analgesics, and chewing gum are all examples. For marketers of convenience goods, there are two major concerns. Since the consumer engages in little search or deliberation, name recognition and product distribution are critical. Makers of Tylenol, for example, prominently place their brand on eye-level shelves in pharmacies and other stores where medicine is sold.

A second type of consumer product is a **shopping good**. Shopping goods are products in which the consumer engages in a significant amount of search to compare competing brands on selected attributes, such as price, style, or features. Televisions, computers, and cameras are all common examples of shopping goods. Marketers of shopping goods must differentiate their brand from their competitors' on the attributes that are important to their customers. Salespeople often play a major role in helping the consumer learn about alternative brands and ultimately make the purchase. To some degree, salespeople calling on referral physician offices or pharmaceutical representatives play a similar role as they help inform referral physicians about alternative practices to which they could send patients or different therapies that might be suitable.

A final category of consumer goods includes **specialty items**. Specialty products are those that the consumer specifically seeks out. Often the consumer is very loyal to a particular brand and will go to great lengths to find that particular item. While specialty items vary from one individual to another, common examples might include a Rolex watch, Joy perfume, or an Apple IPOD. Table 8-1 shows a representation of consumer products.

Industrial Goods Classification

Industrial products have two broad levels of classification. **Production goods** are those that are used to become part of a final product. Raw materials fit into this category. A second type of industrial goods is known as **support goods**. These are items used to assist in the producing of other products. Support goods can include buildings, accessory equipment, and supplies. A CT scanner would be considered a support good, as would a desk used in an office, or paper clip attached to a billing invoice.

Table 8-1	Categorization of Products		
Criterion	Convenience	Shopping	Specialty
degree of search effort	little	compares alternatives	seeks specific brand
price	relatively inexpensive	moderate	usually expensive
differential advantage	little on product	often varies by product	identity
key marketing mix component	distribution	product or price	product (brand)
customer loyalty	little	prefers a brand but will substitute	highly loyal
frequency of purchase	frequent	infrequent	very infrequent

Service Classifications

Services can be classified primarily by how they are delivered: whether by people or equipment.[6] FIGURE 8-1 shows the two major distinctions and examples of each. Services that are primarily equipment-based have fewer problems with inconsistency. Health care services are primarily delivered by professionals and skilled labor.

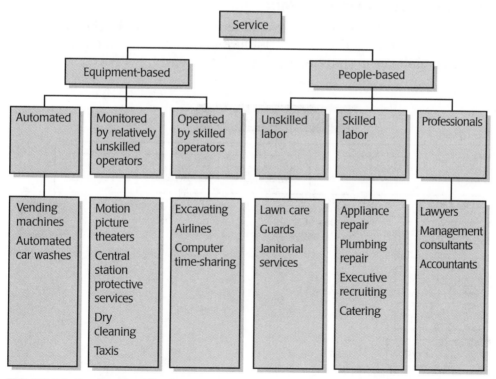

FIGURE 8-1 Service Classifications

Source: Reprinted by permission of *Harvard Business Review*. Service Classifications from "Strategy Is Different in Service Businesses" by D. R. E. Thomas, Vol. 56, No 4. Copyright © 1978 by the Harvard Business School Publishing Corporation; all rights reserved.

In the health care industry there is also another common delineator of services. This categorization pertains to the tax status of the organization either as a for-profit or a nonprofit entity. During the 1980s, health care saw a rapid rise in the number of for-profit health care organizations, such as National Medical Enterprises, Hospital Corporation of America, and US HealthCare. The major distinction of these services pertains to the distribution of excess revenues (profits) over expenses. In for-profit businesses, some portion of profit often is directed to shareholders. In nonprofit service organizations, excess revenues are redirected back to the organization to continue the maintenance of the service.

■ Managing the Product

The remaining discussion in this chapter will use the terms "product" and "service" interchangeably. In cases where there are variations in the marketing implications, the differences between products and services will be noted.

Developing the Product Line and Mix

All businesses must decide which products and services to offer. The **product mix** is the entire range of products a firm offers. FIGURE 8-2 shows a portion of the product line of a large community hospital that provides some tertiary services. This chart

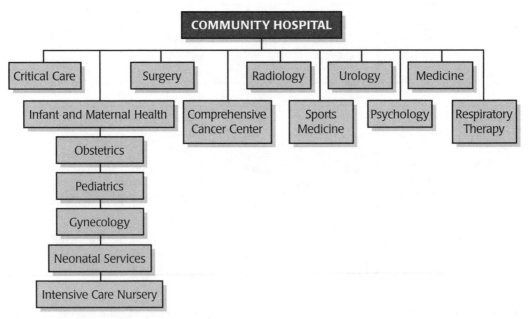

FIGURE 8-2 Community Hospital Product Mix

shows several distinct **product lines**, which are groups of related services. For example, the product line in Infant and Maternal Health contains the services of obstetrics, pediatrics, gynecology, neonatal care, and an intensive care nursery. In determining the product mix, companies must determine the breadth and depth of the product mix. The **breadth** refers to the number of different product lines in the mix. As can be seen in Figure 8-2, the hospital has a reasonably well-developed product line, consisting of such services as a comprehensive cancer center, sports medicine, and respiratory therapy. **Depth** refers to the number of product items within each product line. FIGURE 8-3 shows the depth of the product line in the comprehensive cancer center. Significant depth is represented by the number of services offered within this program, which range from invasive procedures such as oncological surgery to supportive assistance with social services. A real-life example is St. Francis Hospital, in Roslyn, New York, (www.stfrancisheartcenter.com), which specializes exclusively in the diagnosis and treatment of heart disease. Although this is a narrow product line, the program has significant depth by including services such as a community outreach program that brings cardiac screening to low-income residents living in medically underserved areas. The hospital operates a cardiac fitness center and offers regional employers a corporate education and screening program. St. Francis also offers an educational outreach program to teach children healthy eating and exercise habits.[7]

Most companies manage multiple product lines and items. In these circumstances, companies must guard against **cannibalization**—when a company's own products steal market share from other products within the company's product line. A hospital, for example, might open a free-standing emergency department only to find that it steals patients from the hospital's main emergency department. The major rationale used to allow for cannibalization is that it is better to offer the product oneself than for a competitor to enter the market with the same product. A company would market the product to appeal to a different market segment that would not have a major impact on other product lines.

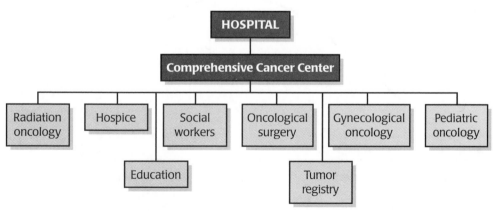

FIGURE 8-3 Depth in the Product Line

The Product Life Cycle

The marketing implications and considerations for any product vary depending on how long the product has been in existence, the number of competitors, and the level of sales or revenue the product is generating. Central to understanding the marketing of products, then, is the concept of the product life cycle. The **product life cycle** refers to the stages a product goes through as it exists in the market from its first introduction to its final withdrawal.[8] FIGURE 8-4 shows the four stages of a generalized product life cycle: introduction, growth, maturity, and decline. In this representation the X axis represents time, and the Y axis represents gross revenues or sales.

Introduction

The first stage of the product life cycle, introduction, occurs when the product is first rolled out into the marketplace. This might be considered the present market position of sub-acute care facilities. These organizations, often nursing homes and skilled nursing facilities, are for those patients who no longer need acute care. One thousand such centers were operating in 1994 with a projected tenfold increase by the end of this decade.[9] As seen in FIGURE 8-5, sales start slowly in the introduction stage and gradually increase. Looking at Figure 8-5, one can see the early stage of the life cycle of ambulatory surgical procedures between 1980 and 1984 before it began the rapid rise. At this stage of the life cycle, there are distinct considerations for each element of the marketing mix.

Product

The key consideration in the introduction stage of a product is quality. Product quality must be at the level that meets customer expectations. A product whose quality suffers

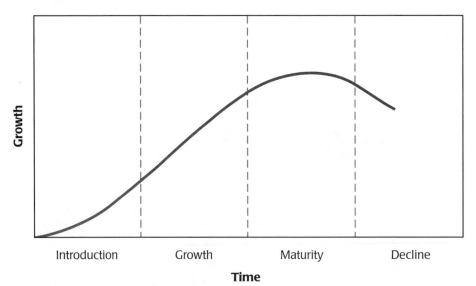

FIGURE 8-4 The Generalized Product Life Cycle

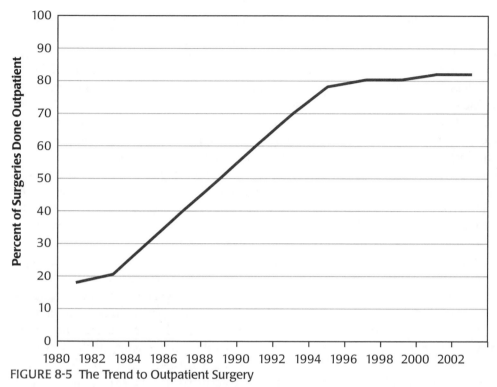

FIGURE 8-5 The Trend to Outpatient Surgery

Source: The Lewin Group Analysis of American Hospital Association Annual Survey data, 1980–2003 as displayed in The Lewin Group, Inc. (2002) Cutting Edge Costs: Hospitals and New Technology, *American Hospital Association Trend Watch*, Vol. 4, No. 4, May 19, 2003, www.hospitalconnect.com. Reprinted with permission.

at this stage of the life cycle will have a difficult time reaching the growth stage. Early buyers who try the product will become dissatisfied and will discourage prospective buyers. Any repeat purchase probabilities by these early buyers will be quickly eliminated.

In service marketing, the introduction stage of the life cycle is particularly difficult. Since much of the service delivery involves a process and personnel, internal controls become of paramount importance. In introducing an industrial medicine program, for example, a hospital must have procedures in place to provide quick follow-up with the employee assistance professional who processes the paperwork for a company's injured employee. If the system fails, it will be difficult to get that employer to sign a second-year contract for the industrial medicine program.

Price

At this stage of the product life cycle, pricing follows one of two primary strategies. One is a **skimming price** strategy, involving a high initial price relative to competing products or substitutable services. Or, the organization can roll out the new product and price it lower than the competition, using a **penetration price** strategy. There are advantages and disadvantages to each approach.

One advantage to a high initial price is that, for any new product or service, there are often some early buyers who want the product, no matter what the price. These buyers are less price sensitive. Following the skimming strategy allows the organization to achieve a greater margin on these early buyers and to recoup the cost of developing the new product. As competition enters the market, the price subsequently can be reduced. A second major advantage to a high initial price is image. The high price sets off the product as a premium good or a status item. In health care there is some strong logic to this rationale. Since services are intangibles, price is one way consumers can infer the quality of the service, since price is a tangible element. For physicians, the initial pricing of a service sets up the profiles for Medicare and Medicaid reimbursements, as well as for other third-party carriers. As a result, a higher price allows for a more remunerative level of reimbursement from these agencies.

With services, there is another strong reason supporting a skimming strategy. Services require personnel and processes. Often, in spite of an organization's best efforts, there is a shakeout period in which processes for delivering the service must be reworked once actual demand is established. The admitting procedures for a day surgery program, for example, might need to be streamlined. In such cases, when complicated systems or multiple departments are involved in the delivery of the service, a high price acts as a safeguard to discourage too much start-up demand. The organization can use the initial high price as a spigot to control the flow of demand until there is confidence that the systems, personnel, and supporting facilities are in place to meet customer needs.

The disadvantages of a skimming strategy are obvious. If the organization needs to have some economy of scale to deliver the service efficiently, a high price discourages demand. A skimming strategy also may entice competitors to enter the field. A potential competitor watching the premiums being charged by a new managed care organization (MCO) may decide it can offer a similar plan at a lower price in the marketplace and still earn a reasonable return.

The advantage of a penetration strategy is that it keeps the competition out and encourages demand. St. Michael's Medical Center, in Newark, New Jersey, introduced a 20-minute heart check for women. The service included an electrocardiogram, cholesterol check, blood pressure check, and computerized health test risk appraisal. The introductory price was only $25. After an introductory period, the price was raised to $40.[10] The major limitation of penetration pricing, however, is that setting a low price requires a good understanding of what it costs to produce the product. The organization must understand the per-unit cost to ensure that the low initial price covers the per-unit cost, in addition to providing a return to the company. In a health care business, an accurate per-unit cost of delivery has always been a difficult figure to obtain. In such instances, a low-cost strategy can entail some real financial risks for an organization.

Promotion

Promotion is an essential component to consider in the introduction stage. For a truly new product or service, the company must develop **primary demand**, or interest in purchasing this new class of service. A new product requires significant promotional effort to educate the market about a product's capabilities. GlaxoSmithKline, an international pharmaceutical manufacturer, for example, spent significant promotional dollars educating neurologists about a new migraine headache medication. Advertisements in clinical publications, displays at the annual meeting of the American Academy of Neurology, and personal calls in physicians' offices—some of the tactics that were used by GlaxoSmithKline—are all key promotional components in the introduction stage of the life cycle of the new drug product.

Place

The distribution issues in the introductory stage of the product life cycle are somewhat limited. The key challenge is to obtain some initial exposure for the product.

Growth

In the growth stage of the product life cycle, as shown in Figure 8-4, sales of the product begin to increase rapidly. For example, between 1982 and 1988 there was a 128% increase in ambulatory outpatient surgery procedures, as depicted in Figure 8-5. By 1996 the number of procedures grew to over 31.5 million per year.[11] As can be seen in Figure 8-5, although only 21% of all surgical procedures in the United States were done on an outpatient basis in 1984, the number today is closer to 80%.[12] An early sign that one is entering this stage of the life cycle is the appearance of competitors. Once other providers enter the market, the key challenge is to generate **selective demand**, which is preference for the company's product or service. The marketing mix issues regarding the product life cycle also begin to shift.

Product

A key decision for organizations at this stage of the life cycle is whether to expand the product mix. Organizations will often expand the product line by offering a variation of the original product. Apple, for example, offers less expensive versions of its IPOD, which has less storage than the original. The purpose of these new variations is to expand the product's appeal to new market segments.

Promotion

While in the introduction stage, the promotional concern was to generate awareness. Now with competitors, the purpose of promotion is to develop product preference. Advertising must create brand awareness. For example, when the first MCO enters a particular community, its major promotional objective is to educate people about this new "managed care" plan. Once other competitors enter the market, each MCO advertises its particular name to generate selective demand.

In the growth stage of the product life cycle, personal sales become more important. Once there is market competition, the competitors battle for middleman support. With the introduction of DAT recorders, for example, each manufacturer's sales force works aggressively to convince retailers to carry its particular brand. So too, in health care, this same personal sales emphasis is occurring with managed care plans. Each plan has a sales force offering its products to large employers. Most health care providers know that employers offer their employees only a limited choice of health plans, just like most retailers carry only a limited number of brands in any particular product category.

Price
The pricing decision in the growth stage depends on the initial price at which the product is offered, and whether the company is broadening its product line. It is difficult to raise the price for a product after its introductory offering. In health care, many health maintenance organizations (HMOs) raised their prices after they reviewed utilization rates. Too large a price increase without a substantial change in the product quality, however, can lead to significant buyer dissatisfaction in any business.

Place
A major emphasis of marketing strategy in the growth stage is on the distribution component of the marketing mix—solidifying the loyalty of the middleman. Hospitals, for example, have often faced this dilemma when a competing hospital established a similar medical or surgical service, such as cardiovascular surgery.

Maturity
In this phase of the life cycle, sales begin to slow. An indicator of the mature stage is when the marginal competitors begin to exit the business line. This happens in many communities with an aging population. Selected hospitals in particular communities may leave the pediatric business, for example. In the mature stage of the life cycle, the key objective is to maintain the existing customer base. Some additional growth in sales can occur as the remaining competitors fight for the business of those who have left the market.

Product
There are few major product decisions at this stage of the life cycle. Most companies have a relatively full product line. The key product issue is to develop some new lines that can help reposition the organization to return to the earlier stages of introduction and growth. Kaiser Permanente's recent developments in California can be viewed as a strategy to move back up on the growth curve of the life cycle in the face of maturity. Having existed for many years in this market, the Kaiser HMO is a mature product within California. In 1994, Kaiser began offering a point-of-service plan that allows its subscribers a choice—they can receive their health care from a Kaiser provider, or, for the payment of an additional deductible, they can receive care from a non-Kaiser physician.[13] Kaiser now offers a plan with a $1500 deductible, while Aetna offers a plan with a $5000 deductible, both of which are targeting young, single adults.

Price

At the mature stage of the life cycle, pricing becomes far more competitive. Typically, at this stage, there is aggressive price discounting, which contributes to the exit of some marginal competitors.

Promotion

Promotion at this stage involves retention of existing customers. In traditional industries, coupons or promotional games are often used to keep existing customers coming back. McDonald's, for example, offers different promotional products to children as a way to maintain customer loyalty. In the health care setting, such games or promotions would be considered unacceptable. Some institutions, however, have set up senior citizen clubs as a way to tie this population to a particular facility.

Place

The distribution decision at this stage is relatively simple—the profitable channels are maintained and marginal outlets are dropped. At this point, for example, a health care organization may decide to close some free-standing emergency departments in locations that haven't developed a reasonable return.

Decline

The decline stage of the life cycle is difficult for any organization; it must recognize that the service cannot continue to grow. Services in the decline stage of the product life cycle can consume a disproportionate share of management time and financial resources. There are relatively few options. The most difficult option is to *drop*, or eliminate the service. There may be significant emotional attachment to the service within the organization. A hospital's board of trustees, for instance, might note that from its early days, the hospital always offered pediatric services.

A second option is to *contract* with another party to provide the product or service. In health care, for example, some companies might agree to run a hospital's emergency department or rehabilitation department under a contract.

A final option is to *harvest* the service.[14] This involves paring out the aspects of the service that are truly not profitable and offering a reduced version of the service for loyal customers. In the pediatric example, the hospital could decide to offer a pediatric clinic for primary case consults, but drop its inpatient beds.

Product Life Cycle Issues

The product life cycle is a useful management concept for determining where a service is positioned in the marketplace and what external influences, such as competitors, might affect strategy. Yet, there is no exact way for an organization to determine where a respective service or product is in the life cycle. Nor do all life cycles necessarily have the shape of that shown in Figure 8-4.[15]

Alternative Product Life Cycles

FIGURE 8-6 displays four other common product life cycles. One life cycle is for a **high learning product** that requires a significant introductory period.[16] These represent rather complicated services for which the immediate benefit might not be seen by the consumer. These types of products often require significant buyer education. A high learning product might include services of a physiatrist. Studies have shown that few people understand what a physiatrist does, including members of the medical profession, who lack the knowledge of this medical specialty's capabilities. Thus, a rehabilitative medicine service staffed by a physiatrist can be viewed in some markets as a high learning product. Significant time must be spent educating potential referral physicians about the value of this service, compared to dealing with orthopedists or physical therapists.

A second variation shown in Figure 8-6 represents the **low learning product** for which the benefits are clearly seen by the consumer.[17] This product has a short introductory period and enters competition rapidly. These products generally are not technologically sophisticated, so that there is lower complexity and a lower cost of entry for the

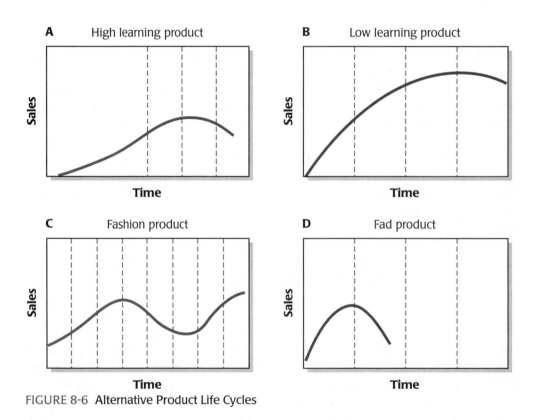

FIGURE 8-6 Alternative Product Life Cycles

competition. A walk-in medical center can be considered a low learning product. Consumers see these as convenient places for care for minor medical problems. The benefits of reduced waiting time compared to a hospital emergency department, as well as the "no appointment needed" approach, has led to rapid acceptance of this concept.

A third life cycle shown in Figure 8-6 represents the fashion product, in which there is a decline and an eventual reemergence of the product. The name of this curve is related to the fashion styles that often disappear, only to reemerge years later in modified form. Some fashion magazines were touting bell bottom slacks as the fashion statement of 1993. Yet, bell bottoms were tossed out of most closets at the end of the 1960s. The width of men's ties and the length of hemlines vary in the fashion life cycle.

Figure 8-6 also includes the fad product. There are really only two stages to the fad life cycle: introduction and decline. Pet rocks, wall walkers, and toe socks are all examples of past fads. These items are quickly adopted by consumers for their novelty value, and competitors often enter quickly to capitalize on the sales growth. Yet, as quickly as the sales occurred, the fad can end, once it reaches saturation. The shape of this life cycle can tell the fortunes of many companies. A company fortunate to enter the life cycle early can reap significant financial gain. A competitor entering the fad market too late can find itself with a warehouse full of rocks that no one wants for a pet. In the health care industry, fads occur, often with regard to vitamins and treatment approaches. At one time, for example, bran was cited as a preventative for heart disease. This led to the rapid proliferation of bran additives in many products. After a relatively short time period, however, and the publication of several medical studies questioning the validity of the claim, the bran fad disappeared.

Length of the Life Cycle

It is difficult to affect the length of the product life cycle. In health care, the major factor that moves a service rapidly from introduction to decline is technology. As was seen in Chapter 2, Figure 2-8 shows the impact of new technology on the life cycles of the preceding products over which there has been an improvement. The life cycle of X-rays as an imaging device was fairly long. Yet increased imaging performance became available through the advent of nuclear imaging, which led to X-ray technology becoming mature in terms of performance (and most likely sales). The past 15 years, however, have seen rapid development in imaging technology with the result of shorter product life cycles in terms of the existing technology. With increasing developments in health care, the impact of new technologies on existing business lines is real. Consider the shifts of revenue that have occurred with the developments of drug-eluting stents. Duke University Medical Center in Durham, North Carolina, believes the introduction of this new product has significantly impacted the number of cardiac bypass operations done at its facility from 1100 in 2002 to 950 in 2003.[18] Introduction of new technologies makes long-term strategic management of revenue streams a challenge in health care.

The Life Cycle of Hospitals

In health care management, the life cycle phenomenon is real. FIGURE 8-7 shows the classic life cycle of inpatient acute-care hospitals in the United States from 1965 to 1985. As hospitals reduce beds and convert unused facilities, few would argue that the inpatient side of the hospital business is in the decline stage of the product life cycle.

Product Life Cycle Concerns

While the product life cycle is one of the most common conceptualizations used within marketing, it is not without its limitations. A major criticism is that there is no standard life cycle and that many products defy the life cycle sequence.

A second concern is whether the product life cycle relates to the product class (automobiles), the product form (full-size sedans), or the specific product (Mercury Marquis). The product life cycle treats each product as a new form or a new product class when, in fact, the product may just be a new brand of a product at the growth or maturity stage. This factor may lead to different life cycle strategies.[19] A third concern is that the product life cycle is tied closely to sales. It is often difficult, however, to relate some marketing activities directly to their impact on sales.

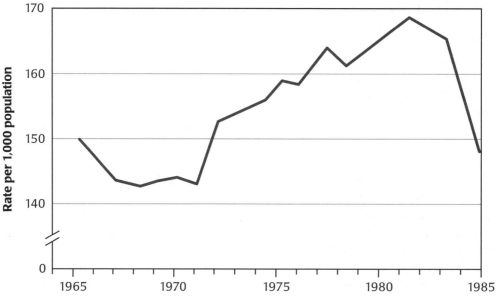

FIGURE 8-7 **The Declining Hospital Life Cycle** (discharge rate in nonfederal short-stay hospitals)

Source: National Center for Health Statistics, 1985 Summary, *National Hospital Discharge Survey*. Advance data from *Viral and Health Statistics*, No. 127, DHHS Pub No. (PHS) S6-1250 (Hyattsville, MD: Public Health Service), September 25, 1986.

Modifying the Product Life Cycle

While it is impossible for marketing managers to alter the external factors, such as demographics or new technology, that affect the product life cycle, there are three strategies they can consider to stretch the life of the product they control. These strategies include product modification, market modification, and repositioning the product.

Product Modification

The strategy of **product modification** involves actually altering the product in some fashion by changing its quality, features, performance, or appearance. A hospital may decide to add more services to its industrial medicine program. A membership at a local health club could become part of the standard package, thereby actually improving the service.

Market Modification

An alternative approach to stretch the life cycle is **market modification**, in which the company tries to increase the use of the product by creating new uses or new users for it. Promoting more frequent use of a product is common in traditional industries. Brushing your teeth after every meal has long been touted as important by toothpaste manufacturers. There are some strong ethical concerns, however, about promoting the more frequent use of health services. In fact, this aspect of health care advertising was an early concern voiced by opponents of the practice. Physicians believed that the advertising of medical services would lead to unnecessary utilization or demand from consumers for an advertised clinical service that may not be appropriate for all of these consumers.

Create New Uses

This strategy involves identifying new ways to use the product. Arm & Hammer baking soda is an example of a product that has stretched its life cycle very successfully with this strategy. Arm & Hammer baking soda is advertised as a refrigerator deodorizer, toothpaste, cat litter refresher, and also as a baking product. In health care, identifying new uses for medications has become common. A particular drug is often found to be beneficial for the treatment of unrelated problems. As noted earlier, Retin-A is a topical cream originally intended for treatment of severe acne. This product's life has been stretched considerably since put to new use as a topical for early-stage skin cancers, as well as an anti-wrinkling preventative for the skin.

Find New Users

Seeking out new target markets is a third way to stretch the life of a product. In the rehabilitative medicine department of the Cleveland Clinic, a seat was developed to assist patients who were wheelchair-bound. This seat (and the process to create it) was originally intended for patients who came to the clinic. To stretch the life cycle of the product, the clinic considered selling the process and technology to other large medical centers for use with their patients.

Repositioning the Product

In offering a service or product, a company must first decide how it wants to position the product in the market. **Product positioning** involves how a product is perceived in the minds of consumers relative to defined attributes and competing products. There are several alternatives a company can consider in the initial product positioning. Target market strategies can include mass market, niche, and growth market strategies.

As noted in Chapter 2, with a mass market strategy, the company tries to attract larger market segments by positioning the product so it appeals to the largest number of customers in the market. A medical group, for example, may offer primary care services at a number of sites in the community, planning to attract the largest volume possible to utilize the service.

Within the mass market strategy, a firm can follow either an undifferentiated or differentiated approach. In using an undifferentiated strategy, the service is positioned to appeal to the larger segments. In a differentiated strategy, services are developed to meet the individual needs of the multiple segments that comprise the total market.

A niche strategy involves selecting a narrow segment or segments of the market. Shouldice Hospital, in Toronto, Canada, received significant attention when it specialized in short-stay hernia repairs. The hospital introduced this service not only within Canada, but also in the United States. The target market was corporate executives who could fly to Canada for treatment but needed to return to their jobs as soon as possible. Today MedCath might be considered a corporation following the niche strategy as it targets the cardiovascular segment of the market (www.medcath.com). MedCath has built facilities in Dayton like the Dayton Heart Hospital; in Tucson, the Arizona Heart Institute; the Louisiana Heart Hospital, Lacombe, Louisiana; all facilities focus on cardiovascular problems and disease.

A growth market strategy involves targeting those segments that are going to expand. Prior to the changes in reimbursement, many hospitals targeted oncology as a growing market segment. Demographics, technology, and advances in treatment led many facilities to establish comprehensive cancer programs since this area generated significant revenue by using many services within a hospital's product mix in the diagnosis and treatment of the disease. In the 1980s, however, the government began to change how hospitals were reimbursed for the inpatient care they provided. Historically, hospitals were paid based on the costs incurred during the length of stay for the treatment of a medical problem. This was called cost-based reimbursement. During the 1980s, the government moved to reimbursing hospitals for the treatment of a disease or medical problem at a predetermined rate, regardless of the length of stay or services utilized in the treatment of a condition. Medical problems were categorized into diagnosis-related groups (DRGs). This change in reimbursement meant that an intensive medical service, such as oncology, would no longer be so profitable if it required significant resources. The change to DRGs required the hospital to be efficient, since charges for excessive treatment would no longer be reimbursed by the government. As

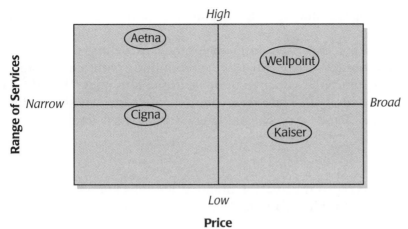

FIGURE 8-8 Multidimensional Scaling Map

reimbursements shift, this only underscores the need to continue to monitor the environment as part of an ongoing marketing analysis.

Assessing Product Position

One way to assess the position of a service in the minds of consumers is through the use of multidimensional scaling (MDS). With this statistical technique, perceptual maps can be developed of a hospital's position relative to competing institutions. In a typical MDS situation, consumers are asked to provide paired similarity ratings of services or hospitals. All possible combinations are provided. Consumers rate desired attributes in order of importance. An MDS map such as that shown in FIGURE 8-8 then can be developed. These maps help to visualize the service gaps and also show how the competitive set of alternatives is positioned for consumers.

Branding

When offering any product, a company needs to decide how it will be branded. A **brand** is any name, term, colors, or symbol that distinguishes one seller's product from another.[20] A brand name can be spoken, such as the names Chevrolet, GlaxoSmithKline, or Crest; or it can be recognized, such as the apple for Apple Computer or the greyhound for the Greyhound Bus Company. A **trade name** is the commercial name under which a company does business.[21] A **trademark** is a brand name or trade name given legal protection. Services use a service mark in the same way.

To be protected, a trademark must have a distinctive meaning, must be used in interstate commerce, and not be confused with other registered trademarks. Service names cannot be registered unless they describe a particular business, nor can terms that are primarily descriptive, such as "medical services," be registered.[22] In health care, most organizations use their trade name as opposed to a brand name. Yet as more health care organizations produce alternative plans and products, brand names are becoming more common.

Branding is important to consumers because it helps them to identify the product as coming from a particular source. There is a growing recognition of the added value a brand name gives a product through associations made by the consumer. This added value is referred to as **brand equity**.[23] The Mayo Clinic's trade name has significant brand equity. The clinic uses this name on its health newsletter, which is sold by subscription to consumers.

Branding Strategies

There are several strategies a company can use in branding a product or service. These are referred to as multiproduct, multibrand, reseller, or mixed strategies.

Multiproduct Strategy

In using a **multiproduct branding strategy**, the company places one brand name on all the products in its line. This strategy is common to companies such as Honda, which puts its name on its cars, lawn mowers, motorcycles, and home generators. This is also common strategy for health care organizations. A hospital puts its name on the outpatient surgery center, its walk-in emergency centers, and its industrial medicine program. The rationale for this approach is the use of brand equity. Knowing the brand name, consumers have confidence that the new product should work as well as other items in the line. Honda cars are reliable; therefore, so are Honda lawn mowers. Using a well-known name should lead to reduced promotional expenses in any new product introduction.

The risks for a multiproduct strategy, however, are significant. Because the organization uses one name for all items in the line, each new product puts the brand equity at risk. Companies that follow this strategy must ensure that the new product meets the quality standards for which the company is known. Otherwise, a failure in one item may negatively affect other similarly branded products.

Multibrand Strategy

In a **multibrand strategy** the company places a different name on each item. This approach is followed by Proctor and Gamble, which manufactures four different laundry detergents (Tide, Cheer, Ivory Snow, and Oxydol) and toothpastes such as Crest and Gleam. Companies follow this strategy when they are manufacturing products that appeal to different market segments. For example, a specialty health clinic, which has historically been known for sophisticated, high-technology care, may enter the primary care market by opening satellite clinics. Establishing those satellites under a different brand name may by advisable because the historical image of the group is so strong in one particular aspect of care. Extending to primary care may seem inconsistent, or consumers may think the new clinics will not be price competitive. The downside to a multibrand strategy is that each brand must establish consumer recognition. Promotional costs thus tend to be higher and the introductory period of the life cycle may take longer.

Reseller and Mixed Strategies

In a **reseller strategy**, one company sells its product under the name of another company. Sears Roebuck sells Craftsman tools and Kenmore appliances. Sears has no manufacturing facilities—these products are made by other companies and sold under the Sears name. Companies use this strategy when the reseller appeals to a strong segment of the market, or, if the reseller's market segments are different from the manufacturer's. In a mixed strategy, a company offers a product under the name of the reseller and under its own brand name. Michelin makes tires that are sold under its own name and that are also marketed under the Sears name.

Co-branding

A relatively new branding strategy in health care is **co-branding**, whereby the organization markets its name along side another brand name. This strategy has occurred outside of health care for some years. For example, Ford has marketed its Explorer with the Eddie Bauer brand; Lexus advertises its seats with Coach Luggage. The advantage is the synergistic effect of two positive brand names. An additional effect that has also been cited is to maximize the marketing budget of the organization by creating partnerships. When the partners are properly matched, this can stretch the marketing budget effect of both organizations. Yale New Haven Hospital, for example, partnered with VHA Inc., Bayer, Eli Lilly, New Haven Savings Bank, Southern New England Telephone, WTNH Channel 8, and AstraZeneca to help underwrite its Women's Heart Advantage Program in March 2001 to encourage women to with possible symptoms of a heart attack to seek immediate and appropriate medical care. In its first year, the program received more than 500 calls a month to its Women's Heart Line, saw awareness of heart disease as women's number one killer rise from 26% to 39%, and saw the percentage of women discussing heart disease with their doctor increase from 12% to 17%.[24]

In offering any new product or service to the market, a major concern is gaining initial product acceptance. A key component is the product's first buyers. If a product cannot obtain initial buyer interest, it will never reach the growth stage of the life cycle.

The Diffusion of Innovation

Consumers differ in the amount of time they require before adopting a new product. The rate at which a product is adopted by the market is called the **diffusion of innovation**. Research in rural sociology and marketing has shown that consumers can be classified in one of five categories, based on the time at which they adopt a product.[25] Shown in FIGURE 8-9, these categories include: innovators, early adopters, early majority, late majority, and laggards. The characteristics of these groups also differ.

Innovators. These consumers are the first to adopt a new product. Innovators tend to be risk takers who are highly educated and who use multiple information sources.
Early Adopters. These are people who are leaders in their social setting. They tend to be respected by their peers and are turned to for information by slower

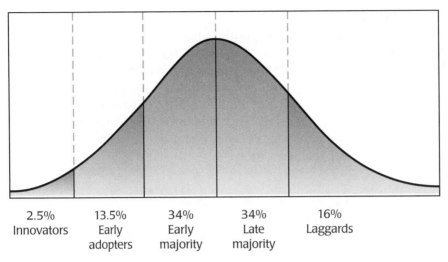

| 2.5%
Innovators | 13.5%
Early
adopters | 34%
Early
majority | 34%
Late
majority | 16%
Laggards |

Time of Adoption Innovations

FIGURE 8-9 The Diffusion of Innovation

adopting groups. Early adopters act as opinion leaders and are above average in education.

Early and Late Majority. These two groups represent the bulk of the population. The early majority are deliberate decision makers who have many informal social contacts. The late majorities are far more skeptical of new products and are below average in social and economic status.

Laggard. This group represents the last people to adopt. They have a strong fear of debt and are price conscious. Their sources of information are primarily family and close friends. This group tends to be tradition-bound.[26]

Most companies develop profiles of the innovators and early adopters. This strategy has been closely followed by health care company sales forces who try to identify which nurse or physician groups might be the most likely to adopt and have the greatest influence on their hospital staffs. Companies send these groups information on new products or invite them to conferences where new product announcements are made. Lyons has suggested four tips for identifying physician opinion leaders:

1. Be a detective. Question physicians to identify the roles colleagues play. Whom would they call to determine what is going on?
2. Find the power brokers, both formal and informal leaders.
3. Focus on the dominant, long-standing referral patterns and potential threats. Reviewing patterns can help identify who has the power.
4. Identify the main leader who assumes the role of motivator.[27]

Factors Affecting Adoption

There are several factors that determine the speed at which a new product is adopted by consumers. These are: relative advantage, compatibility, complexity, divisibility, and communicability.[28]

Relative Advantage

This dimension refers to the perceived benefit or advantage that a new product has over existing products, or over substitutable goods in the market. The more the product has a noticeable and valued relative advantage, the quicker it will be adopted. Health care providers quickly recognized the benefits of arthroscopic surgery on recovery time for simple knee operations. In a short period of time, the hospital lengths of stay for these procedures dropped as surgeons adopted this new invasive technique.

Compatibility

A product that is compatible with existing values or customs will be adopted more quickly than one that is not. Among older consumers, the early adoption of microwave ovens was rather slow. The manner in which foods are cooked in microwaves was inconsistent with long-used methods and recipes.

Complexity

A product's complexity will affect its rate of adoption. More complex products are accepted at a slower rate.

Divisibility

A product's divisibility is the degree to which the product can be tried on a limited basis. In consumer product marketing, divisibility can be offered through the use of samples. In health care services this is more difficult to achieve. Many hospitals have offered educational seminars as a way to help consumers experience the hospital staff and the nontechnical components of the service.

Communicability

The easier a product's benefits can be communicated, the quicker the rate of adoption. In a health education workshop, the best form of communication to generate corporate interest in enrolling employees in a new health plan would show that lower health care costs are possible.

■ Conclusions

The product component of the marketing mix is the element around which other strategic decisions are made. An organization must initially determine the breadth and depth of its product or service mix. Compared to products, services have some unique elements which, by their very nature, make their marketing more challenging. In either instance, it is essential to recognize the life cycle position of a product or service and the range of strategic options available at each stage. Complicating the life cycle analysis is the reality that the life cycle has various forms. Regardless of the form, however, the health care organization must make decisions regarding product positioning and branding. As the health care marketplace becomes increasingly competitive, the challenge for all organizations will be to facilitate the diffusion of their new market entries.

■ Key Terms

Nondurable Good
Durable Good
Services
Customer Contact Audit
Consumer Goods
Industrial Products
Convenience Goods
Shopping Goods
Specialty Items
Production Goods
Support Goods
Product Mix
Product Lines
Breadth
Depth
Cannibalization
Product Life Cycle
Skimming Price

Penetration Price
Primary Demand
Selective Demand
High Learning Product
Low Learning Product
Product Modification
Market Modification
Product Positioning
Brand
Trade Name
Trademark
Brand Equity
Multiproduct Branding Strategy
Multibrand Strategy
Reseller Strategy
Co-branding
Diffusion of Innovation

■ Chapter Summary

1. Products and services differ in terms of tangibility. Services can also be distinguished by five Is; intangibility, inconsistency, inseparability, inventory, and interaction.
2. Consumer goods can be differentiated by the amount of effort and manner of search the consumer uses in purchasing the product. Industrial goods are classified as either production or support goods. Service distinctions depend on whether they are delivered by people or by equipment.
3. When establishing the product element of the marketing mix, a company must decide its product mix, product line, and its breadth and depth.
4. All products and services can be described as having a life cycle consisting of four stages: introduction, growth, maturity, and decline. While there is a generalized product life cycle, variations also exist.

5. The length of the product life cycle is affected by uncontrollable forces such as technology and demographics. An organization can impact its sales in each life cycle stage relative to the competition through the effectiveness of its marketing mix strategy.

6. In the early stages of the product life cycle, a new entrant can price high to skim only the most likely buyers, or penetrate the largest market by pricing low.

7. Organizations can stretch the life cycle in the mature phase through either product or market modification.

8. An organization's brand name, if well known and regarded, can have value or equity in the marketplace. In deciding upon the brand name, a firm can pursue a multiproduct, multibrand, reseller, or mixed strategy, co-branding.

9. Acceptance of a product is the result of its diffusion through the population. Individuals differ in terms of the rate at which they accept new products.

10. The rate of adoption of a new product is affected by perception of relative advantage, compatibility, complexity, divisibility, and communicability.

■ Chapter Problems

1. A large academic medical center was interviewing candidates for the position of marketing director. One interviewee was a vice president of marketing for a large consumer food product firm. During the interview, the interviewee was asked what skills he had for the position. He responded, "I've sold products all my life and have been successful. Marketing a food product is no different than marketing a hotel, airline, or hospital." Explain to this candidate how this view might be naive.

2. How would you array the following organizations in terms of the depth and breadth of their product lines: (a) a solo-practice family practitioner who does not deliver babies, (b) a multi-specialty group practice that provides primary care at five satellite locations, (c) an academic medical center, and (d) Shouldice Hospital in Toronto, which specializes in short-stay surgery for hernia repair.

3. Listed below are three different organizations at various stages of the product life cycle. Explain the strategy considerations they might undertake for the specific marketing mix variable listed.

Organization	Life Cycle Stage	Marketing Mix Variable
1. Prucare, a managed care plan entering a new metropolitan area	Introduction	Promotion
2. HealthStop, an urgent care clinic offering minor ED treatment	Mature	Product
3. Community Hospital, a 234-bed facility with seven pediatric beds	Decline	Product

4. Explain how the advertising copy for a managed care plan would look if it were trying to develop primary demand. How would the advertising copy change to develop selective demand?

5. A large community hospital, River Valley, has recently begun to acquire physician practices. At issue is whether to rename each acquired practice "River Valley Associates" or to leave each name alone. What are the trade-offs River Valley should consider in this decision?

6. A company has decided to offer a health savings account plan to its employees. This new option is the first such type of coverage available in the market. Based on the factors that affect the diffusion of innovation, how might the company best accomplish the successful roll-out of this new health coverage option?

■ Notes

1. V. A. Zeithaml, A. Parasuraman, and L. L. Berry, "Problems and Strategies in Services Marketing," *Journal of Marketing* 49, no. 2 (Spring 1985): 33–46.

2. M. J. Bitner, B. H. Bloom, and M. S. Tetreault, "The Service Encounter: Diagnosing Favorable and Unfavorable Incidents," *Journal of Marketing* 54, no. 1 (1990): 71–84.

3. E. Sheuing, "Conducting Customer Service Audits," *Journal of Consumer Marketing* 6, no. 3 (Summer 1989): 35–41.

4. W. E. Sasser, R. P. Olsen, and D. D. Wyckoff, *Management of Service Operations* (Newton, MA: Allyn & Bacon, 1978).

5. This original classification was proposed by M. T. Copeland, "Relation of Consumer Buying Habits to Marketing Methods," *Harvard Business Review* 1, no. 3 (1923): 282–289.

6. D. R. E. Thomas, "Strategy Is Different in Service Businesses," *Harvard Business Review* 56, no. 4 (1978): 158–165.

7. R. Weiss, "A Hospital That Is All Heart," *Health Progress* 74, no. 9 (1993): 60–61.

8. A comprehensive discussion of the product life cycle has been presented by D. R. Rink and J. E. Swan, "Product Life Cycle Research: A Literature Review," *Journal of Business Strategy* 5, no. 4 (Spring 1985): 218–242.

9. A. Waldman, "Subacute Care: Spreading the Word," *Healthcare Marketing Report* 12, no. 8 (1994): 6–8.

10. M. Luallin, "The 20-Minute Heart Check," *Marketer's Guidepost* (Spring 1994): 1, 8.

11. "Health Care in America: Trends in Utilization," U.S. Department of Health and Human Services, Centers for Disease Control, DHHS Pub. No. 2004-1031.

12. HMR Clips, *Healthcare Marketing Report* 12, no. 8 (1994): 6–8.

13. A. Waldman, "Kaiser Expands Choice with New Co-Op Products," *Healthcare Marketing Report* 12, no. 9 (1994): 6–7.

14. L. P. Feldman and A. L. Page, "Harvesting: The Misunderstood Exit Strategy," *Journal of Business Strategy* 5, no. 4 (Spring 1985): 79–85.

15. See W. E. Cox, Jr., "Product Life Cycles as Marketing Models," *Journal of Business* 40, no. 4 (1967): 375–384; and J. E. Swan and D. R. Rink, "Fitting Marketing Strategy to Various Product Life Cycles," *Business Horizons* 25, no. 1 (1982): 72–76.

16. C. R. Wasson, *Dynamic Competitive Strategies and Product Life Cycles* (Austin, TX: Austin Press, 1978), 53–64.

17. Ibid., 66.

18. Philip L. Ronning, "Lessons Learned from Heart Hospitals," *COR Healthcare Market Strategist 5*, no. 1 (January 2004): 9–15.

19. N. K. Dhalla and S. Yuspeh, "Forget the Product Life Cycle Concept," *Harvard Business Review 54*, no. 1 (1976): 102–112.

20. D. Bennett, *Dictionary of Marketing Terms* (Chicago, IL: American Marketing Association, 1968), 18–19.

21. E. N. Berkowitz et al., *Marketing*, 6th ed. (Boston: Irwin/McGraw-Hill, 2000), 325.

22. D. Cohen, "Trademark Strategy Revisited," *Journal of Marketing 55*, no. 3 (1991): 46–59.

23. For a detailed discussion of brand equity, see D. A. Aaker, *Brand Equity* (New York: The Free Press, 1991).

24. William Gombeski, Clayton Medeiros, Robert Serow, and Kelley Tice, "The Buddy System," *Hospitals and Health Networks*, Hospitals Connect.com (November 12, 2003). (http://www.hhnmag.com/hhnmag/hospitalconnect/search/article.jsp?dcrpath=AHA/PubsNewsArticle/data/031202HHN_Online_Gombeski&domain=HHNMAG#anchor450147).

25. This concept was presented by E. Rogers, *Diffusion of Innovations* (New York: Free Press of Glencoe, 1962), 81–86.

26. E. M. Rogers, *Diffusion of Innovations*, 3rd ed. (New York: Free Press, 1982), 246–261.

27. M. F. Lyons, "Trying to Get a Fix on Your Medical Staff? Sometimes, It Pays To Go Underground," *Medical Staff Strategy Report 3*, no. 2 (1994): 6–7.

28. These factors are drawn from S. L. Lampert, "Word-of-Mouth Activity during the Introduction of a New Food Product," in *Consumer Behavior Theory and Application*, ed. J. U. Farley, et al. (Newton, MA: Allyn & Bacon, 1974), 82; and J. R. Mancuso, "Why Not Create Opinion Leaders for New Product Introductions," *Journal of Marketing* 33, no. 3 (1969): 20–25.

Price

Learning Objectives

After reading this chapter you should be able to:

- Appreciate the many factors that affect pricing decisions
- Recognize the array of alternative pricing strategies available to health care marketers
- Calculate break-even pricing
- Learn the positioning value of price

■ The Meaning of Price

In its simplest form, **price** is the level of monetary reimbursement a firm demands for its goods or services. From a marketing viewpoint, the price also represents the economic value that the buyer provides to the producer in exchange for a product or service. A company's main priority is to establish a price that corresponds to the level of value that the consumer perceives in the service being offered. Yet, price is far more than just an economic indicator of a product's worth.

In establishing a price, companies realize that the established price has a perceptual or positioning value for the service.[1] Higher prices often connote better quality. Yet in establishing the price, a company must also consider the competitive dynamics of the marketplace. Price can affect consumer demand, as well as competitor response. As a result, the pricing decision is a major aspect of marketing strategy. In this discussion of price, it is important to recognize that the price of a product or service goes by many names. Companies such as Toro charge a *price* for their lawn mowers, physicians charge *fees* for their services, and universities charge *tuition*.

In the health care industry, the issue of price was rarely a marketing concern. Pricing was based on predetermined reimbursement formulas. Often, in deciding price, the main issue was determining where the reimbursement might be most favorable.

Considerations of competition or consumer perception of value were not factored into the strategic discussion of price. The health care environment of today, however, makes the pricing of services as challenging as product pricing in traditional industries. Health care organizations operate under a complex environment in which there is direct contracting, health savings account, a return to fee-for-service, and still the existence of managed care. In addition, many states have made pricing information available on the Internet. All these factors make pricing strategies difficult to formulate. Health care providers must be ever sensitive to what the buyer will consider a value for the medical or health service being provided. Competitive considerations have become a key component of the pricing decision, as the number of competing managed care players in the marketplace continues to increase. Based on coverage and deductibles, the old dictum that the consumer doesn't pay for health care is also no longer valid. A recent study has demonstrated that pricing is a particularly effective strategy for increasing hospital profitability when increases are made selectively rather than across the board.[2] Health care providers must consider the response of individual consumers and employers to likely charges and fees.

Moreover, in an age where price is a visible component of the marketing mix, states have begun to put pricing information on Web sites so that consumers can see how hospitals vary on the charges for particular services. No different than comparison shopping for other goods and services, the environment for price competition has dramatically increased. In 2005, the state of Wisconsin made available a Web site called Price Point, which compares hospitals on 60 common medical procedures (www.wipricepoint.org/).[3] Similar sites are available in Florida, South Dakota, and California. According to an article in the *Wall Street Journal*, physicians are also facing such scrutiny. Aetna has a tool on its Web site that helps consumers estimate the costs of office visits and certain medical tests based on different geographical areas.[4]

■ Establishing the Price

Establishing the price for a product or service effectively is a multistep process. Organizations must: (1) identify the constraints to their pricing policy; (2) determine their objectives; (3) estimate demand and revenue; (4) determine the cost, volume, and profit relationships; (5) select a pricing strategy; and (6) consider the positioning element to their final price.

Identifying Constraints

Ideally, one might suggest pricing a product high. Obviously, the higher the price, the greater the potential for profit. Yet in any pricing decision, several constraints must be recognized to temper the final price level established.

Demand

A major factor in establishing price is recognizing the demand for the product or service. Products in great demand can command a higher price. An interesting example of high demand and thus ultimately high-priced products was the introduction of the drug-device combination, drug-coated stent. The introductory price for this product was around $3000, approximately two to three times that of a traditional stent. However, its promise of a reduction in the incidence of restenosis was a major benefit to the payer, the insurance company, which as a result did not have to pay for as many bypass surgeries.[5]

Newness in the Life Cycle

In Chapter 8, the concept of the product life cycle was reviewed. Pricing considerations change over the length of time a product exists in the competitive market.[6] Pricing in the early stages of the life cycle depends on several variables. If the company has a limited capacity to meet demand, or if it needs to recoup investment costs prior to competitors entering the market (for a truly new service), it may select a higher price. If, however, an organization needs to generate volume to achieve an economy of scale, or if it wants to minimize the likelihood of competitive entries, it will establish a lower price level.

Typically, the newer a product is in the life cycle, the higher the price that can be charged. When a company holds a patent on a product—such as is common in the pharmaceutical industry—the greater the likelihood it will price the product high. Health care is a service-driven industry, with little ability to establish proprietary rights to what is being provided. This lack of sole providership has made higher pricing more difficult. Many states, however, have required filing a certificate of need or a determination of need, for example, when a hospital was establishing a new service that required significant capital expense. Once granted to a hospital, this certificate often served as a form of patent or franchise, since the state regulatory agencies try to cap the number of health care providers offering similar services. The regulators determined that duplication of services would lead to greater health care costs. In terms of competitive strategy, however, one can see that increasing the number of competitors would drive prices down.

Single- vs. Multiple-Product Pricing

Many organizations have more than one product or service in their product line. In pricing these products, a company must evaluate whether the products are **complementary**, in other words, whether the purchase of one product or service will affect the purchase of another item in the line. Organizations can employ multiple pricing strategies when they have complementary products. These are discussed more fully later in this chapter.

Production Cost

A fourth constraint in the pricing decision is the cost of production. A company must determine whether it has high fixed costs or high variable costs to consider in its pricing decisions. A more detailed discussion of the nature of production costs and the types of production costs is provided later in this chapter.

Channel Length

Pricing decisions cannot be made independent of consideration of the channel of distribution described in Chapter 10. The producer of a product or service, which is provided through resellers, must determine what the final price will be to the end consumer as the product is marked up throughout the distribution channel. Each member of the channel provides services and adds to the cost, and thus price, of the service at the next level.

Market Structure

Every pricing decision must reflect, to some degree, the nature of the market structure. As noted in Chapter 3, there are four basic types of market structure: pure monopoly, oligopoly, monopolistic competition, and pure competition.

A pure monopoly involves one seller who sets the price for a unique service. This situation existed historically in the communications industry when AT&T, at one time, was the sole provider of telephone service in the United States. It is still a common form of market structure in the energy industry, where one company supplies all of the local or regional demand for electricity or natural gas. There is no direct price competition in such a market. Usually, pure monopoly markets result in government or regulatory price control or review. Even in this type of market structure, however, a company must consider whether there are **substitutable goods**, or other products that can satisfy the same basic needs. For example, when the price of electricity rose in many northeastern states in the 1970s, many consumers switched their home heating source to natural gas or oil.

In an oligopoly—a market structure where a few companies control a majority of industry sales—there is often great awareness of competitors' pricing policies. There tends to be a price leader who dictates the direction of price levels. In the airline industry, for example, one company will occasionally raise fares and hope the others will follow suit, rather than induce a price war that erodes all sellers' margins. Similar situations have been reported in the health care industry when hospitals merge. It has also been reported that the price increases tend to be greater among for-profit hospitals when there are mergers than among nonprofit mergers in oligopolistic market conditions.[7]

Monopolistic competition exists in markets where many sellers offer substitutable products. These producers want their offerings to be viewed as unique and different from the competition. This shifts the focus of competition and consumer buying decisions away from price. In recent years, hospitals have focused on advertising their particularly unique services and amenities in an effort to create more of a monopolistic competition in the health care market.

As noted earlier, pure competition involves markets with many small producers and many small buyers—the typical market structure faced by many physicians in their office practices. There is relatively easy entry and exit from these markets, and buyers are supposed to have perfect information. This last characteristic tends not to exist in the real world. In a purely competitive market, price levels would be set by the market.

Pricing Objectives

In determining its pricing strategy, an organization must first specify its pricing objectives. There are several objectives that are relevant to pricing programs.

Profit

A common objective for many organizations is to price in a way to maximize profits. In following this objective, companies will utilize a skimming price strategy, especially in the introduction stage of the product life cycle, as discussed in Chapter 8. This strategy may be workable in the short term. An 11% across the board increase in hospital prices would typically generate a 25% increase in a hospital's operating profits.[8] The problem with a skimming strategy, however, is that while short-term profits can be maximized, the high price may encourage competitors to offer a similar service at a lower price and thereby capture market share. The original company that tried to maximize profits might end up with a small position in the market.

Sales

A second pricing objective is to maximize sales or volume. In following this objective, companies often employ a penetration pricing strategy, which involves setting a low price (as noted in Chapter 8) relative to the competition or to substitutable services. Sales are maximized. The value of this approach is apparent when the firm must meet some economies of scale. Morton Plant Health System in Clearwater, Florida, for example, lowered the price of mammography services from $55 to $39. The health system decided it could make up the price difference in higher patient volume. Between March and December 1993, 11,651 mammograms were performed, compared to 4199 in 1992.[9]

Unlike a skimming strategy, this approach discourages competition. Following the sales objective, however, requires a good knowledge of the cost curves. Generating sales that lead to a dollar loss will be a short-lived approach for any company.

Market Share

Many companies set their pricing strategy around the objective of gaining market share. This strategy is common in two different types of market conditions. In the early stages of competition for a new product or service, a market share objective is often important to achieve economies of scale to support the operation's overhead. This condition is true for managed care plans that have slashed premiums.[10] A second condition in which market share is often the objective is in industries that have no real growth. In these instances, the opportunities for increased revenue will come only from increasing market share relative to a competitor. Today, many acute care hospitals are aggressively competing with each other for managed care contracts in order to increase market share.

Image

The image a company wants to project is often tied up with its pricing objectives. One pricing strategy is called **prestige pricing**, in which a high price is established relative to the competition, or to the true cost of producing the service. The reason is to project an image of exclusivity or value. This strategy is common to products that are hard to differentiate in any other tangible way, such as liquor. Alternatively, Wal-Mart stores set their pricing strategy as one not to be undersold. Their image is that of a place where the price-conscious consumer shops.

Stabilization

A fifth pricing objective is to establish a price level that will encourage a similar response from competitors. Although overt agreement among competitors to set prices is illegal, a stabilization pricing objective can result in maintaining margins while encouraging competition on other elements of the marketing mix. This is especially true if the pricing strategy considers attributes important to consumers, such as convenience and quality.

Estimating Demand and Revenue

An essential step in establishing any price level is to estimate the demand for the company's product. A key aspect of this phase of pricing is to prepare a **demand schedule**, or summary of the amounts of a product that are desired at each price level. Understanding consumers' price sensitivity at various levels is where marketing research plays a critical role.[11]

In determining consumer response to price, marketers try to assess the degree of **price elasticity**, or change in demand relative to a change in price, which exists in the marketplace. Consumers are said to be price elastic when the percentage demand for a product exceeds the percentage change in price. Consumers are price inelastic when the percentage change in demand does not exceed the percentage change in price. FIGURE 9-1 shows the price elasticity of consumer demand as the monthly premium for a managed care organization (MCO) is lowered. Based on the curve, one can see that the demand is relatively price inelastic as the monthly premium is decreased from $200 per family per month to $170 (D2) per family per month. The number of subscribers

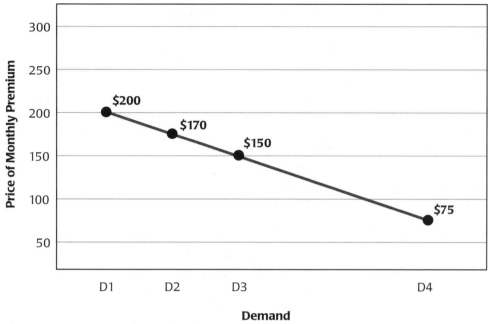

FIGURE 9-1 Price Elasticity for an MCO

increases dramatically as the premium begins to drop from $150 to $75 (D4). At this point demand might be considered price elastic. Researchers have found that patient price sensitivity differs, and utilization (thus it is elastic) differs not only by customer type but also by type of service. Preventive care and pharmaceuticals have been found to be price elastic.[12] The more that a marketer can position a product so that it is perceived as unique, the greater the likelihood that demand will be price inelastic. A company that positions itself as a high-quality provider can charge higher prices. Price elasticity is reduced when the customer perceives higher quality in the service.[13,14]

Cost and Volume Relationships

In establishing the price for a product, marketers must take into consideration the nature of the organization's costs. There are three cost concepts to consider: fixed costs, variable costs, and total cost. **Fixed costs** are those costs that do not change based on the volume of product or service delivered. For example, a hospital that buys a piece of laboratory equipment would incur a fixed cost for the equipment. Regardless of whether one or a hundred tests are performed with the equipment, the cost of the machinery is fixed. **Variable costs** are those costs that vary with the amount of the service delivered. Nursing personnel salaries are considered a variable cost. For example, if patient volume declines, the number of full-time-equivalent nurses can be reduced. **Total cost** represents the total expense that the firm bears in delivering and marketing its service. Total cost represents the combination of fixed and variable costs. With these concepts in mind, companies can consider the relationship between cost and volume in establishing prices.

Cost-Plus Pricing

One of the simplest approaches to setting price is the cost-plus method, in which the selling price represents the total cost of the service, *plus* some additional amount for profit. While simple in methodology, cost-plus pricing does not consider the differences between fixed and variable costs.

EXHIBIT 9-1 shows the cost/price relationships that must be recognized. In a high fixed-cost organization to total cost, the major consideration is to price for volume. With high variable costs compared to total cost, an organization must price for margin.

Consider the example of the airline industry, in which fixed costs are a high percentage of total costs. Its major concern is to price in such a way to ensure the coverage of fixed costs. As a result, the airline offers significant consumer fare discounts in order to cover fixed costs, if consumers purchase tickets well in advance of their scheduled travel times. This point is shown as T1 in FIGURE 9-2. As the airline comes closer to covering its fixed costs (T2), prices rise; the additional revenue generated now contributes to profit. Finally, departure time arrives, and the airplane is ready to leave the gate (T3). Because an empty seat is a wasted seat, it is not long before the airline reduces the fare for a consumer willing to hop on the plane as a last-minute standby.

This same type of pricing as a reflection of production costs is followed by arts organizations. These entities provide subscriber discounts if tickets are purchased several months prior to the performance. Ticket prices rise as the date of the show draws closer. Then, many theater groups will offer significant customer discounts for last-minute rushes for seats as the curtain rises. Similarly, Rick Scott, chief executive officer of Hospital Corporation of America, a Nashville-based organization that owns over 200 hospitals in the United States, has discussed the possibility of discounted midnight surgery. Recognizing the high fixed cost of an unused operating room suite, this approach could result in some surgeries being scheduled during off-hours at a lower price. The target market might be self-paying individuals or those whose insurance coverage carries high deductibles.[15] FIGURE 9-3 shows the implications of loading

Exhibit 9-1   Cost/Price Relationships

High Fixed Cost/Total Cost = Volume Sensitive

High Variable Cost/Total Cost = Margin Sensitive

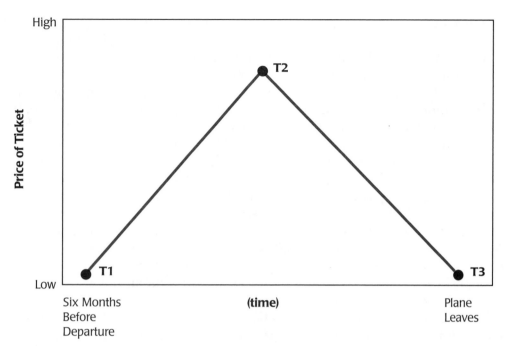

FIGURE 9-2 Covering Fixed Cost: The Airline Case

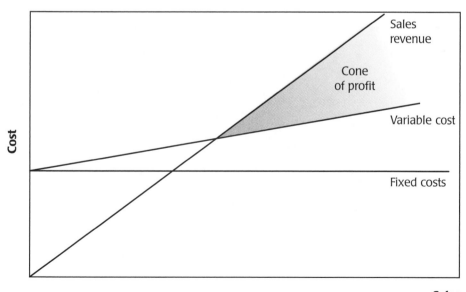

FIGURE 9-3 Profit Effect of Volume Loading

volume with a high fixed cost structure (hospitals) and the resultant reasoning behind the strategy suggested by Rick Scott in discounting surgery at midnight. Increasing sales revenue has a dramatic implication since there is little variable cost in the business.

Consider this cost-plus scenario: An airline wants to price its tickets at 50% above the cost of each flight. The cost of a flight (maintenance, salaries, landing rights, etc.) is $5000. In addition, the cost of meals, snacks, and beverages is $2 per passenger. If 150 seats on the plane are occupied, the total cost of the flight is over $5000 (150 × $2 = $5300). Adding 50% profit would yield a total cost of over $5000 (50% × $5000 = $7500). Since this cost is based on the assumed volume of 150 passengers, the price per ticket would be $7500/150 = $50.

If, however, only 100 passengers show up for the flight, total cost does not change very much. As described, the fixed cost represents a higher proportion of total cost. Yet, in this instance, total revenue changes dramatically. With only 100 passengers, the airline's total revenue for the flight is $5000 ($50 per ticket × 100 passengers). The airline would not cover the total cost of the flight, which is $5200 [$5000 + ($2 × 100)].

The opposite of a high fixed cost–to–total cost ratio is the firm whose variable costs are a higher proportion of the total cost of production. With these companies, small increases in margin can result in significant increases in profit. Look at FIGURE 9-4 to see the dramatic shift in the cone of profit in a low fixed cost, high variable cost business. In this situation it is not so much volume that drives the profitability of the business but a shift in margin that can lead to a dramatic increase or decrease in overall profitability.

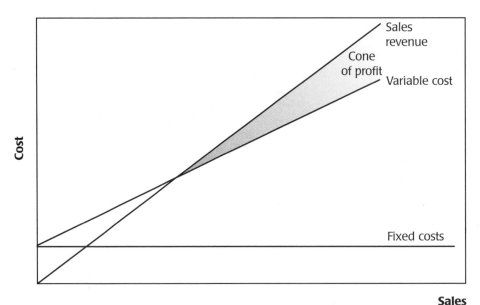

FIGURE 9-4 Profit Effect of High Variable Cost

Break-Even Analysis

An alternative concept that considers the level of sales required at a given price to cover total costs is referred to as **break-even analysis**. Using this price-setting method, a company determines the break-even point needed to cover total costs. This point is derived by the following equation:

$$\text{B. E. P. (break-even point)} = \frac{\text{Total Fixed Cost}}{[\text{Price} - \text{Variable Cost}]}$$

The break-even point is that point of volume where total revenue equals total cost.

Consider the example of the free-standing surgery center shown in Table 9-1. In this case, the average price per procedure is $500. Because of the contractual arrangement with MCOs, a 10% discount is required. Annual fixed costs total $500,000, and variable costs are $200 per procedure. The volume of procedures now necessary to operate the facility at break-even point is 2000. Consider what happens if a higher price or lower discount were possible. At a charge of $500 with no discount, the break-even point drops to only 1667 procedures to cover costs and break even.[16]

At this point it is important for the free-standing surgery center management to recognize the linkage between the break-even point and market share. Identifying varying break-even volumes, the organization should consider what percentage of the market it can attract, and what discount levels are required by buyers (managed care

Table 9-1	Free-Standing Surgicenter: Cost Structure
Factors	Costs ($)
Break-even analysis	
Average price per procedure	500
Average discount or allowance (10%)	− 50
Net price per procedure	450
Annual fixed cost (depreciation, interest, utilities, management, etc.)	500,000
Variable cost per procedure	200
Break-even computation	
Net price per procedure	450
Variable cost per procedure	−200
Contribution margin per procedure	250 (A)
Fixed cost	500,000 (B)
Break-even number of procedures (B divided by A)	2000

Source: Keith B. Pitts, "Pricing and Reimbursement Strategies," *Topics in Health Care Finance,* Vol. 12, No. 1 (Fall 1985), pp. 24–31.

plans). In this way, an organization can assess the likelihood of generating revenue and the pressures on the ultimate price. For example, if the low price represents a competitive market price—most other competitors discount surgery $75—this constraint must be considered. Yet, if this price level represents a break-even volume of almost 75% of all surgery cases, the venture might be considered too risky to enter.

Marginal Cost Pricing

Marginal cost pricing is based on the concept that the price per additional procedure must equal or exceed the cost of an additional procedure. In Table 9-1, the $200 per procedure variable cost equals the marginal cost of each additional procedure.

To understand a marginal cost pricing approach, consider the data shown in Table 9-2, which evaluates the marginal, or variable, cost per procedure. As is common today, assume that the surgery center negotiates with an MCO. This managed care plan guarantees at least 600 procedures, at $325 per procedure. This price exceeds the marginal cost ($200), but it is below the level of the full price with the discount as shown earlier in Table 9-1. Complicate this scenario by assuming that the MCO purchases 100 procedures at the higher price. Table 9-3 shows the impact of increased volume at reduced price and the profitability of entering into the contract. This marginal cost approach is useful in considering appropriate pricing strategies to attract large-volume purchasers.

Table 9-2	Free-Standing Surgicenter: Variable Cost Analysis		
Expenses	Full Cost	Fixed Cost	Variable Cost
Salaries	$350,000	$140,000	$210,000
Fringe benefits	50,000	20,000	30,000
Supplies	160,000	6,000	154,000
Maintenance and repairs	10,000	8,000	2,000
Utilities	30,000	28,000	2,000
Administrative and general	40,000	38,000	2,000
Housekeeping	20,000	20,000	—
Property taxes	10,000	10,000	—
Depreciation	130,000	130,000	—
Interest	100,000	100,000	—
Total	$900,000	$500,000	$400,000
Number of break-even procedures	2000	2000	2000
Cost per procedure	$ 450	$ 250	$ 200

Source: Keith B. Pitts, "Pricing and Reimbursement Strategies," *Topics in Health Care Finance,* Vol. 12, No. 1 (Fall 1985), pp. 24–31.

Table 9-3	Free-Standing Surgicenter: Impact of Volume Increase		
	Break-even at 1000 Procedures	Impact of 500 Additional Procedures	Total Income at 1500 Procedures
Revenues			
Current	$900,000	$ —	$ 900,000
Incremental (600 @ $325)	—	195,000	195,000
Lost revenue (100 @ $450)	—	− 45,000	− 45,000
Total	900,000	150,000	1,050,000
Expenses			
Salaries	350,000	52,500	402,500
Fringe benefits	50,000	7,500	57,500
Supplies	160,000	38,500	198,500
Maintenance and repairs	10,000	500	10,500
Utilities	30,000	500	30,500
Administrative and general	40,000	500	40,500
Housekeeping	20,000	—	20,000
Property taxes	10,000	—	10,000
Depreciation	130,000	—	130,000
Interest	100,000	0	100,000
Total	900,000	100,000	1,000,000
Net income	$ 0	$ 50,000	$ 50,000

Source: Keith B. Pitts, "Pricing and Reimbursement Strategies," *Topics in Health Care Finance,* Vol. 12, No. 1 (Fall 1985), pp. 24–31.

Markup Pricing

Markup pricing involves calculating the per-unit cost of producing the service or product and determining the markup percentages needed to cover the cost of selling and profit. This pricing scheme is often used by wholesalers and retailers. The formula for markup pricing is:

$$\text{Price} = \frac{\text{Service Cost}}{(100 - \text{Markup Percent})/100}$$

For example, if a physician pays $6 for lab tests and needs a 40% markup to cover costs, the price billed to a patient's insurance company for the test would be:

$$\text{Price} = \frac{\$6.00}{(100 - 40)/100}$$

In 2004, California passed a law that requires hospitals to show their list prices for what they charge for their full range of services and products. It has revealed a dramatic difference across hospitals for the same service. For example, a chest x-ray (two views, basic) has been found to cost $120.90 at Scripps, LaJolla, to $790 in Sutter General to $1519 at Doctor's Hospital in Modesto. Doctor's Hospital of Modesto was highlighted in an earlier study in 2003 when it was found to mark up its gross charges 1092% over its costs, meaning the hospital would bill a patient $10,920 for a procedure that would cost the facility $1000.[17] In the late 1960s hospitals were fairly straightforward in terms of using markup pricing but shifted to a more complicated formula as health maintenance organizations (HMOs) entered the market and negotiated discounts. Now, many hospitals are trying to return to a more reasoned markup pricing approach.[18]

Target Pricing

A fourth pricing strategy, **target pricing**, involves setting price to provide a targeted rate of return on investment for a standard level of service delivery or production. For example, a hospital may have an average rate of occupancy of 60%. The hospital might compute a target price for services directly paid with the following formula:

$$\text{Price} = \frac{\text{Investment Costs} \times \text{Target Return on Investment (\%)}}{\text{Standard Volume}}$$

Target pricing is common in production firms that are capital intensive. A major limitation to this method, however, is that price is set with no consideration of market demand, and thus, all the volume needed to generate the target return might not be forthcoming.

Demand-Minus Pricing

A final pricing strategy that is becoming more relevant for health care providers with the advent of managed care is **demand-minus pricing**, which involves determining what price the market is willing to pay and working backwards to compute costs. This pricing concept focuses on a major difference in pricing considerations between financial officers in health care organizations and marketing professionals. Typically, health care prices have been set, based on the costs the facility estimated in providing the service. In fact, 20 years ago, hospitals were reimbursed under a procedure called *cost-based reimbursement*. Subsequent reform dictated that hospitals would be paid for services based on diagnosis-related groups (DRGs). This reimbursement mechanism paid a price to treat a disease. Yet, in fact, hospital reimbursement under the DRG system was based on average historical costs.

Under the prevailing managed care models, health care organizations are competing for contracts. Employers and individual consumers who enroll in individual health plans care little about what it costs to provide the service. Rather the determining factor is the buyers' own respective price ceiling, or limit, that they are willing to pay. Past distinctions of inpatient charges, outpatient charges, and the like are irrelevant to the consumer. Health care providers must identify through market research the maximum price a buyer is willing to pay for a bundle of services. The organization must then calculate the markup percentage it needs to cover selling expenses and desired profits. Then, the maximum permissible cost can be computed through the following formula:

$$\text{Maximum Service Cost} = \text{Price} \times [(100 - \text{Markup Percent})/100]$$

Dallas Medical Resource (D.M.R.) is using this pricing strategy with participating hospitals. D.M.R. is a nonprofit corporation comprised of nine major Dallas health care providers and major Texas employers. Employers set prices, and the providers decide whether they can meet them. Fina, Inc., a Dallas-based, integrated oil and chemical company, proposed a global price for coronary artery bypass procedures, hip and knee replacements, and neck surgery. The D.M.R.–affiliated hospitals accepted this market price.[19]

Pricing Strategies

There are several types of pricing strategies that firms can use. Many of those discussed in the following pages have not been applied previously to health care, but this is changing as the health care regulatory environment and marketplace evolves. Health care organizations that sell managed care products and services in the marketplace are behaving more like retailers.

Price Lining

One price strategy is **price lining**, in which products in a line are priced within a distinct price range that is significantly different from the prices of substitutes in the next range. The purpose of this strategy is to give the consumer the impression that quality differences exist between the price lines. This pricing strategy works best under conditions where the consumer has little prior experience with the product or service or lacks the expertise to evaluate the service objectively. For many years, for example, Sears Roebuck operated with three distinct price lines of *good*, *better*, and *best* for its home appliances and household items.

Price lines make it easier for consumers to shop because they can consider the level of product quality they want to buy. For price lining to be effective, however, consumers must perceive a significant difference between the items in each line in terms of quality. When making changes in price lines, marketers must be aware of the fact that a change in one aspect of the line can affect the entire price line.[20]

Odd Pricing

A second pricing strategy has been referred to as **odd pricing**, in which items are priced at just below whole dollar amounts. Perusing the shelves of any supermarket, one will notice the vast array of items marked with prices ending in 5, 7, or 9. Several reasons have been posited for odd pricing. One rationale suggested is that of pluralistic ignorance—one retailer does it because the other competitor is following this strategy. There is no real logic to the approach, however. A second, more plausible, explanation for odd pricing pertains to in-store theft. Odd prices require the cashier to make change for the customer. In so doing, the clerk must record the sale on the cash register and enter the cash drawer in the presence of the customer. If the item were priced at $1 or $5, the customer might just hand the clerk a bill of the correct amount and leave the store. The cashier could then just not record the sale and pocket the money. A third reason suggested for odd pricing is that it gives the impression that the item has been discounted from a higher price.[21] For example, $4.99 suggests a markdown as opposed to $5.

The final explanation for odd pricing is based on a theory of how consumers shop. **Item budget theory** suggests that consumers set out with a predetermined price that they are willing to pay for a particular item. Any item just below this predetermined price will be deemed acceptable. If the item is priced even slightly above that amount, however, it will be considered too expensive. For example, a consumer decides to shop for a new business suit and decides to pay no more than $400. Seeing a suit priced at $420, the consumer would find the price unacceptable. Priced at $395, however, the suit would fit within the shopper's budgeted amount.

For health care providers, this last explanation of odd pricing based on item budget theory is extremely relevant for pricing health care services in today's marketplace. Through marketing research, providers must determine the item budgeted amount that a consumer feels is acceptable for a monthly health plan premium, or for a routine mammogram not covered by insurance.

One-Price versus Flexible Pricing

With a **one-price policy**, the company charges the same price to all customers who buy the service under the same set of conditions. Discounts may be provided for the timing of the purchase or the level of volume; however, all customers have the opportunity to avail themselves of these discounts. This policy instills customer confidence, and it is also easy to administer.

A second variation is the **flexible pricing policy**, in which customers are charged different prices based on their ability to negotiate or on their respective buying power. This strategy is common in the automobile industry where, based on the ability to haggle, a customer might get a lower price than another person purchasing the same car. Recently, because many consumers find this strategy uncomfortable, some automobile dealers have begun promoting one-price policies. Flexible pricing is common in industrial settings where the consumer's buying power can often result in lower prices. The major concern here, however, is to ensure the legality of the pricing policy according to the Robinson-Patman Act, as described in Chapter 3.

Prestige Pricing

A fourth pricing strategy described earlier in this chapter is prestige pricing, in which items are deliberately priced at a high level to connote uniqueness or value. This pricing strategy goes against the typical economic logic of the rational buyer who purchases more as the price declines. The demand curve for prestige pricing is shown in FIGURE 9-5. As can be seen, at price level P1 demand is D1. Yet as the price rises to P2, demand increases rather than decreases to D2. At some point, however, if the price should increase to too high a level (P3), demand will again decrease to a low level again (D1).

Prestige pricing is a strategy often followed for products or services where it is difficult to distinguish real quality differences or where the perceived risk of purchasing is high.[22] For many years, for example, L'Oreal hair coloring has been promoted on the basis of "It costs more, but I'm worth it." Again, the risk of health care services might provide some logic to prestige pricing, along with the fact that it is hard for the average consumer to discern the quality differences of the service delivered. The only limiting constraint to prestige pricing as discussed at the beginning of this chapter is that the price must not be so high as to generate little demand.

Leader Pricing

Leader pricing is a strategy of attractively pricing an item in the product line and aggressively promoting it to encourage consumers to purchase it and also other items in

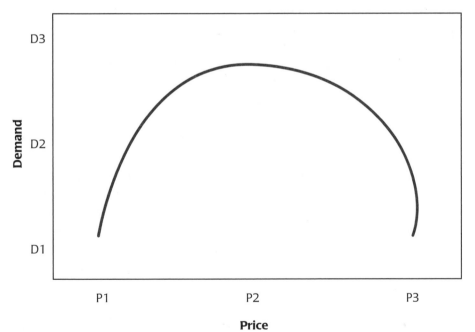

FIGURE 9-5 Prestige Pricing Demand Curve

the line at the same time. This strategy is often implemented by grocery stores. Popular brand-name items are priced low to get consumers into the store, who then complete their grocery shopping by purchasing items priced at more favorable margins for the retailer.

For leader pricing to be successful, the consumer must recognize the promoted price to be a significant value, and the item must be desired.

Bundled Pricing

Bundled pricing or packaged pricing involves selling several items or services together for one total price.[23,24] This strategy has been common in health care for occupational and industrial medicine programs. Companies are offered an array of services—such as health education for employees, pre-employment physicals, job hazard analysis, and toxicology support—for a set price per employee.

For price bundling to be effective, the savings on the bundle must be seen as a real value as opposed to buying the services individually.[25] The University of Alabama at Birmingham provided an example of bundled pricing within its joint replacement center. Patients are able to "purchase" a three-night package that includes staying in a room designed similar to a high quality hotel, arriving the night before surgery. They receive gourmet meals in a communal setting along with other joint replacement patients, and a special nursing staff member is assigned to them.[26] Internationally, this approach is being increasingly used. For example, in Asia, bundled pricing is a common strategy of Gleneagles Hospital of Singapore (owned by Parkway Hospital System). This hospital provides a bundled price of $10,500 for a six-day stay for a total knee replacement (www.gleneagles.com.sg/). At Bangkok Hospital, a coronary artery bypass graft off-pump with a 5–7 night stay and a follow-up is approximately $8500 (U.S.) with free pick-up service at the airport (www.bangkokhospital.com/). Mouwasat Hospital in Dammam has an extensive package pricing program it touts on its Web site in the Mideast (www.mouwasat.com.sa/).

Package Deals

Mouwasat started package deal prices in 1997 for the most common surgical procedures and deliveries (normal and Caesarean section). The package deal price will be applied when the patient is admitted for any surgical procedure [that] comes under a package deal. The following are some of our package deal programmes:

- *Maternity and delivery programme*
- *Comprehensive medical screening*
- *Pre employment screening*
- *Pre school screening*
- *Breast screening*
- *Well women and men programmes*[27]

Thus the bundled price approach for health care services appears to be a viable and consistent strategy across the globe. It also appears to be one that may well gain in attractiveness for patients in the United States who might seek care outside of this country from highly skilled medical professionals who can offer their services in a very price-competitive, high-quality setting.

In the "unbundled pricing," a company breaks down the price of the items to be purchased individually. Increasingly in health care, providers are offering customers the opportunity to tailor the product line by offering both pricing strategies.

Going-Rate Pricing

Going-rate pricing is a pricing strategy that involves setting prices relative to the prevailing market price with less consideration for internal costs or margin requirements. This strategy has been common in oligopolistic industries where there are only a few sellers who sell relatively similar items. This situation somewhat describes the hospital competitive environment of the 1970s before many institutions tried to differentiate themselves in terms of the services provided.

Discounts

In many situations, companies often provide discounts, or price reductions, to buyers. There are four common types of discounts: volume, functional, seasonal, or allowances.

Volume or Quantity Discounts

Volume discounts are provided to buyers who purchase the service or guarantee to utilize the service at some predetermined level. Studies have demonstrated that MCOs and HMOs have been effective in gaining discounts based on their effectiveness to shift volumes of patients or channeling patients.[28,29] Legally, volume discounts must be offered equally to all buyers. To offer volume discounts, the seller must be able to demonstrate that there are real cost savings that can be achieved if the service is utilized at some specified volume level.

Functional Discounts

Functional discounts on price are offered if the buyer agrees to perform or take over particular functions involved with the product or service. For example, if a manufacturer agreed to provide onsite space for the administration of routine employee exams or for a nurse practitioner to meet with employees, this might be factored into a discount. An employer might also receive a discount if it agrees to distribute all health plan promotional material internally to its employees.

Seasonal Discounts

These are price reductions provided when the product is purchased out of season. The objective of a seasonal discount is to smooth out demand. Hotels offer special discounts on weekends when business travel use is light. Golf equipment manufacturers will run winter sales to stimulate demand in off-peak times in order to keep the production line operating.

Allowances

Allowances refer to other reductions from the standard price. Occasionally, companies will offer trade-in allowances to customers who bring in an older item for the purchase of a new one. Manufacturers often offer allowances to resellers who agree to use certain promotional material like end-of-aisle displays of the product within their stores.

Positioning Value of Price

Price plays a major strategic role in the positioning of the product, service, or organization. In establishing the price level, companies must consider the competitive environment and the position where they would like their service to be priced relative to the competition. Second, a company must consider how much focus will be placed on price in promoting the service.

FIGURE 9-6 displays four broad options for price positioning. There are two axes defining these quadrants. The horizontal X axis refers to whether the price to be charged will be high or low relative to the competition. The vertical Y axis refers to whether the price will be an active or passive part of the promotional strategy. When price is active, promotional efforts will call attention to the price level. When price is passive, the promotional effort focuses on other attributes of the product or service.

Quadrant A represents situations where prices are high relative to the competition and price is a very active part of the strategy. This approach is useful in situations

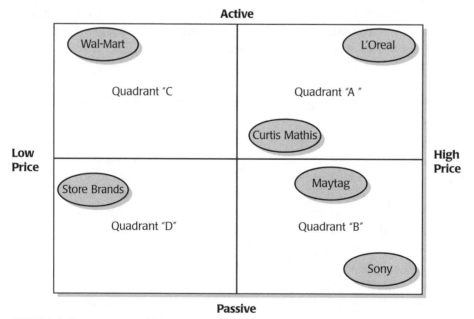

FIGURE 9-6 Positioning of Price

Source: Adapted from Tellis, G. J., Creative Pricing Strategies. Reprinted with permission from the *Journal of Medical Practice Management,* Vol. 3, No. 2, pp. 120–124, © 1988 Greenbranch Publishing, PO Box 208, Phoenix, MD 21131, (800) 933-3711.

where it is hard to differentiate the product on tangible dimensions or when promoting a prestige image for the product. Curtis Mathis televisions have been promoted as "The most expensive television set money can buy." L'Oreal hair coloring was mentioned earlier as a prestige-priced item.

Quadrant B involves situations where price is set high but kept a passive element in the marketing mix. Maytag appliances, for example, are premium-priced relative to competitors' products. Maytag, however, does not mention price but focuses instead on the reliability of its product. Maytag advertising often displays the lonely company repairman who is never called for repairs. The implication is that Maytag products never need fixing. Sony audio and video equipment is also priced higher than the competition. Again, Sony focuses on sound and visual quality and advanced technology as its differential advantage.

The third quadrant, C, involves setting a low price and being very aggressive in promoting it. Wal-Mart aggressively promotes its low-price position, which is a common position for many discounters.

The last quadrant, D, unusual for many marketers, entails assigning a low price but not promoting it. In traditional businesses, this is very uncommon. In health care, however, this strategy has been used for services that an organization might be mandated to provide, but for which they did not want significant demand. Many hospitals have often posted notices regarding the availability of free care, if economically necessary. Few institutions, however, would want to promote this option.

■ The Coming Challenge for Pricing

In the United States, more information, or greater transparency, about health care prices is the challenge for the coming century. While individual states have moved with greater frequency to requiring hospitals to post price information around common procedures, now there are calls on the federal level for such information. In May 2005, the Hospital Price Disclosure Act (HR 1362) was proposed to make 25 of the most common outpatient procedures done in hospitals and their prices available on the Internet.[30] While the initial reception by provider organizations and even Congress has been less than enthusiastic, as states move toward having this information, the federal government will follow suit or the law at this level will be moot. Over time, it is likely that similar information will then be required of other providers within the health care system, physicians, MCOs, ambulatory surgical centers, mental health care providers, and the like.

■ Conclusions

Price is a major aspect of marketing strategy. As the health care industry moves from a reimbursement environment into a retail economy where products and services are offered to consumers, the pricing considerations common to traditional businesses such as Pillsbury and Sony will become more prevalent. The strategic and positioning implications of price cannot be ignored when developing the organization's marketing strategy.

■ Key Terms

Price	Target Pricing
Complementary Products	Demand-Minus Pricing
Substitutable Goods	Price Lining
Prestige Pricing	Odd Pricing
Demand Schedule	Item Budget Theory
Price Elasticity	One-Price Policy
Fixed Costs	Flexible Pricing Policy
Variable Costs	Leader Pricing
Total Cost	Bundled Pricing
Break-Even Analysis	Going-Rate Pricing
Marginal Cost Pricing	Volume Discounts
Markup Pricing	Functional Discounts

■ Chapter Summary

1. The price an organization establishes has an economic, perceptual, and positioning value to the firm.
2. Multiple factors—such as demand, life cycle, product line, and channel structure—all affect the pricing decision.
3. Organizations can pursue several different pricing objectives that affect their strategy. These are profit, sales, market share, image, and stabilization.
4. An important consideration in pricing is determining the amount of sales needed in order to break even. This figure is based on the total fixed cost, variable cost, and price charged.
5. In addition to break-even pricing, firms can follow a cost-plus pricing, marginal cost pricing, markup pricing, target pricing, or demand-minus price-setting policy.
6. In establishing price lines, it is essential to have noticeable differences in perceived quality for the distinct lines.
7. Odd pricing is based on item budget theory, which assumes a consumer predetermines the amount to be spent on an item.
8. Prestige pricing is counter-intuitive to the economic logic of a rational buyer. Too high a price, however, will lead to a decline in demand.

9. Bundling, or selling several medical services together at one set price, is becoming a common strategy in health care.
10. There are several ways an organization can reduce the price for a product. Discounts can be based on volume, function, seasonality, or an allowance.
11. Price has an important positioning value depending on how active or passive a role it plays in the promotional strategy, and on the level of the price relative to the competition.

■ Chapter Problems

1. Explain how a pharmaceutical company's pricing for a nonproprietary drug might change if the objective was: (a) profitability, (b) sales volume, (c) market share.
2. Two medical organizations have recently examined their cost structures. The first group is a radiology practice with a significant investment in diagnostic imaging equipment. The second group is a single-specialty pediatric practice. The cost analysis reveals the following distribution:

	Radiology Group	Pediatric Group
Fixed Cost	70%	20%
Variable Cost	30%	80%

Explain the implications of these differing cost structures of each medical group in terms of contracting with MCOs.
3. An MCO marketing manager reduced the MCO's premium by 10% and saw a 20% increase in the number of subscribers. He then thought that if the premium were reduced by another 20%, he would see a 40% increase. What is your analysis of this reasoning?
4. An ophthalmology practice is deciding whether to offer prescription eyeglasses for sale in-house. The new service would require the training and hiring of additional personnel, inventory for glasses and frames, and some minor space alterations. The utilized space in the office would be a charge allocated to the program. The costs for this new service are:

Variable Costs (electricity, labor, supplies)	$80 per completed pair of eyeglasses
Total Fixed Cost	$36,000

How much volume does the group need to break even if they charge $100 per pair of eyeglasses? If they charge $200?
5. Assume that in Problem 4 the total market for eyeglasses in this community is 2400 pair. What are the market share implications of a $100 price? A $200 price?

6. A health club decided to offer a yearly membership. Separate fees were to be charged for nutrition counseling, tennis court usage, and aerobic instruction. How might this organization implement: (a) a prestige pricing strategy? (b) a bundled price strategy? (c) price lines?

7. What type of price positioning strategy would you recommend for a medical group that: (a) has customer service features such as weekend appointment hours that distinguish it from the competition, and (b) wants to entice wealthy South Americans to seek treatment in the United States? What is your rationale for each recommendation?

■ Notes

1. Several studies consider the perceptual aspect of price. See: J. Jacoby and J. C. Olsen, eds., *Perceived Quality* (Lexington, MA: Lexington Books, 1985); V. A. Zeithaml, "Consumer Perceptions of Price, Quality, and Value," *Journal of Marketing* 52, no. 3 (1988): 2–22; and J. Wind, "Getting a Read on Market-Defined Value," *Journal of Pricing Management* (1990): 5–14.

2. William O. Cleverley, *Effective Hospital Pricing Strategy*, (Worthington, OH: Cleverly & Associates, 2003).

3. "Wisconsin Launches WEB site That Compares Hospitals Prices," *IHealth Beat* (February 17, 2005), (www.ihealthbeat.org/index.cfm?Action=dspItem&itemID=109137).

4. *IHealth Beat*, op. cit.

5. Mark Speers, "A Pricing Strategy for Combination Products," *Medical DeviceLink* (May/June 2004), www.devicelink.com/mx/archive/04/05/speers.html.

6. For a discussion of pricing issues over the life cycle, see P. M. Parker, "Price Elasticity over the Adoption Life Cycle," *Journal of Marketing Research* 29, no. 3 (1992): 358–367.

7. Geflen Melnick, Emmett Keeler, Jack Zwanziger, "Market Power and Hospital Pricing: Are Nonprofits Different?" *Health Affairs* (May–June 1999): 167–173.

8. Michael Nugent, "The Price Is Right: For Optimal Price Setting, You'll Need a Strategic Focus That Adjusts for Recent Industry Trends," *Healthcare Financial Management* (December 2004).

9. R. L. Cohen, "Retail Strategy Works Wonders for Hospital Mammography Promotion," *Healthcare Marketing Report* 12, no. 8 (1994): 12–13.

10. C. Sardinha, "HMOs, Hoping To Win Market Share, Slash Premium Hikes to New Lows," *Managed Care Outlook* 7, no. 2 (1994): 1–2.

11. For a good review of methods used to measure sensitivity and price, see T. T. Nagel, *The Strategy and Tactics of Pricing* (Englewood Cliffs, NJ: Prentice Hall, 1987).

12. Jeanne S. Ringel, Susan D. Hosek, Ben A. Vollard, and Sergej Mahnovski, "The Elasticity of Demand for Healthcare: A Review of the Literature and Its Application to the Military Healthcare System," (National Defense Research Institute, Rand Health, 2002).

13. Y. K. Shetty, "Product Quality and Competitive Strategy," *Business Horizons* 30, no. 3 (1987): 345–352.

14. K. B. Monroe, "Buyer's Subjective Perception of Price," *Journal of Marketing Research* 10, no. 1 (1973): 70–80.

15. D. Jones, "Election Gives Hospital Giant More Clout," *USA Today*, November 11, 1994, B1, B2.

16. This discussion and that of marginal pricing is based on K. B. Pitts, "Pricing and Reimbursement Strategies," *Topics in Health Care Financing* 12, no. 1 (Fall 1985): 24–31.

17. Kay McVay, "What Price Health Care? Hospital Charges Fueling Health-care Crisis," *San Francisco Chronicle* (July 11, 2003), http://www.sfgate.com/cgi-bin/article.cgi?f=/c/a/2003/07/11/ED83885.DTL.

18. Lucette Lagnado, "California Hospitals Open Books, Showing Huge Price Differences," *The Wall Street Journal* (December 27, 2004), pp. A1, A6.

19. "Dallas Project a Model for Physician-Hospital Collaboration," *Hospital Integrated Strategy Report* 2, no. 1 (1994): 8–10.

20. S. Petroshius and K. B. Monroe, "Effects of Product-Line Pricing Characteristics on Product Evaluation," *Journal of Consumer Research* 13, no. 4 (1987): 511–519.

21. Z. V. Lambert, "Perceived Price as Related to Odd and Even Price Endings," *Journal of Retailing* 51, no. 3 (Fall 1975): 13–22.

22. G. J. Szybillo and J. Jacoby, "Intrinsic versus Extrinsic Cues as Determinants of Perceived Product Quality," *Journal of Applied Psychology* 59, no. 1 (1974): 74–78.

23. J. Guiltinan, "The Price Bundling of Services: A Normative Framework," *Journal of Marketing* 51, no. 2 (1987): 74–85.

24. D. Paun, "When To Bundle or Unbundle Products," *Industrial Marketing Management* 22, no. 2 (1993): 29–34.

25. G. J. Tellis, "Beyond the Many Faces of Price: An Integration of Pricing Strategies," *Journal of Marketing* 50, no. 4 (1986): 146–160.

26. Robert C. Ford and Myron D. Fotler, "Creating Customer-Focused Health Care Organizations," *Health Care Management Review* 25, no. 4 (Fall 2000): 18–33.

27. www.mouwasat.com.sa/Dynamic/Package/package.asp.

28. Alan T. Sorensen, Insurer-Hospital bargaining: Negotiated Discounts in Post-Deregulation Connecticut," (March 30, 2001) working paper.

29. M. Pauly, "Managed Care, Market Power, and Monopsony," *Health Services Research* 33, no. 5 (December 1998): 1439–1440.

30. Phil Kadner, "Law Would Force Hospitals to Post Prices on Internet," *Daily Southtown* (May 6 2005) (www.dailysouthtown.com/southtown/columns/kadner/x06-pkd1.htm).

Distribution

Learning Objectives

After reading this chapter you should be able to:

- Understand the concept of channel structure and the alternative channels available

- Know the varying levels of distribution intensity and the considerations in implementing each alternative

- Understand the concept of vertical marketing systems and their application in health care

- Describe the nature of channel leadership and the source of channel power

- Recognize the application of retailing in health care strategy

Place, which refers to distribution, is a basic component of the marketing mix. It represents how and where the product is accessed by the consumer. The path a product takes as it travels from the manufacturer to the consumer is referred to as the **channel of distribution**. In both service and product marketing, marketers have several key decisions to make involving the channel of distribution and the place component of the marketing mix, such as: how the product should be distributed, who within the channel should perform specific functions, how much coverage of the market is needed, and ultimately how the channel can be controlled.

■ Alternative Channels of Distribution

All businesses must decide how many other organizations are needed to distribute their product or service. The channels companies use vary in length, with length referring to the number of intermediaries. A *direct* channel is one in which no one stands between the producer of the product and the ultimate consumer. FIGURE 10-1 shows a direct channel (a). In health care, the most direct channel is between the primary care physician and the patient. However, in recent years, new direct channels are also

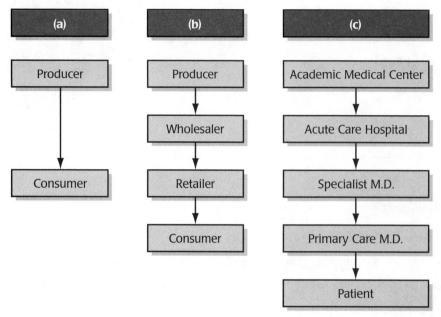

FIGURE 10-1 Channels of Distribution

appearing. QuickMedx care sites are located in Cub Foods stores, Target stores, and Best Buy retail outlets in Minneapolis, Minnesota (www.minuteclinic.com/). They offer a limited menu of tests and treatments with a price range between $18 and $45.[1] Using a direct channel in health care has not been limited, however, to primary care services. Lifeview Imaging in Fullerton, California, provided full body scans to patients who could direct schedule with the office. A full scan in January 2004 was $450, or $849 for two people.

An *indirect* channel may have several intermediaries between the producer and the ultimate consumer. For example, Proctor and Gamble (P & G), a consumer products company located in Cincinnati, Ohio, uses the middle channel (b) in Figure 10-1 for the distribution of its many products. An academic medical center that provides sophisticated tertiary services might have an indirect channel with several intermediaries (c), as shown in Figure 10-1. The community hospital, the specialist, and the primary care physician all are involved in early stages of diagnosis, intervention, and care before the patient is referred to the academic medical center. In traditional product marketing, the intermediaries within the channel will vary as to whether they take ownership or title to the goods as they move through the channel. In health care, taking title is not an issue for channel consideration.

The Web channel is a new and powerfully emerging alternative within health care. Some leading organizations have actually utilized this channel to provide second opinions as can be seen on the Web page of the Partners Health Care system in EXHIBIT 10-1. The full site can be viewed at https://econsults.partners.org/. In 2002 it was estimated

Exhibit 10-1 Partners Web Portal

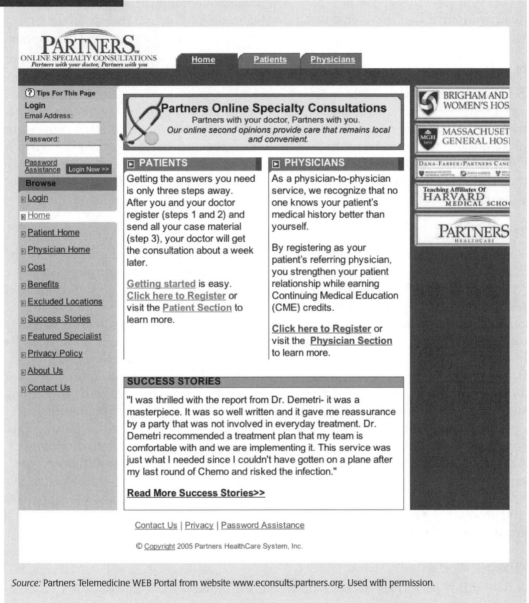

Source: Partners Telemedicine WEB Portal from website www.econsults.partners.org. Used with permission.

that over 5000 patients had availed themselves of this channel in seeking second opinions online. The vast majority of these patients had been searching for information on cancer.[2] The Cleveland Clinic featured "remote second opinions" on the front page of its Web site in Fall of 2005 (www.clevelandclinic.org).

Functions in the Channel

A common view that consumers have had of traditional industries is that the middleman, or intermediary, adds cost or little value to the product. In reality, though, most intermediaries perform several valuable functions or **utilities** in the channel of distribution.

Place

A major function of any intermediary is the place value provided to the product or service, by making it more accessible to the consumer. A primary care clinic that offers after-hours care or weekend appointment hours would be offering significant place value to the consumer. Another example is the outreach strategy of U.S. Health Corporation in Columbus, Ohio. The multihospital system operates a medical van that visits two inner-city Columbus high schools to bring prenatal care to pregnant students.[3]

Time

The time utility refers to the fact that many intermediaries store the product until the consumer wants to purchase the item. A department store, for example, may stock some bathing suits for sale throughout the entire year. As a result, a consumer does not need to maintain an inventory in anticipation of future need. Instead, the customer can purchase close to the time the item is required. The value to consumers is that they can use their money for other purposes, and the retail store can carry the cost of the inventory. Stores that sell manufacturer overloads or distressed merchandise offer little time value. Since items are not regularly stocked, the customer must purchase them when offered. The store cannot guarantee that the manufacturer overrun of bathing suits available in January will also be available just before the summer months.

In health care organizations, there is a time value provided regarding the ancillary support goods often needed such as durable medical equipment or pharmaceuticals. Any business organization must recognize that the more of each utility it provides, the greater its cost structure. The objective, however, is to provide a level of each utility that the customer values sufficiently enough to pay the additional cost. A primary care group that has its own onsite pharmacy may have a higher cost structure than a group that provides no such convenience.

Possession

A third utility performed in the channel of distribution is that of possession or financing. In traditional businesses, some intermediaries will provide credit, allowing the customer to take the product and pay over time. So too, in health care, some intermediaries vary regarding the provision of possession utility. Many urgent medical care centers that were established in the 1980s as for-profit enterprises required patients to pay for services at the time of delivery. If health insurance was going to reimburse these patients, they had to seek this reimbursement after payment to the urgent care center. Most hospital emergency departments will, however, bill the patient's insurance company directly, and for the uninsured patient, some will provide services regardless. The patient then works out a repayment schedule with the financial office of the hospital.

Hospitals have begun to recognize the value of this utility. Since 1991, MasterCard and Visa credit cards have been accepted in 5000 hospitals and in 40,000 physician offices. Many hospitals offer designated health care credit cards under a program by Health Charge Corporation in Skokie, Illinois. This company offers a charge card in the hospital's name, for which the patient can apply upon admission. At discharge, the self-pay portion of the visit is placed on the charge.[4]

Form

The fourth utility provided by some intermediaries is that of form or alteration, in which the intermediary actually changes the product for the customer. Some intermediaries provide customization of the product. In a traditional industry, form utility might be found when a department store alters a suit to better fit an individual. Similarly, form utility might occur at the Rehabilitation Hospital of the Pacific, a 100-bed inpatient acute care rehabilitation facility in Honolulu, Hawaii. This organization has the capabilities to redesign orthotic devices to better conform to the rehabilitation needs of their patients.

Functional Shifting

In spite of criticism often leveled at the middleman, it is important to recognize the concept of **functional shifting**, which involves the movement of different functions such as credit and sorting, between the producer of a product or service and its intermediaries or the customer. The intermediary can be eliminated but then the function has to shift to some other entity in the channel. For example, if the intermediary is eliminated and no longer provides customer credit, then either the customer must assume the credit requirement or the manufacturer must provide the credit.

An extreme form of functional shifting has been described by Trombetta. In the late 1970s, Goodyear established a plant in Lawton, Oklahoma. Area physicians were unwilling to grant any price concessions when approached by the company. Goodyear proceeded to assume the medical functions by setting up its own hospital, medical staff, and labs.[5]

Channel Management

In designing the channel of distribution there are several factors to consider, including determining the degree of distribution required, gaining channel cooperation, and dealing with conflict.

Ultimately, in the deliverance of a service or product, an organization must decide how available the product or service will be to customers. This issue might involve questions of the number of satellite facilities or primary care offices that would be staffed by physicians who participate in a prepaid plan. Secondly, there is always a question of whether any intermediaries who will be involved in the service will cooperate in how the service is delivered. Hospitals, for example, have always been concerned about getting physicians to admit to their hospitals. Managed care organizations (MCOs) and preferred provider organizations often need to convince physicians to join the plan as participating physicians. Both of these situations involve channel cooperation.

Finally, whenever two or more separate entities are involved in the delivery of a service, there is the potential for conflict. Conflict has often existed between hospital administrators and their medical staff. Conflict is now common between administrators of a MCO and the clinicians. Thus, channel management is a major consideration in the establishment of the place component of the marketing mix.

■ Intensity of Distribution

For any channel formation, the provider of a product or service must first decide how intensive the distribution should be. This **channel intensity**, as it is called, will then determine how available the product is to the ultimate consumer. In traditional businesses, there are commonly three forms of distribution intensity: intensive, selective, and exclusive. FIGURE 10-2 shows examples of the three distribution strategies regarding intensity. There are several factors that determine the ultimate selection of any specific strategy.

A major consideration in the selection of an intensity alternative is the consumer and how much effort consumers will expend searching for a particular product or service. The more effort they are willing to expend, the more an organization can be selective or exclusive in its intensity. A second consideration is control. The more control the manufacturer wants over the intermediary, the more it would choose the strategy of exclusivity. Retailers, for example, who carry products also carried by their competitors, find less reason to be attentive to the demands of the manufacturer, since the manufacturer is not offering them a product that the competition doesn't have. Market coverage is another consideration. The greater the desired coverage, the more the strategy leans toward intensive distribution with more outlets for distributing the service.

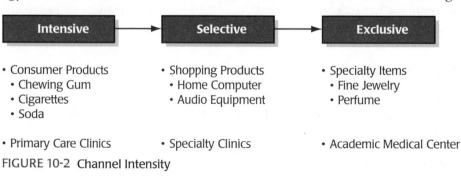

FIGURE 10-2 Channel Intensity

Intensive Distribution

This strategy is typical of consumer goods manufacturers. In intensive distribution, the product is available in a large number of outlets. This strategy applies to products such as soda or chewing gum; the consumer exerts no effort to find these and knows that there are many available outlets for such products. The traditional view in health care was that patients had their own personal physicians and would accept no substitutes. Increasingly, however, convenience has become a major customer concern, a dimension that affects the amount of effort patients will expend in seeking care from a particular primary care physician.

As a result, many primary care groups have used more intensive distribution efforts by providing multiple satellite facilities and extended hours. Hospitals, too, have not overlooked the growing need to increase intensity of distribution. David Ginsburg, executive vice president for planning and program development at Presbyterian Hospital in Manhattan, commented regarding his organization, "In 1977, Presbyterian had one address, and basically one location. In 1987, we already have twenty different addresses, and we expect in the next century to be even more decentralized."[6] In fact, by 2005, the hospital and health system has more than 25 locations beyond the main hospital.

Exclusive Distribution

The opposite of intensive distribution is exclusive distribution, in which the product or service is offered in a highly restricted number of outlets. Manufacturers of luxury products, which often have high margins, follow this strategy. Rolls Royce, for example, has few auto dealerships in the United States, in the belief that the customer who wants a Rolls Royce will be willing to travel to make the purchase. In the same regard, the manufacturer—by limiting the number of dealerships—can exhibit strong control over these intermediaries. Because a Rolls dealership is exclusive, the manufacturer can place certain demands on it regarding service levels, parts inventory, and sales training. In health care, exclusive distribution has existed for the providers of highly specialized medical services. Historically this was a common position for many health care providers. Joslin is a world renowned provider for diabetes treatment and research. In 1996, its distribution strategy was exclusive; patients had to travel to Boston to receive services and to access the expertise of the Joslin. Joslin has now broadened its distribution strategy as can be seen on its Web page entitled "Delivering Joslin Healthcare Solutions around the Globe" (www.joslin.org/Business_Index_2622.asp).

Selective Distribution

An intermediate intensity strategy is that of selective distribution. As noted in Figure 10-2, this approach involves fewer retailers than the intensive approach and is particularly attractive to manufacturers of shopping goods. At this distribution level the consumer compares alternatives on selected attributes and compares the value. Intermediaries are restricted to those whom the manufacturer believes will provide the best product support. By providing some selectivity among intermediaries, the manufacturer can require them to meet certain objectives. Nikon, Sony, and Ping are three companies that follow selective distribution. Nikon does not sell its cameras in every outlet where cameras are sold. Rather they use selected outlets that see Nikon cameras as a differential advantage and present them more favorably to customers than Kodak or Minolta cameras. Sony follows a reasonably selective distribution approach for its products. Ping distributes its golf clubs only through golf professionals. While there may be two golf pros in one community, both know that if the customer wants Ping clubs they cannot buy them at the local sporting goods store or golf retailer.

In health care, the use of selective intensity strategies has increased. Historically, the Mayo Clinic in Minnesota and the Ochsner Clinic in Louisiana followed an exclusive intensity approach. Consumers wanting to use the services of either facility had to travel to Rochester or to New Orleans, respectively. Now, as customer requirements have changed, both facilities have increased their distribution intensity. The Mayo Clinic has opened satellites in Jacksonville, Florida; Scottsdale, Arizona; and has purchased groups throughout Wisconsin, Iowa, and Minnesota in more than 60 locations. Mayo even staffs an office in Mexico City to help its international patients in Latin America access Mayo services. The Mayo Clinic also operates primary care clinics in the manufacturing facilities of the John Deere Corporation. The Ochsner Clinic, a 600-person physician group based in New Orleans, has 24 clinic locations throughout southeastern Louisiana.

■ Vertical Marketing Systems

Among traditional organizations and now in the health care industry, the longstanding concept of a channel consisting of separate organizational entities, such as a manufacturer, wholesaler, and retailer, is undergoing change, with a noticeable growth of vertical marketing systems. **Vertical marketing systems** can be defined as channels in which the intermediaries are integrated so their functions are performed at the most efficient place within the channel.[7] Ideally, in a well-run vertically administered system, conflicts and differing goals should be eliminated so that the system performs well.

Several factors have been cited as driving vertical integration in health care:

1. Production cost savings
2. Transaction cost savings and improved coordination of services (i.e., continuity of care)
3. Overcoming market imperfections
4. Management and internal factors
5. Environmental changes that affect market conditions, production technologies, and transactional relationships.[8]

In this framework, transaction cost savings center on economies in the transfer and use of information across different care points. Market imperfections relate to regulatory constraints or market power on the side of the buyer or seller. Vertically integrated systems can help achieve countervailing power.

Vertical marketing systems can be formed by any entity within the channel. One approach to creating these entities is through **forward vertical integration,** in which operations are acquired or developed that are closer to the final buyer in the channel of distribution. For example, Health Dimensions, in San Jose, California, has vertically integrated forward. The hospital foundation operates health clinics in schools that provide primary care services to the community. An alternative strategy is to develop a vertical marketing system by backward integration, acquiring operations that are farther from the consumer. In this instance, the Ochsner Clinic vertically integrated backward by adding its Baton Rouge site several years ago. The multispecialty group practice of physicians purchased a small hospital in the community by which to deliver inpatient services. Table 10-1 shows a variety of vertically integrated health care organizational forms relative to the five factors previously mentioned.

In traditional industries, there are three common forms of vertical marketing systems: (1) corporate, (2) administered, and (3) contractual.

Corporate Vertical Marketing Systems

A **corporate vertical marketing system** combines both the production and distribution of a product or service under one corporate ownership. Companies can achieve this result by integrating either forward or backward depending on the position from the channel that they evolve. Levi-Strauss, for example, was originally a manufacturer of clothes. The company created a corporate vertical marketing system by integrating forward and opening its own retail clothing stores to sell its merchandise. A similar strategy has been used by the University of Michigan Hospitals of Ann Arbor. This tertiary center has almost 30 locations around the state of Michigan outside of Ann Arbor. FIGURE 10-3 shows several alternative vertical marketing systems.

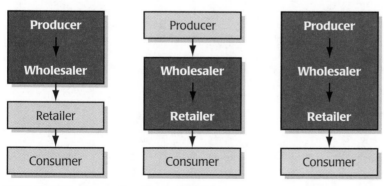

FIGURE 10-3 Alternative Marketing Systems

Table 10-1   Alternative Health Care Integration Forms

Form of Vertical Integration	Determinants	
	Production Cost Savings	Transaction Cost Savings
1. Closed-staff-model HMO (common ownership, fully integrated value chain)	Primarily through utilization management of inpatient care	Continuity of care through integration of facilities and medical staff
2. IPA-model HMO (separate ownership; contracting between the "plan" and physicians, hospitals; contract-based integration of value chain)	Utilization management; less-rigorous utilization management incentives than in closed-staff HMO	Still essentially market in contracting between plan and physicians, hospitals
3. Insurer-sponsored PPO (separate ownership; contracting on preferred vs.closed-panel or exclusive basis; contract-based integration)	Minimal; achieved primarily through unit cost reductions stimulated by price discounting	Replaces repeated contracting with one-time costs of establishing preferred provider network
4. Integrated hospital-multispecialty physician group practice (shared governance of the hospital and clinic, partially integrated value chain)	Not a prominent factor	Continuity of care benefits; referral and practice network; increased congruence of hospital and physician goals
5. Hospital-based ambulatory primary care group practice (shared-equity investment by hospital and physician group; internal staffing of semi-autonomous unit; partially integrated value chain)	Minimal factor	Some continuity of care gains due to tightened referral network between the hospital and primary care physicians (PCPs)
6. Local-market-based managed care product (formation of "quasi-firm" by short-term general hospital, multi-specialty physician group, skilled nursing facility, and insurance carrier; partially integrated value chain)	Primarily through overall "case management" of utilization	Managed care via case manager, partially supplants arms-length market contracting; enhanced pre- and post-discharge services (visit, planning for hospital, ambulatory care, and long-term care); link to insurer enhances continuity between delivery and financing of care
7. McKesson's "value-adding partnership' (VAP) (with manufacturing, distribution, retailing, third party insurance, and consumers for prescription drugs) (separate ownership of value chain components, contract-based integration)	Dramatic reductions in cost of order processing; reduced costs of restocking orders through conscious redesign of shelves	Enhanced monitoring though computer database of clinical-biological effects of alternative drug combinations

Overcoming Market Imperfections	Management and Internal Factors	Environmental Conditions
Response to physician market power	Internal "culture" linking organizational and physician interests	Cost sensitivity of purchasers; necessary supply of physicians
Potential for more competitive physician pricing through contract and capitation incentives	Contracting largely supplants internal hierarchy	
Simulates competitive market's price network	Minimal	Similar to Form 4
Minimal factor	Internal culture linking hospital and physician interests	Minimal factor
Minimal factor	Example: an internal corporate joint venture	Excess hospital bed capacity; increasing supply of PCPs
"Backward" integration by insured into delivery, exerts buyer bargaining power on providers to reduce costs of services	Can deliver the product through variety of tightly or loosely "coupled" market or ownership mechanisms	Cost sensitivity of purchasers; excess supply of physicians; limited reimbursement for long-term care; (health) insurance underwriting cycle
Minimal factor	Create management culture that monitors competitive dynamics throughout value chain and fixes weaknesses as they occur; use of computer systems and information technology for order entry, packing, shipping, shelf design (e.g., for quality assurance) (drug combination)	Increasing competition from large drug store chains; eroding market share of independent drug stores served by McKesson

Source: From Conrad, D. A. and Dowling, W. L., Vertical Integration in Health Services: Theory and Managerial Implications from *Health Care Management Review*, Vol. 15, No. 4, pp. 18–19, 1990.

FIGURE 10-4 shows examples of several vertical marketing systems being developed in health care. These systems are called **integrated delivery systems,** in which health care is coordinated and is delivered at the level of intensity needed. One of these

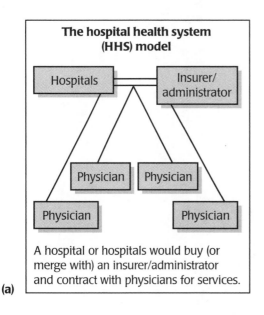

The hospital health system
(HHS) model

A hospital or hospitals would buy (or merge with) an insurer/administrator and contract with physicians for services.

(a)

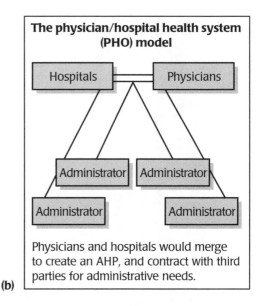

The physician/hospital health system
(PHO) model

Physicians and hospitals would merge to create an AHP, and contract with third parties for administrative needs.

(b)

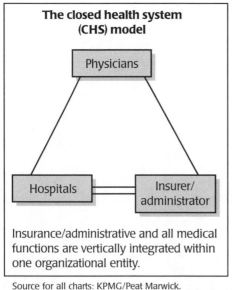

The closed health system
(CHS) model

Insurance/administrative and all medical functions are vertically integrated within one organizational entity.

(c)

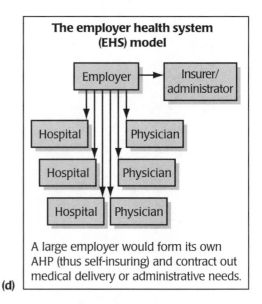

The employer health system
(EHS) model

A large employer would form its own AHP (thus self-insuring) and contract out medical delivery or administrative needs.

(d)

Source for all charts: KPMG/Peat Marwick.

FIGURE 10-4 Four Models of Integrated Delivery Sytems in Health Care

Source: Steve Findlay, "How New Alliances Are Changing Health Care," *Business and Health* (October 1993), pp. 28–34.

systems, referred to as a closed health system model, is comprised of physicians, hospitals, and an insurer all vertically integrated in one system in which the functions are delivered at the optimum point and centrally managed.

In Miami, Florida, Affiliated Health Providers consists of eight hospitals with multiple physician group practices. This network plans to contract with several insurers to be able to assume risk.[9] This enables the network, in conjunction with the insurance companies, to act as a prepaid health care plan. The physicians in the hospital will be responsible for managing the care and will accept the premiums for the coverage of that care from subscribers. This arrangement is represented in Figure 10-4 as the closed health system.

Administered Vertical Marketing System

An **administered vertical marketing system** occurs when there is coordination between members of the distribution channel but there is not common ownership. Typically, when one member of the distribution channel is more powerful, an administered vertical marketing system can occur. Scott Lawn Products is an administered vertical marketing system. Because of the manufacturer's power with its successful product line, it can demand its intermediary to give it better floor space, differential emphasis in selling, and adherence to pricing guidelines. In some administered vertical marketing programs, the manufacturer may take over the functions of pricing items, checking inventory levels, and servicing the account.

Administered vertical marketing systems are the growing form in health care. Increasingly, hospitals are employing their own physicians and staffing their own outpatient facilities and diagnostic centers. As the health industry moves to contracting for care, hospitals have integrated forward, with the objective of owning the referral flow of patients. In a similar fashion, the Kaiser Foundation Health Plan, a multispecialty, prepaid group model health maintenance organization (HMO) in Chula Vista, California, vertically integrated backward and has opened its own hospitals in several communities rather than trying to negotiate discounts from community hospitals. An interesting administered program was attempted by Mt. Sinai Hospital in Chicago in 1986. Primary medical centers owned and operated by Mt. Sinai were placed in Zayre department stores in the Chicago metropolitan area.[10] Figure 10-4 shows a variation of an administered vertical marketing system appearing in health care—the physician–hospital organization model, in which the physicians and hospitals merge and contract with third parties for administrative needs. The hospital health system model is also presented in Figure 10-4; in this variation, the hospital and insurer merge and contract for the care to be delivered by providers. The most advanced state of the administered vertical marketing system in health care may be that represented in Figure 10-4 as the employer health system model. In this instance, the administered program is formed by the employer, who then contracts out for care and administration of health needs. In Minneapolis–St. Paul, 20 employers formed a coalition representing 80,000 workers. These employers contracted with one consortium of providers to take care of their employees' health needs.

Contractual Vertical Marketing Systems

This form of vertical marketing systems consists of either a cooperative or a franchise. **Cooperatives** are agreements between members of the distribution channel who exist on the same level. For example, several retailers may band together in a retailer co-operative to act as a large purchasing group and to extract discounts or other concessions from suppliers. The Independent Grocers Association is a retailer cooperative of small grocery stores that bulk purchase from manufacturers.

In health care, a recent version of a cooperative marketing system is the National Cardiovascular Network, formed in 1993. Forty-one top heart programs were invited to join a cooperative venture to offer discounted, high-quality services at all-inclusive rates under contract to large employers and MCOs.[11] **Franchising**, one of the fastest-growing forms of a vertical marketing system, is a contract that links elements of the manufacturing and distribution of a product or service.[12] Automobile dealerships are franchise arrangements, as are McDonald's restaurants and many Holiday Inn hotels. In these cases, independent businesses have signed agreements with the franchiser to deliver the product or service in a defined fashion. The franchisee pays a fee for the opportunity to deliver this service, and there is often a yearly payment as a function of the revenue generated by the outlet. Similarly, the franchiser often provides national advertising support, guidance for conducting the business, and ongoing training and product development. A relaxation response program developed under the auspices of Harvard University Medical School at Deaconess Hospital of Boston is being franchised to other medical centers around the country for $80,000.[13]

While franchising has been a fast-growing segment of the economy, it has not escaped criticism. A major issue has been the terms of contracts that exist for many franchisees. A growing number of lawsuits by franchisees cite nonsatisfactory performance by the franchiser, or an overselling of the possibilities of the business. A common complaint voiced by franchisees is that the franchiser promises a level of sales that is found to be unachievable. Or, the franchiser promises to provide advertising or marketing consulting support, but does not follow through with this promise.

■ Channel Leadership

In many distribution channels there is often one member who is considered the channel commander. The **channel commander** can dictate or control the activities of the other members of the channel of distribution.

The manufacturer can be the channel commander when its product is very popular. P & G, for example, has several brand-name products that are well recognized and have significant market share. Ivory soap and Crest toothpaste are just two of

P & G's many brands that retailers know are important to carry in their grocery stores. In this way P&G can control certain aspects of its product merchandising. A manufacturer can also be channel commander by providing intermediaries with significant rewards.

A wholesaler can be the channel commander if the product must be distributed to a large number of manufacturers or to a large number of retailers. In these instances, the consolidating function of the retailer becomes a key element in the distribution of the product. In the alcoholic beverage industry, Foremost McKesson is a wholesaler that exerts significant leadership in the channel of distribution.

The retailer is the channel commander when it has a strong image or extensive market coverage. K-Mart has a large number of outlets across the United States. As a large purchaser and ultimately distributor of products, manufacturers must consider K-Mart's needs when the retailer places an order.

This framework of a channel commander also applies in health care. M.D. Anderson is an internationally known cancer center in Houston, Texas, and is part of the University of Texas medical institution. As a result of its strong reputation, this organization can act as a channel commander in terms of cancer treatment. Similarly, in areas with several community hospitals, the intermediary (the physician) is often the channel commander. In the managed care environment, large managed care companies (Wellpoint, Anthem) and their power were described in the oligopolistic market condition in Chapter 3. These large entities increasingly play the part of wholesalers coordinating the needs of the many employers in the community with the services of available providers. Many of the larger managed care plans such as Cigna or Aetna can play the role of a channel commander and negotiate effective discounts with hospitals or physicians.

Using Power

There are several sources of power a distribution channel member can use to control other members of the channel.[14] Five specific sources have been identified: coercive power, economic power, rewards, referent power, and expertise.

Coercive

One negative source of power is coercive power. Threats can be effective in modifying behavior if they can be implemented. A manufacturer might threaten to pull its popular product from the shelves, or a retailer might withhold the kind of merchandising attention the manufacturer would like for its product. Typically, most members of the distribution channel prefer not to use this form of power since it has little positive impact on building long-term channel relationships. A hospital might threaten the physicians with the possibility of recruiting additional practitioners if the physicians do not comply with the hospital wishes. Yet the gains from this approach would, no doubt, be short-term if physicians developed an alternative organization or switched hospital allegiance.

Economic

A second form of power is economic power. If one member of the channel has significantly more economic resources than another, that firm has the power. General Motors can exert significant power over small manufacturers that supply it with auto parts. A large multispecialty health clinic could convince a small two-person medical group to sell its practice to the clinic or face stiff competition. Columbia/Hospital Corporation of America–Healthtrust in its heyday wielded great economic power with its suppliers. In February 1994, Columbia renegotiated several purchasing contracts and announced it would pay $160 million instead of the $220 million previously negotiated for these services.[15]

Reward

Power can always be gained by providing other intermediaries with a significant incentive to cooperate. In traditional industries, the margins or profit provided can be a useful mechanism for gaining cooperation. In March 1994, Cigna Companies of Bloomfield, Connecticut, an insurance and HMO company, rewarded Torrance Memorial Medical Center of Torrance, California, by shifting 40,000 covered lives to this hospital from South Bay Hospital in Redondo Beach. Torrance agreed to offer a broader array of services than South Bay Hospital. The loss of business for South Bay Hospital was estimated to be 20% of its daily census.[16]

Referent

This form of power refers to the name or reputation of the organization. As was noted previously, an organization that has brand-name recognition in the marketplace can exhibit significant power over smaller competitors or intermediaries.

Expertise

Having a recognized expertise in a particular area is a fifth valuable source of distribution channel power. There are several rankings published that can provide a hospital with the appearance of expertise power. *U.S. News & World Report* annually publishes a ranking of major tertiary hospitals on 12 clinical specialties. The U.S. Department of Health and Human Services is now providing a detailed analysis of quality ratings in terms of clinical care for hospitals. Consumers can search by city and sort for particular clinical care areas. FIGURE 10-5 shows how four hospitals do in terms of the percent of patients given an angiotensin converting enzyme inhibitor for left ventricular systolic dysfunction. Individuals in the Denver market can compare hospitals in this market relative to the average for all hospitals in the United States on several similar standards of clinical care. In this way a hospital may ultimately have some expertise power.

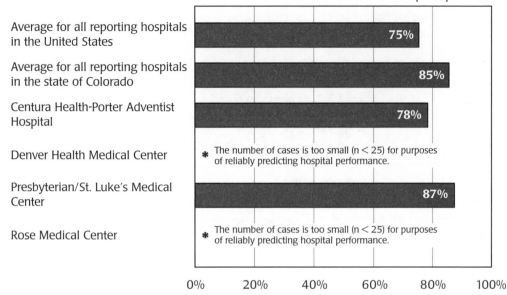
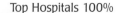

Average for all reporting hospitals in the United States	75%
Average for all reporting hospitals in the state of Colorado	85%
Centura Health-Porter Adventist Hospital	78%
Denver Health Medical Center	* The number of cases is too small (n < 25) for purposes of reliably predicting hospital performance.
Presbyterian/St. Luke's Medical Center	87%
Rose Medical Center	* The number of cases is too small (n < 25) for purposes of reliably predicting hospital performance.

These Hospitals represent the top 10% of hospitals nationwide. Top hospitals achieved a 100% rating or better.

FIGURE 10-5

Percent of Heart Attack Patients Given ACE Inhibitor for Left Ventricular Systolic Dysfunction (LVSD)
The rates displayed in this graph are from data reported for discharges January to December 2004.

Source: U.S. Department of Health and Human Services, Centers for Disease Control, 2004, Washington, DC.

■ Selected Concepts from Retailing

There are many aspects of the distribution of health care services that involve basic aspects of retailing. In examining the distribution element of the marketing mix, then, concepts such as the retail positioning matrix, the retail mix, and the wheel of retailing can aid a health care organization in strategy development.[17]

The Retail Positioning Matrix

The **retail positioning matrix** shown in FIGURE 10-6 is a concept developed by the Chicago-based management consulting firm, MAC, Inc. (now called Gemini).[18] This matrix is a model for retail positioning based on the breadth of the retailer's product line and the value added. The breadth of the product line can be defined as the number of different products and services offered by the company. The value added refers to such things as location (7–Eleven, Health Stop neighborhood urgent care centers), the prestige or

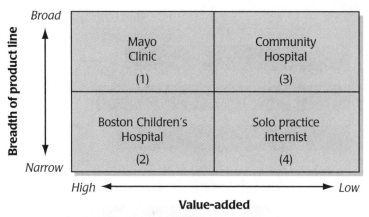

Value-added

FIGURE 10-6 Retail Positioning Matrix

Source: Steven G. Hillestad and Eric N. Berkowitz, *Health Care Marketing Plans: From Strategy to Action,* 1991: Jones and Bartlett Publishers, Sudbury, MA. www.jbpub.com. Reprinted with permission.

name recognition of the organization (Neiman Marcus or the Mayo Clinic), the product reliability (McDonald's), or personal service offered by a personal financial advisor or a medical group that might offer extended hours or even house calls.

In using this matrix, an organization can position itself in any of four quadrants. Whereas all organizations attempt to build a loyal base of customer support, the retail positioning matrix suggests that the medical organization can accomplish this goal through several alternative strategies.

1. The Mayo Clinic position is one of four options. Organizations in this quadrant have a broad product line and a high degree of value-added. Organizations in this quadrant typically offer many services and are recognized as prestige organizations.
2. High value-added with a narrow product line can also be provided by organizations such as Boston's Children's Hospital and Tiffany's. The jewelry retailer is known for premium jewelry and a strong customer service orientation.
3. The position of the community hospital is similar to that of Wal-Mart. These organizations provide a reasonable range of products and services but not at the margins achieved by those with the prestige name and service delivery.
4. Low value-added with a narrow range is common to DSW Shoes and the solo-practice internist. Both entities provide a narrow product line in a setting that is sometimes inconvenient because of limited sites.

In positioning an organization, no one quadrant is necessarily better than the others. The chosen position must offer an identity in the market relative to the competitors. Organizations can shift between quadrants in this matrix, but the implications of moving up the value-added dimension are clear. Typically, there is a need to provide more services to the market. A lower value-added position implies fewer services and reduced prices to the market. Organizations should consider reviewing the following five steps to position themselves successfully in the market:

1. *Strategic Direction*—An organization must decide whether to be a full-service or partial (narrow) service provider.
2. *Current Positioning*—The organization must understand its current composition, using quantitative and qualitative information.
3. *Competitive Positioning*—Primary and secondary data should also be employed to understand competitors' positions.
4. *Alternative Evaluation*—An organization should compare its current position with competitors to identify gaps, weaknesses, and strengths.
5. *Plan Development and Implementation*—The position selected should reflect the organization's attributes and conventions. The chosen position must be re-selected with a consistent marketing mix.[19]

Retail Mix

In developing a position for the organization, retailers can vary the components of the **retail mix**, which includes the goods and services the organization offers, the distribution of these services, and the communication strategies implemented.[20] FIGURE 10-7 shows the components of the retail mix with the health care alternatives.

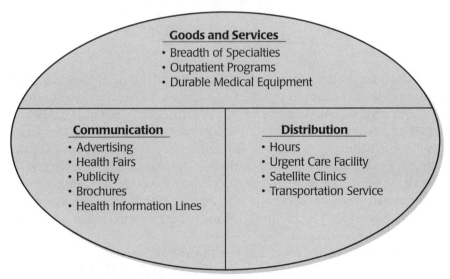

FIGURE 10-7 Health Care Organization's Retail Mix

Goods and Services

The goods and services component pertains to the breadth and depth of the product line, the prices, and the level of service delivery. A multispecialty clinic may offer traditional medical services as well as a pharmacy and other retail services in its mix. Within the goods and services mix is the service component. Organizations vary in the amount of services or even products that they provide to the customer. Some retailers, for example, provide home delivery, credit, extended hours, and personal shopper assistance. Park Nicollet Health Services in St. Louis Park, Minnesota, operates stores in several facilities. These outlets sell eyeglasses, fitness products, pharmaceuticals, durable health products, and books. In 2001, this retail operation generated $50 million in revenue for the organization.[21] Likewise, some medical organizations will fill out insurance forms for seniors, have an onsite pharmacy service, and rent durable medical equipment in an attempt to be more customer service oriented.

Pricing, as noted in Chapter 9, is becoming a more critical factor in health care as organizations move away from cost-based pricing to value pricing. Health care organizations are increasingly dealing with the issue of markup, which refers to how much should be added to the cost of the service before it is offered to the final consumer. As in retailing, health care is experiencing the growing phenomenon of service discounting. Hospitals have had to offer discounts to MCOs in order to get contracts to provide certain services. This situation involves the retailing concept of "maintained markups," which represents the amount of the markup received from the original markup, less the final price at which the product or service is sold. In retailing, discounting a product is referred to as a "markdown."

In determining its goods and services mix, the organization must identify which elements to offer, and how this mix will affect the relative position, as noted in the retail positioning matrix.

Distribution

The number of locations, the hours open, and the transportation of products are all part of the distribution side of the retailing mix. The location decision for most physicians has historically focused on convenience for the practitioner. Most medical office buildings are located adjacent to inpatient facilities. In metropolitan areas, this location is usually downtown where there are few residential developments. As a result, facilities are finding ways to bring patients to the service. Columbia-Presbyterian Hospital in New York City has a satellite practice in midtown Manhattan with a shuttle that brings patients to the medical center in Washington Heights. Site location is a key element for any organization. The facility's location directly affects the profile of the customer who uses the organization.

Acknowledging the importance of location, health care organizations are turning to Geographic Information Systems. These systems overlay maps with demographics databases. Overlook Health System in Summit, New Jersey, plans to use such programs to plot physician office sites with the addresses of employees. The organization hopes to position itself appropriately for direct contracting.[22]

Some retail organizations have based their competitive strategy on the distribution component of their retail mix. 7-Eleven convenience stores have multiple locations in any one community where they compete. This organization's goal is to have the customer drive no more than 10 minutes to access one of its stores. So too, in health care, convenience is becoming an important component for customers. Multiple primary care satellites with convenient parking play a major role in the mix of value provided to the patient.

In the retail setting, it is easy to observe another trend in terms of hours of availability. Many supermarkets are now open 24 hours a day in response to the changing household demographics with both spouses working throughout the day. Many primary care physicians are scheduling office hours on weekends and evenings in response to the time-compressed consumer.

Communication

The communication component of the retailing mix includes advertising, personal selling, public relations, catalogs, and brochures. The 1980s saw a growing acceptance of health care advertising. Some hospitals also expanded their retail mix with the addition of physician relations personnel who call upon staff physicians as well as on potential referral services. Brochures have played a major role in hospital advertising. Some academic medical centers have expanded these brochures to resemble catalogs with detailed descriptions of services, access numbers, and biographical sketches of the personnel who deliver the service. All of these communication components provide additional value-added by delivering more information to the marketplace.

Related to the communication component is the issue of store layout and atmosphere. Retail research has demonstrated that the ambience of the retail setting can affect employees as well as customers.[23] Historically, many medical organizations viewed the atmospherics purely as an expense. Now many facilities are paying greater attention to the layout and design of the space in which the services are delivered.

The Wheel of Retailing

There are always new retailing forms that enter the market and seem to replace or capture some of the core business of an existing entity. The **wheel of retailing** describes the process of how new retail forms enter the market and how they evolve over time.[24] FIGURE 10-8 depicts this evolution.

According to this concept, the retail outlet enters the market at position 1 with low status, low price, and low margin. McDonald's first began with two brothers operating a hamburger stand in California. Operated as a drive-in restaurant, it had no seats for customers and a limited menu of hamburgers, French fries, and shakes. Over time, the restaurant added services and other outlets. McDonald's began to expand, by offering fish sandwiches on its menu and tables for customer seating in multiple

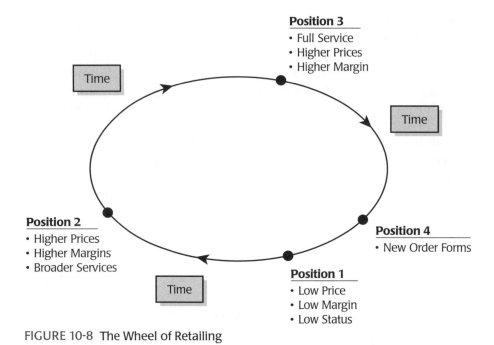

Position 3
- Full Service
- Higher Prices
- Higher Margin

Time

Time

Position 2
- Higher Prices
- Higher Margins
- Broader Services

Time

Position 4
- New Order Forms

Position 1
- Low Price
- Low Margin
- Low Status

FIGURE 10-8 The Wheel of Retailing

locations. At position 3, McDonald's no longer differs from the restaurants and diners from which it originally stole market share. McDonald's restaurants exist around the world. Services have been expanded to include morning bingo games for seniors at some locations, and birthday parties for kids. Menus have broadened to include pizza, salads, and even Mexican food. Some outlets offer home delivery. Margins and prices have also increased. At position 4, the wheel of retailing concept predicts that a new low-margin, low-price, low-status organization will enter the market. In the hamburger business, a relatively recent entrant is "Just Burgers." The wheel begins to turn anew.

The wheel concept also can be applied in health care. Consider how it has turned for many former solo-practice primary care groups or hospitals. The solo-practice physician adds a partner, opens a number of satellite offices, expands into offering other clinical specialties, and becomes a multispecialty group practice. Margins increase, prices rise. Over time, another practice opens in the community offering low-cost, convenient primary care in the shopping mall, and the wheel turns again.

■ Conclusions

The channel of distribution is a central consideration in the formulation of health care marketing strategy. Understanding the flow of patient volume and the intermediaries who affect this flow is at the foundation of the marketing mix plan. Channels can be controlled and influenced by a variety of alternative strategies and depend on the respective power of any entity involved in the channel. As many health care organizations establish vertically integrated marketing systems, concepts common to traditional retail settings will play a more important role.

■ Key Terms

Channel of Distribution	Administered Vertical Marketing
Utilities	System
Functional Shifting	Cooperatives
Channel Intensity	Franchising
Vertical Marketing Systems	Channel Commander
Forward Vertical Integration	Retail Positioning Matrix
Corporate Vertical Marketing	Retail Mix
System	Wheel of Retailing
Integrated Delivery Systems	

■ Chapter Summary

1. The channel of distribution is the path a product takes as it moves from producer to end user, or the path a patient takes as he or she moves through the health care system to the appropriate level of care.
2. Within the channel of distribution, intermediaries (middlemen) provide value in the form of utility. While the intermediary can be eliminated, the function is only shifted elsewhere in the channel.
3. In establishing the channel of distribution, organizations must decide the level of intensity of service delivery—or how available their service will be to consumers.
4. In order to control the channel of distribution and obtain greater efficiencies, organizations can integrate either forward or backward.
5. The growing formation of integrated delivery systems in health care is a vertical integration strategy.
6. In any distribution channel, there is often a single entity or leader who can dictate or control policies with its intermediaries.
7. There are several sources of power available to any distribution channel member. These sources can take the form of economic power, rewards, referent power, coercion, or expertise.
8. Organizations can be positioned perceptually in terms of the breadth of their product line and the perceived value-added.
9. Health care organizations, like retailing businesses, have a retail mix that includes their pricing policies, distribution, services, and communication tactics.

10. In service industries, new market entrants tend to start as low margin, low status. As they mature and grow, this low-entry position is left open to new retail forms.

■ Chapter Problems

1. In recent years, two nationally known health care providers established satellite facilities a great distance from their main clinic locations. The Mayo Clinic, of Rochester, Minnesota, opened facilities in Arizona, Florida, and throughout Iowa, Wisconsin, and Minnesota. The Cleveland Clinic also opened two facilities in Florida. Explain the changes in distribution intensity these actions represent.
2. Explain the vertical integration options and directions for the following providers: (a) a major academic medical center such as the University of Iowa, (b) a five-person general surgery group, and (c) a manufacturer of durable medical equipment.
3. In a recent contract negotiation session between a group of physicians and a managed care health plan, the parties disagreed about the level of reimbursement that the physicians would receive for treating subscribers. The physician group is the largest such organization in the community and represents 75% of all primary care providers in the area. What sources of power does this group wield in negotiating a managed care contract?
4. In examining Figure 10-6 containing the retail positioning matrix, explain how the community hospital in its present position (quadrant 3) could reposition itself to quadrant 2, and to quadrant 1.
5. Utilizing the wheel of retailing concept, explain the evolution in market growth of a neighborhood urgent care medical center that treats minor emergencies.

■ Notes

1. Scott McStravic, "The Boutique Brouhaha," *COR Healthcare Market Strategist* 4, no. 3 (March 2003): 1, 10–14.
2. Daniel Costello, "Virtual Second Opinions," *Los Angeles Times* (December 12, 2002), www.latimes.com/features/health/la-second30dec30.story).
3. E. Chapman and T. Wimberly, "Looking Upstream," *Healthcare Forum Journal* 37, no. 3 (1994): 18–21.
4. S. Gelfond, "Don't Leave Home Without Your Health Card," *Health Week* 5, no. 3 (1991): 29–30.
5. W. L. Trombetta, "Channel Systems: An Idea Whose Time Has Come in Health Care Marketing," *Journal of Health Care Marketing* 9, no. 3 (1989): 26–35.
6. B. Holcomb, "Hospital HYPE," *New York* (August 3, 1987): 30–35.
7. L. W. Stern and A. I. El-Ansary, *Marketing Channels*, 4th ed. (Englewood Cliffs, NJ: Prentice Hall, 1991).

8. D. A. Conrad and W. L. Dowling, "Vertical Integration in Health Services: Theory and Managerial Implications," *Health Care Management Review* 15, no. 4 (Fall 1990): 12.

9. S. Findlay, "How New Alliances Are Changing Health Care," *Business & Health* 11, no. 10 (1993): 28–34.

10. R. Contreras, B. Greenspan, and R. C. Leventhal, "Medical Care in the Discount Aisle," *Journal of Health Care Marketing* 9, no. 3 (1989): 58–61.

11. G. Borzo and B. McCormick, "Cardiovascular Network Receives Federal Approval," *American Medical News* (1993): 4.

12. J. A. Tannebaum, "Franchise Fever," *The Wall Street Journal*, October 16, 1992, R14–R15.

13. I. Albert, "Unconventional Medicine . . . The Other Half of a Continuum," *Strategic Health Care Marketing* 11, no. 7 (1994): 6–8.

14. J. Gaski, "The Theory of Power and Conflict in Channels of Distribution," *Journal of Marketing* 48, no. 3 (Summer 1984): 9–29.

15. L. Scott, "Suppliers Feeling Effects of Columbia," *Modern Healthcare* 24, no. 11 (1994): 22.

16. "The Dynamics of Power in Healthcare," *Integrated Healthcare Report* (November 1993): 1–7.

17. An early article suggesting the linkage of retailing concepts in health care was T. Paul and J. Wong, "The Retailing of Health Care," *Journal of Health Care Marketing* 4, no. 4 (Fall 1984): 23–35.

18. This discussion is derived from W. T. Gregor and E. M. Firars, *Mass Merchandising: Retail Revolution in Consumer Services* (Cambridge, MA: Management Analysis Center, 1982).

19. E. F. Goldman, "The Power of Positioning," in *Responding to the Challenge: Health Care Marketing Comes of Age*, ed. P. D. Cooper (Chicago, IL: Alliance for Health Care Marketing and Strategy, 1986), 109–111.

20. W. Lazer and E. J. Kelley, "The Retailing Mix: Planning and Management," *Journal of Retailing* 37, no. 1 (Spring 1961): 34–41.

21. Mindy Thompson, "Retail Strategies," *Healthcare Financial Management* (August 2003): 73–40.

22. J. Morrissey, "Geographical Software Aids Executives," *Modern Healthcare* 25, no. 2 (1995): 34.

23. M. J. Bitner, "Servicescapes: The Impact of Physical Surroundings on Customers and Employees," *Journal of Marketing* 55, no. 1 (1992): 57–71.

24. This theory was first proposed by M. P. McNair, "Significant Trends and Development in the Postwar Period," in *Competitive Distribution in a Free High-Level Economy and Its Implications for the University*, ed. A. B. Smith (Pittsburgh, PA: University of Pittsburgh Press, 1958), 1–25; and M. McNair and E. May, "The Next Revolution of the Retailing Wheel," *Harvard Business Review* 56, no. 5 (1978): 81–91.

Promotion

Promotional strategies that companies use to communicate their messages to the marketplace have four basic components: (1) advertising, (2) personal selling, (3) publicity, and (4) sales promotion. At the heart of all of these tools lies communication. With any promotional strategy, the ultimate goal is to communicate to a market. Before examining each of the four basic promotional tools of marketing, however, this chapter will first consider how communication occurs, and discuss the elements necessary for communication to take place.

■ The Communication Model

There are several factors that contribute to effective communication. Many of these essential components can be affected by a company's strategies and tactics. Successful communication with a target market depends upon the effectiveness of the major components of communication, as shown in FIGURE 11-1.[1] The components within this diagram include:

1. A *sender*, which can be a person or company who wants to communicate a messag~
2. A *receiver*, the target of the communication
3. The process of *encoding* or developing the message

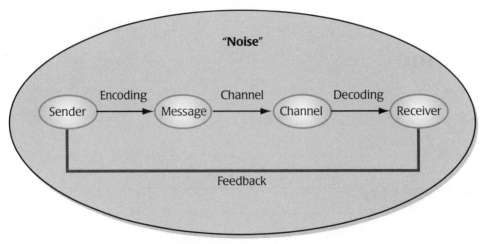

FIGURE 11-1 The Communication Process

4. The *message*, which is what is to be communicated
5. The *channel* by which the message is sent
6. The process of *decoding*, or interpreting the message encoded by the sender
7. The element of *noise*, which includes external factors that affect how the message is interpreted
8. *Feedback*, which provides the sender with an assessment of the effectiveness of the communication between sender and receiver

Each of these elements determines whether effective communication occurs.

The Sender

The sender of the message is often referred to as the source. The sender can be a person, a company, or a spokesperson representing someone else. The *spokesperson* is the person in marketing communications who delivers the message. In an advertisement, the spokesperson can be a famous baseball player, for example; in personal selling, the spokesperson is the company's sales representative.

An important element for the senders, or spokespersons, of any message is their *source credibility*, which is the target market's perception that the sender can be believed. Elements that contribute to source credibility are dimensions such as trustworthiness, knowledge or expertise, experience, and to some degree the source's likability.[2] During the mid-1970s, an actor named Robert Young played the role of a physician, Dr. Marcus Welby, on a well-liked television drama. Young's acting role translated into a high degree of medical source credibility, which resulted in his being hired in 1978 to promote the positive benefits of Sanka, a brand of decaffeinated coffee. Similarly, famous movie actor John Wayne promoted Datril 500, a headache remedy, during 1979.

Encoding

Communication cannot occur without the process of **encoding**, which refers to translating the meaning to be communicated into words or symbols. For example, a family practice group might want to communicate that it is a caring organization that will meet the health care needs of the entire family. To encode this message, the group practice might use a picture of a physician caring for a child with the parents looking on. The message is encoded with a series of pictures and possibly a tag line that reads, "Your family's one-stop health source."

For communication to occur, the sender of the message must encode with symbols or words that are shared in a similar way by the receiver. In Chapter 12, on advertising, the issue of pretesting is discussed as a way to ensure that the shared meaning is occurring.

Increasingly in the United States, health care organizations are facing a multicultural marketplace. The interesting and challenging nature of this marketplace is the frequent absence of shared meaning between different cultural groups. As the U.S. marketplace becomes more culturally diverse, health care organizations are responding in their communication pieces. Hospitals such as Providence Memorial Hospital in el Paso Texas, DiMaggio Children's Hospital in Hollywood, Florida, and Methodist Health System in Houston are but a few of the health care organizations today recognizing the increasing cultural diversity within the United States. Each of these organizations have Web sites that can be easily converted to Spanish language encoded to a Spanish language version with the click of an icon. The problems of the past, such as experienced by many US companies when they expanded into the international market will hopefully be avoided as health care marketers recognize the need for proper encoding and decoding. One only need to recognize the problem that can occur when realizing the challenges faced by Chevrolet in attempting to sell their Nova in Latin American countries. This language problem has been experienced in the international marketplace. For many years, Chevrolet tried to market its Nova automobile in Latin American countries, with dismal sales for its efforts. In Spanish, the word *nova* means "no go." Needless to say, promoting a car with this meaning makes gaining market acceptance an impossible challenge.

The Message

The **message** is the combination of symbols and words that the sender uses to transmit. There are several forms a message can take. Some varieties are:

Two-Sided versus One-Sided Message

In a two-sided message, the sender presents both the pros and cons of the service being promoted. Prior research has shown that two-sided messages have a stronger impact on higher-educated consumers. A two-sided message also helps prepare the market for opposing messages, which they may hear about or read in competitors' presentations.

The disadvantage of two-sided messages is that it may make the target market aware of negative product features that it might not have considered.[3]

Comparative Messages

Comparative messages involve direct claims relative to the competition. Prior research reveals that these types of messages work best when the product is noticeably different from the competition. Studies also show, however, that consumers generally find comparative advertising less credible and informative than advertising that just focuses on the product itself.[4] Organizations that engage in comparative advertising must have supportable evidence for any product claims to ward off litigation from the competitor whose product is being compared.

In Canada very detailed and strict guidelines have been established regarding the use and support of comparative advertising claims with regard to comparative advertising of pharmaceutical products. The government has published the "Therapeutic Comparative Advertising Directive and Guidance Document."

The Canadian government has very specific guidelines as to what must be provided as supporting evidence in comparative advertising claims between product to product comparisons.

1. Two clinical trials are required to support a comparison of the onset or duration of action of two products.
2. Alternatively, sponsors should justify and provide information on alternative methods used and data generated to support the comparison. For example, comparative pharmacokinetic/pharmacodynamic studies may be appropriate in this context, provided that a strong correlation can be established between the measured endpoint and the onset duration of the therapeutic effect of the compared products. In no circumstances would extrapolation of the claim beyond the actual conditions of supporting studies be acceptable.
3. Ingredient to ingredient and product to ingredient comparisons
   (1) Comparisons may be drawn with respect to onset and/or duration of action provided sponsors adequately justify the method(s) used, and the data generated, to support the comparative claim relating to onset or duration of action.[5]

Although there are other requirements, the important aspect of these examples is the detailed nature of what is required from advertisers when using comparative claims in advertising messages.

Emotional Appeals

The creation of any message involves determining its level of appeal. Messages can appeal to the product benefits or to emotions. Emotional appeals can take the form of fear, humor, or sentiment. In health care, there is some concern about using fear as an emotional appeal in advertising. Because concern about health is a basic issue for most consumers, a fear appeal could generate unnecessary anxiety or higher utilization rates—all due to an issue that, factually, might be true, but has a very small incidence rate.[6] For example, a medical group might run an advertisement, stating that the presence of a number of symptoms might indicate a heart attack. While there is a factual basis for any one symptom, a consumer would have to experience these symptoms with a degree of frequency combined with other factors before any diagnosis could be made. Such an advertisement could generate a large number of medical claims at a diagnostic clinic. In general, moderate fear appeals have been found to be more effective than either weak or strong appeals.[7]

Sentiment is also used in some health care–related advertisements. Manufacturers of Rogaine® show men looking into the mirror thinking about prior days when they had hair. Usually these reminiscences show them in the company of an attractive woman or as the focus of a party. The advertisement returns to the man looking at his head of thinning hair and announces an available treatment. A similar concern with regard to personal appearance has led to many plastic surgeons placing an attractive person who has undergone cosmetic surgery in their advertisements. Such emotional appeals are viewed by some as testing the boundaries of what is acceptable for promotion within health care. The issue is whether such promotion is medically appropriate or necessary. Yet, since cosmetic surgery is a self-paid procedure, promotion of cosmetic surgery might be considered similar to any other product for which consumers pay directly out of their own pockets.

Occasionally, health care providers use humor to draw attention to negative aspects of a health care service. The advertisement typically will show how improved conditions are in the particular provider's setting. Humor is a useful emotional appeal; however, its major problem is that it is often very individual-specific. Funny to one person may be degrading to another. It is necessary in the use of humor to ensure that the encoding and decoding processes occur. Health care marketers need to exercise great care when using humor in advertising. Since most health care decisions are high involvement issues, as described in Chapter 4 on buyer behavior, consumers treat health care as a serious issue. Like religion, certain issues are less adaptable to humorous appeals. When using humor, it is also important that the theme doesn't so overwhelm the product that it goes unnoticed.[8,9]

The Channel

The **channel** is the means used to deliver a marketing message. It is the foundation of the promotional plan. In the promotional mix, companies can use mass media, personal salespersons, or publicity to communicate their message to the target audience. The latter portion of this chapter will review the advantages and disadvantages of each of these alternative channels in greater detail.

The major difference in channels is whether they involve interpersonal or mass communication. Interpersonal communication involves a salesperson or word-of-mouth communication among members of the target audience. A company can control the salesperson through training and supporting sales literature. Because interpersonal communication occurs between people, however, a company can never ensure total control over how its message is encoded or over the message's content. In health care, this lack of control had been a common source of complaint among physicians who worked for some health maintenance organizations (HMOs). These physicians often believed that the HMO's salespeople, in their enthusiasm to attract new subscribers, made claims that the providers could not deliver upon. In this instance, the physicians believe that the communication is leaving misimpressions in the market. Yet, the sales personnel believe that in their communication they are highlighting the factors that are important in the selection of the health care plan by consumers. Such a source of conflict can indicate a lack of control of this interpersonal channel.

Historically, health care has relied upon word-of-mouth advertising by satisfied patients as its primary promotional channel. One friend telling another friend about a particular physician or a positive experience at a sports medicine clinic has a high level of source credibility. Some organizations try to target specific people who play a vital role in the word-of-mouth process. These individuals are often recognized as **opinion leaders** whose advice or experience is sought out by others. Typically, the opinion leader is someone regarded by peers or social group as having experience or expertise in a particular area. Pharmaceutical companies often try to identify which physicians in the medical group or hospital staff are the opinion leaders whom others turn to for advice. Pharmaceutical sales representatives target these physicians for the initial calls. These physicians might receive advance materials regarding the pharmacological aspects of a new medication.

Decoding

While a sender of a message must encode, the message's receiver must decode, or translate, the message. **Decoding** is the process by which the receiver interprets symbols and words. For communication to be effective, a message must be decoded the same way the sender has encoded. Decoding is based on the attitudes, values, and beliefs of the message's receivers.[10,11] Communication does occur when decoding differs from the encoding; however, the outcomes of this situation are not always positive. For example, the family practice group sent a message showing it as the source of care for the entire family. Yet, the target audience may have decoded the message (the picture and words) depicting the medical practice as a pediatric group. Communication occurred, but not effective communication.

Noise

Noise is anything that interferes with the effective communication of a message. Several sources can produce noise: the message, the channel, the environment, the sender, or the receiver. Noise from any source, however, creates problems.

The message can create noise that distracts the receiver from the intended focus. An advertisement that uses humor, for example, can be quite funny to the receiver. The focus of the message, however, might be lost while the receiver attends to the humor rather than to the service being promoted.

The channel can also create noise. A Harris & Associates poll indicated the physician, as channel, can create noise. In a survey of 2525 women and 1000 men conducted for The Commonwealth Fund, a national health philanthropy, 10% of the female respondents said they didn't discuss a problem with their physician because they found the physician to be squeamish about the issue.[12]

Noise can readily occur when using interpersonal channels. A salesperson who makes a poor presentation due to inadequate preparation or organization can create enough noise to prohibit effective communication.

Channel noise can also exist in mass communication. Advertising on television often faces the problem of clutter, with too many distracting messages. The noise of the medium inhibits effective communication. The environment is often a major source of noise. There are increasingly unfavorable reports about rising health care costs. This noise in the environment may negate an organization's attempt to communicate that it is a cost-efficient provider. Receivers can also create their own noise. Lack of attention or interest greatly inhibits the decoding process.

Feedback

The sender of any message is always concerned whether the message has been decoded exactly as it was encoded. In this regard, **feedback**, which is communication from the receiver to the sender, is essential. Feedback is communication in reverse. When the sender uses an interpersonal channel for a message, feedback is often immediate. A company's human resource director can communicate directly with the managed health care plan indicating that he or she doesn't understand a particular benefit. Feedback is more difficult when using mass communication. Many companies, however, will set up toll-free telephone lines to encourage customer response or feedback. WRNX radio station in western Massachusetts has established a listener call-in line. The audience is encouraged and solicited to call in with their thoughts or preferences regarding the station's song list. Chapter 12 on advertising will examine alternative forms of feedback mechanisms for mass communication channels.

■ The Promotional Mix

The promotional component of marketing involves four basic tools: advertising, personal selling, publicity, and sales promotion. **Advertising** can be defined as any directly paid form of nonpersonal presentation of goods, services, and ideas. **Personal selling** is any paid, personal presentation of goods, ideas, or services. **Publicity** can be defined as any indirectly paid presentation of goods or services. **Sales promotion** is any short-term inducement or offer for a particular product or service. Each of these promotional tools has unique aspects with inherent benefits and weaknesses. Before discussing these aspects, it is important to recognize that an organization might combine one or more of these particular tools to communicate with an intended market.

Advertising

Advertising is distinguished from the other promotional tools in the marketing mix in that it is both paid *and* nonpersonal. The directly paid component of advertising distinguishes it from publicity. Because an organization pays for space in a magazine or for television or radio time, the advertiser has the advantage of control. When paying for the space or time, the advertiser controls to whom the message is sent. This control is achieved wherever the advertiser places the advertisement. An advertisement run on the MTV channel will most likely attract a different audience than an advertisement placed on CNN World News. By directly paying for the space, an advertiser also can control *when* the message is sent. An advertiser can buy time during the 6:00 PM news broadcast, specifying that its advertisement for the hospital will be shown in that time slot. The advertiser also can control *what* is said. Because the advertiser pays for the space, the advertiser can (within the bounds of the law and good taste) create the exact message it wishes to convey. Finally, the advertiser can control *how often* the message is communicated. The frequency of advertising is determined purely by the advertiser's budget constraints. If a health plan wanted to purchase all the time on the Super Bowl broadcast, its greatest limitation would be the cost of the time relative to the advertiser's budget.

Another distinguishing feature of advertising is that it is nonpersonal. As discussed in the model of communication, this may be advertising's greatest limitation because it makes feedback difficult. Another important limitation to advertising is the noise created by the large number of advertisements that bombard the consumer each day. Finally, advertising is limited because most consumers recognize it as a self-promoting communication. In this regard, advertising messages often face credibility problems. Within health care promotional strategy, advertising has become a major focus. In 1990, hospital advertising was $235 million dollars and grew to almost $800 million by 1996. It was expected to reach $1.6 billion by 2000.[13] By 1998 almost half of the roughly 5000 acute care hospitals in the United States were engaged in hospital advertising spending on average $123,000 per hospital.[14]

Advertising Effectiveness

Advertising can be more effective in some situations than in others. Advertising is most effective when buyer awareness about a service is minimal. This is when the differential impact of advertising tends to be the greatest. Advertising also works best when industry sales are rising. Advertising cannot stop a decline in industry sales. No amount of advertising, for example, can change the trend in pediatrics or in inpatient stays for the hospital industry. The factors that affect these aspects of health care—in one case demographics (pediatrics), and in the other technology and reimbursement (inpatient days)—are beyond the influence of advertising.

Advertising also works best when the service features are not normally observable, and advertising can demonstrate the outcome of using a particular service. Health New England, an HMO based in Springfield, Massachusetts, uses outdoor billboards showing a cross-country skier. Its slogan states, "Our definition of an outpatient." Another condition under which advertising works best is when the opportunities for differentiation are strong and advertising can highlight a real point of difference between products. When there is no real differentiation, advertising can do little more than remind the consumer that the brand or service exists in the marketplace. Finally, advertising is effective when the service is new or not commonly advertised. In the early days of hospital advertising, initial campaigns generated significant consumer attention because health care and hospitals were a novel product to advertise. In most communities today, hospital advertising is as common as McDonald's or Burger King promotions.

Personal Selling

The second major tool of the promotional mix is personal selling. The major difference between this tool and advertising is that it is a personal form of communication. The major strength of personal selling is that it allows for direct feedback from the receiver. A message can then be refined or explained in greater detail to correct any misunderstandings or difficulties in interpretation by the receiver. Personal selling also has a greater advantage than advertising in that it provides more direct control over who receives the message. Advertising is a form of mass communication. People who see the message are not always part of the intended audience. With personal selling, a company can target the audience for its communication. Hospitals that use personal selling have reported several benefits, as shown in Table 11-1.

Table 11-1	Benefits of Personal Selling	
Increased Facility Utilization		35.2%
Improved Medical Staff Relations		31.5%
Financial Benefits		26.5%
Increased Market Share		21.6%
Increased Market Presence		17.3%
Increased Organizational Marketing Sophistication		14.2%
Greater Customer Focus		12.3%

(Total Sample: 279 Hospitals)

Source: Adapted from Powers, T. L. and Bowers, M. R., Challenges and Opportunities for Personal Selling, *Journal of Health Care Marketing*, Vol. 12, No. 4, pp. 26–32, with permission of American Marketing Association, © 1992.

As with any promotional tool, however, personal selling also has its limitations. A major limitation is cost. Maintaining an effective sales staff requires expenses far beyond salaries. Costs for a sales staff include individual benefits, travel costs, technical and equipment support and so on. The sales calls a salesperson can make in one day are limited. In health care, sales calls to referral physician offices or companies can be very time-consuming. A salesperson may only be able to make four to six calls per day. Another limitation to personal selling is related directly to the strength of the interpersonal communication. Because sales involves a person, the message may vary as a function of the individual's training, disposition, or style. In these cases, a company can suffer from a lack of uniformity regarding its sales training and communications techniques.

Advertising versus Personal Sales Trade-off

In developing promotional strategy, most companies often face a trade-off in the dollars to be allocated between advertising and personal selling. Table 11-2 shows some of the trade-offs to be made between advertising and personal selling, depending on which tool a company chooses to emphasize in its promotional effort.

The more technologically sophisticated the service, the greater the need for personal selling. A salesperson might be needed to explain the intricacies of a particular diagnostic service or program. A medical center might use a personal sales representative to call on potential referral physicians regarding its hyperbaric medicine program. The uniqueness and newness of any services can warrant significant explanation regarding their use or applicability.

The second criterion shown in Table 11-2—number of potential customers—provides the rationale as to why most consumer product companies use advertising and why industrial firms rely on personal selling. In health care, promoting a primary care group to all households within a particular ZIP code warrants a mass communication strategy such as direct mail. An occupational medicine program, however, might be best promoted with a personal sales effort targeting the companies who have employee assistance personnel.

The third criterion in Table 11-2 relates to the composition of the decision-making unit (DMU). The more people involved in making a corporate purchasing decision, the greater the need for personal selling. When numerous decision makers are involved, each one may have a distinct set of attributes upon which he or she bases a decision. Personal selling is necessary so that the message can be tailored to address each deci-

Table 11-2	Advertising versus Sales Trade-offs	
Sales	Criteria	Advertising
High	Degree of technical sophistication	Low
Few	Number of customers	Many
Complex	Size of decision-making unit (DMU)	Simple
Great	Degree of risk	Little

sion maker's unique concerns. When managed care plans advertise their health plans to prospective enrollees, their ads can promote the benefits covered or the outcomes to be derived. Yet, a personal sales effort is required when the managed care organization persuades a company to offer the plan to the firm's employees. The chief financial officer, the union representative, the company president, and the human resources director may have different concerns that must be addressed before the company accepts the plan. A company that offers significant ancillary services with its product often finds the need to devote more effort to personal selling. In these instances, a salesperson can provide the service or explain its use.

The last criterion when deciding between advertising and personal selling involves degree of risk. The higher the risk, the more personal selling is necessary. This last criterion should make personal selling a key ingredient of most health care organizations' promotional strategy plans. A salesperson can provide the assurance or support that the service or product will meet the customer's expectations. Many academic medical centers have spent significant dollars developing glossy physician referral brochures. Typically, these include photographs of the physicians on staff, their backgrounds, and areas of expertise. While helpful, these brochures have limited impact. Few decisions are riskier for a physician than making a referral. A personal sales call and follow-up with the potential physician from whom the referral will be made will have a greater likelihood of generating a referral.

Advertising versus Sales in Decision Making

In addition to the criteria considered above in the trade-off between advertising and personal selling, these two promotional tools also can vary in impact, depending at which stage the buyer decides to purchase. FIGURE 11-2 displays the levels of impact that advertising and personal selling have at different stages in the buying process.[15] Unlike the buyer behavior model described in Chapter 4, the horizontal axis on this graph has delineated the decision to buy in three basic stages: pre-purchase, purchase, and post-

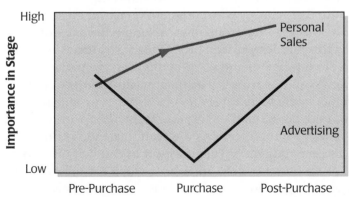

FIGURE 11-2 The Differing Impact of Advertising versus Personal Sales

purchase. In the pre-purchase stage, the consumer searches for information and evaluates alternatives. As seen in Figure 11-2, both advertising and personal selling are of equal significance at this stage. In the actual purchase stage, personal sales is the key—it is the salesperson who closes the sale. Only occasionally can advertising play this role, such as with direct-mail catalogs. Yet even in these instances, the prospective purchaser often seeks out additional information by dialing the toll-free number listed in the catalog.

Finally, there is the post-purchase stage. The consumer selects a particular health plan. Both advertising and personal selling play a role in the post-purchase stage. The importance of this stage is more significant when the buyer chooses between competing alternatives. The consumer often suffers from cognitive dissonance, which is post-purchase anxiety about whether the correct alternative was chosen. The consumer will seek out additional information to reconfirm that the selection was the best alternative. In this stage, the more personal the post-purchase communication, the more satisfied the buyer.

Publicity

This third promotional tool, publicity, is most common to health care organizations. As noted, this form of communication is an indirectly paid form of presentation of goods, ideas, or services. Most publicity is coordinated through the efforts of a public relations department. The public relations department encourages the media to print or broadcast stories about the organization or its accomplishments. The hospital, for example, that is discussed on the nightly news for having saved a person's life does not pay directly for that coverage. Such coverage is usually garnered through the efforts of the public relations director who contacts the media and provides them with the story. Many public relations departments will also develop news or story releases for dissemination to the media for potential publication or broadcast. The indirect payment involves the resources needed to staff a public relations organization.

In Wisconsin, Physicians Plus is a multispecialty medical group that relies heavily on publicity generated through strong media relations. The marketing director sets up media interviews with the group's specialists who comment on nationally reported health care stories. The group also assists reporters in localizing national stories or trends. In five years of following this publicity-driven promotional strategy, the physicians have participated in 49 radio interviews and 71 television interviews, and have assisted in 188 magazine and newspaper stories.[16] The greatest advantage to publicity is its credibility. Most consumers who read a story in a newspaper or magazine or watch a television report do not understand that the organization often worked hard to obtain favorable coverage. These communications are seen, instead, as unbiased presentations about the firm. Yet, the indirect payment aspect of publicity is also its greatest weakness. The organization does not control how or when the message gets out. And, to most media, a story is only good once and then it is old news. Thus, a medical group that works hard to obtain publicity may find its story told on the Saturday evening television news when viewership is light and the target audience who watches the news differs from the desired audience. Because of this lack of control, publicity is only useful as a supplemental tool in the promotional plan. It is the rare promotional strategy that can be fully successful by relying totally on this tool for dissemination of its message.

Negative Information

Occasionally, the publicity that an organization receives is not the result of a planned attempt to have its name or accomplishments mentioned in the media. An area of growing importance for public relations and publicity is how to deal with negative information. Negative information has been found to seriously impact an organization. A recent study within the Veteran's Administration showed the impact directly on patient volume. Twenty-four newspaper articles about adverse patient care at veterans' centers were identified between 1994 and 1999. Patient enrollment was examined at these facilities versus others that did not receive such negative communication, at one year prior, one year after, and three years after the negative communication. Results showed one year before the negative publicity the affected facilities had similar rates of enrollment among veterans. However at one and three years after the negative publicity periods, enrollment rates were significantly lower.[17] There is a growing need for almost every company to prepare a public relations response plan to deal with any unforeseen negative information. The cases in business are classic, from the early days of the Ford Pinto (exploding gas tanks), to Tylenol (product tampering), to the Pepsi-Cola scare (hypodermic needles in the cans). All these cases show the value of being able to respond effectively to negative information.[18]

Public Relations and Marketing Interaction

In many health care organizations, the delineation between marketing and public relations is often unclear. There is a significant overlap between these two functions since both deal with target markets. FIGURE 11-3 shows some overlapping areas of responsibility between marketing and public relations. Circle B within the diagram shows the areas where there is often overlap between both departments. When marketing first appeared as a functional area within the management structure of hospitals, there was significant conflict between marketing and public relations over departmental responsibilities. Both marketing and public relations contribute greatly to the organization's presence among key market segments. The essential ingredient is that there is coordination of the promotional plan by the marketing and public relations departments.

Sales Promotion

The fourth tool in the promotional mix—sales promotion—involves temporary inducements to buy. These efforts can be directed to the end user or to the intermediary who carries a product. Most readers of this text are familiar with the common sales

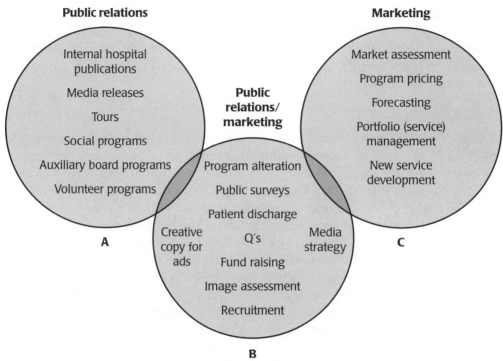

Public relations

Internal hospital publications

Media releases

Tours

Social programs

Auxiliary board programs

Volunteer programs

A

Public relations/ marketing

Program alteration

Public surveys

Patient discharge

Creative copy for ads

Q's

Media strategy

Fund raising

Image assessment

Recruitment

B

Marketing

Market assessment

Program pricing

Forecasting

Portfolio (service) management

New service development

C

FIGURE 11-3 The Marketing and Public Relations Interface

Source: From Berkowitz, E. N., Hillestad, S., and Effertz, P., Marketing/Public Relations: A New Arena for Hospital Conflict from *Health Care Planning and Marketing*, January 1982, pp. 1–10, 1982. Used by permission of Lippincott Williams & Wilkins.

promotions of coupons, sweepstakes, or premiums, each of which will be described briefly later in this chapter. Traditional businesses spend more money on sales promotion than they do on advertising. In health care, limited attempts at sales promotion have been implemented. Some hospitals have used sales promotions to induce consumers into engaging in a health screening activity. Pharmaceutical companies also have used sales promotions to induce trial of medications. Yet, to some degree, the limited use of sales promotion tactics has been due to a concern that such activities might lead to unnecessary utilization of health care services. Although not used to date with any great frequency, it is useful to understand the two broad types of sales promotions that have been incorporated by traditional industries.

Promotions to Consumers

A large number of sales promotions are directed to the end user of the product. There are numerous sales promotion objectives, as shown in EXHIBIT 11-1. For each of these sales promotion objectives, a different promotional tactic might be applied. Following are examples of sales promotions commonly directed to individual consumers.

Exhibit 11-1 Sales Promotion Objectives

1. To encourage trial of the product by consumers
2. To encourage intermediaries to utilize the facility
3. To encourage customers to buy more than one unit of the product
4. To encourage intermediaries to devote more effort in selling the product or service
5. To acquaint customers with service changes
6. To identify new customers
7. To build customer loyalty
8. To encourage customers to switch facilities or providers
9. To gain entry into new markets

Coupons
Coupons are one of the most common forms of sales promotions and one of the few that have been used in health care. Some hospitals have offered coupons for a free blood pressure screening or for a pamphlet on a particular medical problem. Some coupons occasionally will have a discounted offer as part of their appeal. For example, $10 off the price of a mammogram might encourage some first-time triers whose insurance coverage requires a significant co-payment.

Cash Rebates
This sales promotion involves providing consumers with a monetary incentive if they purchase a particular brand. It is an indirect way of discounting a product's price without giving the appearance of a price reduction.

Contests
Contests are sales promotions that require the consumer to participate actively in the promotion. The consumer might have to solve a puzzle or provide a slogan to enter a chance to win. Retail outlets use contests to encourage their customers' return to acquire more game pieces or clues to a puzzle.

Premiums
Premiums are products given to the consumer in return for a particular action. Many premiums are often tied to the product being purchased. Marlboro cigarettes, for example, market a line of western clothes as premiums. These premiums are an attempt to reinforce the image of the rugged cowboy who smokes Marlboros. McDonald's restaurants provide children with small toys related to particular themes, such as pumpkin pails on Halloween.

Samples

Samples are products disseminated to the consumer free or at a greatly reduced cost. Companies frequently manufacture smaller-packaged versions of a product to be promoted as a special trial size. Samples are a valuable form of sales promotion because they allow the consumer to try an item with less risk. Since the product is often given free or at a greatly reduced price, the consumer's investment is minimal. Pharmaceutical sales representatives give physicians samples of new medications as a way to encourage trial use. In 2001 it was estimated that the value of free samples given to physicians was worth over $10 billion.[19] New mothers are often presented with a free sample kit of baby-related products upon discharge from the hospital.

Service businesses are at a disadvantage in terms of sampling. One cannot create a smaller version of the service. Yet it is possible to create a sample by allowing the consumer a free visit or a first-time visit at a greatly reduced price. Sampling, however, is costly. For sampling to be effective, the product or service being tried should be noticeably better than the competition's.

Promotions to the Trade

There is a second level of sales promotions, which is directed to intermediaries within the channel of distribution. For example, traditional businesses such as Proctor and Gamble may direct sales promotion efforts at retailers, with the goal of encouraging retailers to stock more of a particular product in inventory. Two commonly used sales promotions in the distribution channel are allowances and cooperative advertising.

Allowances

A common trade promotion is the allowance, which is a discount based on some particular criterion. For example, a manufacturer might give a case allowance based on a minimum amount of product ordered. Another common allowance is a merchandise allowance, which provides a discount or reimbursement to the intermediary who makes extra merchandising efforts for a particular product or line.

Cooperative Advertising

A second major trade allowance involves sharing or underwriting some portion of the advertising expense with an intermediary. Coca-Cola, for example, might pay Kroger Supermarket up to $5000 per quarter per region for advertisements that highlight Coca-Cola products. This is a form of sales promotion that could be used in health care. A hospital, for example, could pay some of the advertising for a medical group that is a loyal member of the institution. General Electric (GE). has, for example, helped providers who offer mammography services by advertising those programs. At times, GE covers the cost of advertising.[20]

A cooperative advertising program is an acceptable form of a trade allowance. Yet, every organization must be careful that these arrangements are not viewed as tying arrangements, which would violate the Clayton Act (1914). Tying arrangements create situations in which a seller requires the purchaser of one product to also buy another product in its line. These arrangements, which would lessen competition, were specifically forbidden by the Clayton Act.

■ Factors Affecting Sales Promotion Use

There are two main factors to consider when emphasizing one particular promotional tool relative to another in the development of the promotional plan. These factors include the stage of the product life cycle and the channel control strategy.

The Product Life Cycle

At each stage of the product life cycle, there are distinct promotional considerations.

Introduction

A major factor to consider in determining the promotional mix is the stage of the product life cycle. In the introduction stage, as noted in Chapter 8, a key consideration is gaining awareness. At this stage advertising plays a major role. As a mass communication strategy, advertising can efficiently generate early recognition of the service among consumers. In the introduction stage of the life cycle, companies must often develop *primary demand*. This is purchase interest in a product class. Any early publicity to build credibility is of particular value at this stage. Depending on the product, sales promotion can also play a valuable role in this stage. In this regard, service businesses are often limited, whereas a product-based company has the opportunity to disseminate samples of the new item, offering consumers a low-cost way to try the product.

Growth

In the growth stage of the life cycle, competition appears, in which case product businesses try to lock up the channel of distribution. Personal selling efforts are directed to the intermediaries to tie in the buyer. This scenario also works in health care. As more competitors vie for referrals in the cardiac surgery, a physician referral sales force must focus efforts on the primary care referrers to lock up their patient base. At the growth stage of the life cycle, advertising efforts shift from generating awareness to highlighting the differences between competitors. Advertising at this stage develops *selective demand*, which is interest in and preference for the specific brand of product or service.

Maturity

At the mature stage of the life cycle, there are few new buyers. The major goal of promotional strategy is to maintain the buyers the company presently serves. The advertising is done mainly for reinforcement or reminder purposes. In industries where sales promotion is common, these efforts are directed at keeping the present customer base returning. Games or discounts for multiple purchases become more common. Within the airline industry, as business travel began to level off in the recessionary period of the late 1980s, frequent-flyer mileage programs evolved as a new sales promotion tool to encourage repeat business.

Decline

The decline stage of the product life cycle is one where little promotional effort occurs.

Channel Control Strategies

Chapter 10 presented the concept of the channel of distribution. For any organization, the ultimate goal is to control the channel of distribution. There are two basic strategies involving promotional tools that are used to accomplish this; these are referred to as push and pull.

Push

A **push** strategy involves controlling the channel of distribution by working through the channel. FIGURE 11-4 shows the channels of distribution for a typical consumer goods manufacturer and for an acute-care hospital. For the consumer goods company, the product moves to the consumer. For the hospital, the patient moves to the facility. In a push strategy, the manufacturer influences the intermediaries to carry the product. A manufacturer might offer the wholesaler a discount if it orders so many cases of a new brand of soft drink. The wholesaler, in turn, may employ a push strategy by offering the retailer a similar inducement to order. When consumers go to the retailer to buy their regular soft drink, the retailer might encourage the consumer to buy the new brand. Because of the discount provided by the wholesaler, the smart retailer knows it will make more money if the new brand is purchased.

A similar push strategy is familiar in health care. A hospital has a medical staff that also has practice privileges at competing facilities. The hospital administrator

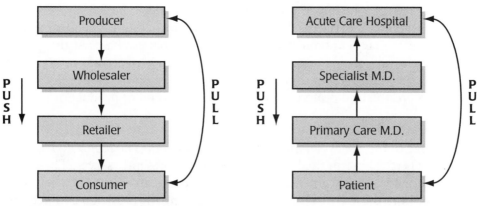

FIGURE 11-4 Push versus Pull Strategies

wants these physicians to admit patients to his or her particular facility. In order to encourage the physicians, the administrator might provide them with preferential parking, free lunches in the physicians' lounge, and office space in an attached medical office building. The goal is that physicians will refer patients to the hospital at which the physicians feel most comfortable. In a related push strategy, pharmaceutical companies in recent years have paid physicians to act as part–time lecturers at meetings attended by physicians. The attendees are other physicians who are provided a free dinner. In 2004, 237,000 meetings and talks were sponsored by pharmaceutical companies that featured such physicians, compared to 134,000 meetings led by company representatives. An internal study done by Merck & Co, a pharmaceutical firm, shows this approach using physician-led discussion groups resulted in doubling the return on investment from company-led meetings.[21] The push strategy was effective.

Pull

An alternative to the push strategy is **pull**. In this strategy, the organization appeals directly to the consumer by bypassing or controlling the intermediary. Again, in Figure 11-4, the manufacturer may find, in trying to introduce a new product, that the wholesaler is not interested in carrying the item in spite of incentives offered. If wholesaler acceptance is not gained, retailer acceptance will be unlikely. As a result, the manufacturer may try to pull the product through the channel by advertising the item to end users. Consumers, seeing advertisements for the new brand, or receiving coupons for a dollar off a two-liter bottle, will seek out the item from retailers. Retailers, seeing consumer demand, will call the wholesalers requesting delivery. Wholesalers, learning of retailer interest, will call the manufacturer to place orders.

Many health care organizations often implement a pull strategy. A tertiary care center might find that local physicians do not want to refer to the medical center. In spite of efforts to generate referrals, patient flow is low. So the medical center begins to promote its new program directly to consumers. Many consumers in Arizona, for example, know about the Arizona Heart Institute. These consumers might bypass their local physician or cardiologist to whom their physician has referred them, in order to seek out care at the Arizona Heart Institute. In the mid-1980s, many hospitals began to establish centers of excellence—specialty clinical programs touted to consumers to generate self-referred business, or to influence the decision making of intermediaries to use the facilities on patient request. However, since the advent of managed care, these entities have entered the channel in many instances between the patient and the primary care provider. It is this member of the channel that is a key entity in directing patients to primary care providers and ultimately other channel members. In this fashion, the patients (end users) were pulled around the intermediaries or traditional referral sources. In July 1993, the American Physical Therapy Association launched an advertising campaign in the *Ladies Home Journal* and *Good Housekeeping* magazines to educate female baby boomers to the benefits of physical therapy. The goal was to have these consumers either request a referral from their physicians to such therapists when they had a problem, or to have these individuals self-refer themselves for an evaluation and possible treatment by a certified physical therapist. [22]

The pull strategy is being used more often in health care, for example, for pharmaceutical products and even for surgical procedures. CooperVision advertised its "Natural Eyes" pigmentation implant procedure in women's magazines to encourage patient requests.[23] Many health care providers question whether the pull strategy does, in fact, work. FIGURE 11-5 shows that many physicians are reporting a dramatic increase in the number of patients requesting specific drugs by name A Kaiser Family Foundation study reported that 44% of the adults who inquired about a particular drug from their physician received the desired prescription.[24] Recent studies by Harvard and MIT reported that advertising of drugs does work. In fact every dollar spent in advertising results in $4.20 in drug sales.[25] The pull strategy is most evident in the direct-to-consumer advertising by pharmaceutical company advertising. Since 1981, spending in direct-to-consumer advertising reached $12 million by 1989 as shown in FIGURE 11-6, but had grown to $3.8 billion by 2005.[26,27] The results of this advertising are powerful. A relatively recent study has found that 80% of patients request a specific medication.

In the second half of 2005, however, the federal government began to raise some cautionary notes regarding the large volume of monies being spent in this pull strategy to consumers. Table 11-3 shows the leading pharmaceutical advertisers and the leading drugs that were being advertised. Some in Congress were beginning to call for

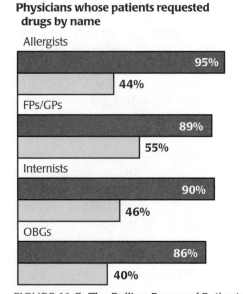

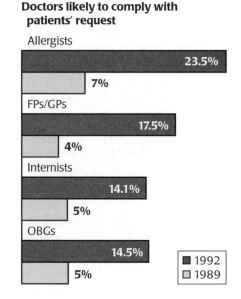

FIGURE 11-5 The Pulling Power of Patients

Source: Reprinted from "Are Your Patients Telling You What to Prescribe?", *Medical Economics*, November 8, 1983, p. 18 with permission of Verispan, LLC (formerly Scott-Levein), © 1993.

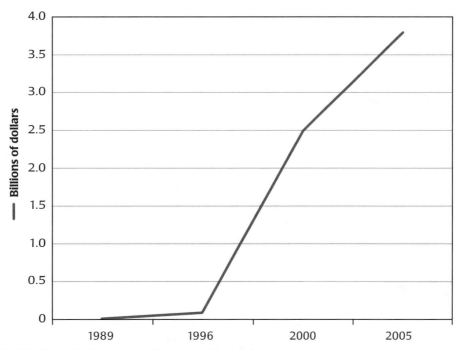

FIGURE 11-6　Direct-to-Consumer Pharmaceutical Advertising

Source: Andrew Robinson, Kirsten Hohmann, Julie Rifkin, Daniel Topp, Christine Gilroy, Jeffrey Pickard, and Robert Anderson, "Direct-to-Consumer Advertising," *Archives of Internal Medicine*, Vol. 164, No. 4 (February 23, 2004), pp. 427–432; Meredith Rosenthal, Ernst R. Berndt, Julie M. Donohue, Richard G. Frank, and Arnold M. Epstein, "Promotion of Prescription Drugs to Consumers," *The New England Journal of Medicine*, February 14, 2002, Vol. 346, No. 7, pp. 498–505.

Table 11-3	Pharmaceutical Spending		
Top Ten Drug Advertisers	Dollars Spent Jan.–Mar. 2005	Most Advertised Drug	Dollars Spent 2004
GLAXOSMITHKLINE PLC	$170 million	Nexium	$242 million
PFIZER INC	$106	Crestor	$214
JOHNSON & JOHNSON	$104	Cialis	$163
SANOFI-AVENTIS	$ 97	Levitra	$148
MERCK & CO.	$ 89	Zelnorm	$124
NOVARTIS AG	$ 62	Prevacid	$122
MERCK/SHERING-PLOUGH	$ 61	Flonase	$119
SHERING-PLOUGH CORP.	$ 53	Celebrex	$114
LILLY ICOS LLC	$ 50	Singulair	$112
ASTRAZENACA PLC	$ 47	Lipitor	$112

Source: Data from Charles Stein, "A Drug-ad Ban Is Tough to Swallow," *Boston Sunday Globe*, (July 10, 2005), D1, D3; Diedtra Henderson, "With Advertising Under Siege Drug Makers Rethink Their Marketing Message," *Boston Sunday Globe* (July 31, 2005), E1, E5.

a ban on all advertising. As these calls were mounted, in the third quarter of 2005, the pharmaceutical companies responded by pulling back drug ad spending, compared to the 28% annual increase seen in 2004.[28,29]

■ Conclusions

Promotional strategy encompasses far more than advertising. Increasingly, health care providers are turning to personal selling and sales promotions as ways to compete more effectively. At the foundation of a good promotional strategy is the understanding of the components essential for effective communication. A sender and receiver must be able to encode and decode often in the midst of significant noise. Successfully communicating can ultimately lead to controlling the channel of distribution for market share. Increasingly, pull strategies are being implemented in health care promotions.

■ Key Terms

Encoding   Advertising
Message   Personal Selling
Channel   Publicity
Opinion Leaders   Sales Promotion
Decoding   Push
Noise   Pull
Feedback

■ Chapter Summary

1. Several factors are necessary for effective communication. There must be a sender, receiver, encoding, decoding, a channel, and feedback. Communication often is affected negatively by noise.
2. Messages can take several forms; they can be one-sided, two-sided, or emotional. Because of the unique nature of health care, emotional appeals to fear must be used with caution.
3. The promotional mix for an organization consists of advertising, personal selling, publicity, and sales promotion.
4. A major advantage of advertising over publicity is in terms of what is said, to whom it is said, how often it is said, and when it is said. Publicity has greater credibility than advertising.
5. Advertising and personal selling each have distinct values. The decision to use one promotional tool more than the other is based on the risk of the decision,

size of the decision-making unit, the complexity of the service, the size of the market, and the geographic dispersion of the market.

6. Advertising and personal selling have differing levels of impact in each stage of the consumer's decision-making process. The more personal the post-purchase contact with the buyer, the more satisfied the buyer.

7. Sales promotion has been an underused tool of the promotional mix within health care. Sales promotion tactics can be directed to consumers or to the trade.

8. In a push strategy, the promotional efforts are directed to the intermediaries in the channel, while in the pull strategy, promotional efforts are directed to the end user.

■ Chapter Problems

1. After a recent presentation of health plans at her company, Julia Brouck joined ABC PPO. The next week she made a visit to a pediatrician in the plan with her son, Arthur, and daughter, Emmy Lou. After seeing the pediatrician, she was told that there was a $15 co-payment for the visits. "I don't understand," Julia said, "I thought all physician visits were free." Explain the potential source of this misconception.

2. At a local hospital, a decision was made to downsize the nursing staff. The local television station sent a reporter and camera crew to interview the administrator regarding the impact of this action on patient care. After 20 minutes filming the interview, the reporter left. That evening a 15-second segment of the interview was shown, which left an unfavorable impression regarding the impact on quality. The administrator wondered what went wrong. Explain how more control could have been used to send out the message about the downsizing.

3. Explain the relative emphasis that would be placed on advertising or personal selling in each of the following situations: (a) a manufacturer of an infusion pump therapy kit for use in hospitals, (b) a hospital offering a nutrition workshop for seniors, and (c) an academic medical center offering a helicopter service for trauma cases within a 200-mile radius of the facility.

4. In recognition of the post-purchase role of promotion, what strategies would you suggest for: (a) a busy hospital emergency room, (b) an executive fitness program that provides health screening and fitness evaluation, and (c) an occupational medicine program that contracts its services to companies?

5. The University of Chicago Hospitals recently ran an advertisement in *The Chicago Tribune*, showing an intensive care nurse employed at the hospital saying, "Personally, I'd be concerned if my health insurance plan didn't offer the University of Chicago Hospitals." Explain the channel control strategy being used with this advertisement, and the logic of the approach.

■ Notes

1. W. Schramm, "How Communication Works," in *The Process and Effects of Mass Communication*, ed. W. Schramm (Urbana, IL: The University of Illinois Press, 1955), 3–26.

2. H. C. Kelman and C. I. Hovland, "Reinstatement of the Communication in Delayed Measurement of Opinion Change," *Journal of Abnormal Psychology* 48, no. 3 (1953): 327–335.

3. C. I. Hovland, A. Lumsdine, and F. D. Sheffield, *Experiments in Mass Communications* (New York: John Wiley & Sons, 1949), 182–200.

4. W. L. Wilkie and P. W. Farris, "Comparison Advertising: Problems and Potential," *Journal of Marketing* 39, no. 4 (1975): 7–15.

5. "Therapeutic Comparative Advertising: Directive and Guidance Document," March 2001, Therapeutic Products Directorate, Government of Canada, part II–11, 12.

6. M. S. LaTour and S. A. Zahra, "Fear Appeals as Advertising Strategy: Should They Be Used?" *Journal of Consumer Marketing* 6, no. 2 (Spring 1989): 61–70.

7. M. L. Ray and W. L. Wilkie, "Fear: The Potential of an Appeal Neglected by Marketing," *Journal of Marketing* 34, no. 1 (1970): 54–62.

8. M. G. Weinberger and C. S. Gulas, "The Impact of Humor in Advertising: A Review," *Journal of Advertising* 21, no. 4 (1992): 35–39.

9. B. Sternthal and C. S. Craig, "Humor in Advertising," *Journal of Marketing* 37, no. 4 (1973): 12–18.

10. H. Hyman and P. Sheatsley, "Some Reasons Why Information Campaigns Fail," *Public Opinion Quarterly* 11, no. 3 (1947): 412–423.

11. J. T. Klapper, *The Effects of Mass Communication* (New York: Free Press, 1960), 166–205.

12. "Are Doctors Sexist? Women Seem To Think So," *Medical Economics* 70, no. 16 (1993): 18.

13. Adam Bruns, "The Changing Image of Healthcare," *Kybiz.com* (www.lanereport.com/issues/january99/coverstory/199.html).

14. Jason R. Cho and Michael Chu, "HMO Penetration, Ownership Status, and the Rise of Hospital Advertising," Working Paper 8899 National Bureau of Economic Research, Working Paper Series, Cambridge, MA (April 2002).

15. E. N. Berkowitz et al., *Marketing*, 6th ed. (Boston: Irwin/McGraw Hill, 2000), 500.

16. A. T. Beal, "How Physicians' Plus Grew into the Video Age," *Marketer's Guidepost* 3, no. 4 (Spring 1993): 1, 4–5.

17. William B. Weeks and Peter B. Mills, "Reduction in Patient Enrollment in Veterans Health Administration after Adverse Medical Events," *Joint Commission Journal on Quality and Safety* 29, no. 12 (December 2003): 652–657.

18. M. G. Weinberger and J. Romeo, "The Impact of Negative Product News," *Business Horizons* 32, no. 1 (1989): 44–50.

19. www.imshealth.com/ims/portal/front/articleC/0,2777,6599_44304752_44889690,00.html.

20. Robin MacStravic, "Reverse and Double Reverse Marketing for Health Care Organizations," *Health Care Management Review* 18, no. 3 (Summer 1993): 53–58.

21. Scott Hensley and Barbara Martinez, "To Sell Their Drugs, Companies Increasingly Rely on Doctors," *The Wall Street Journal* CCXLVI, no. 10 (July 1, 2005): A1, A2.

22. E. DeNitto, "Medical Groups Find Ads Fit the Bill," *Advertising Age* 64, no. 28 (1993): 12.

23. "CooperVision Begins Marketing Eyeliner Procedure for Physicians," *Physician's Marketing* 2, no. 1 (1986): 1.

24. M. Briodie, "Understanding the Effects of Direct-to-Consumer Prescription Drug Advertising," Henry J. Kaiser Family Foundation, Menlo Park, California (November 28, 2001). Available at: www.kff.org/rxdrugs/6084-index.cfm.

25. "Drug Ads Deliver a Few Side Effects," *Boston Globe* (June 12, 2003).

26. Lee Richardson and Vince Luchiisinger, "Direct-to-Consumer Advertising of Pharmaceutical Products: Issue Analysis and Direct to Consumer Promotion," *Journal of the American Academy of Business* 7, no. 2 (September 2005): 110–105.

27. Andrew R. Robinson, Kirsten B. Hohman, Julie I. Rifkin, Daniel Topp, Christine M. Gilroy, Jeffrey A. Pickard, and Robert J. Anderson, "Direct-to-Consumer Pharmaceutical Advertising," *Archives of Internal Medicine* 164, no. 4 (February 23, 2004): 427–432.

28. Charles Stein, "A Drug-ad Ban Is Tough to Swallow," *Boston Sunday Globe* (July 10, 2005), D1, D3.

29. Diedtra Henderson, "With Advertising Under Siege Drug Makers Rethink Their Marketing Message," *Boston Sunday Globe* (July 31, 2005): E1, E5.

Advertising

No element of the marketing mix has been more visible in health care than advertising. In recent years the growth of resources committed to this aspect of the marketing mix has been substantial. In 2005 more than $25 billion dollars was spent annually in health care advertising. Three quarters of this money was directed toward physicians. But, the fastest-growing segment of the industry is in direct-to-consumer marketing. Consumer advertising in health care grew to $4 billion in 2004, 15 times as much as the roughly $260 million spent a decade ago.[1]

"Advertising" may be defined as any directly paid form of nonpersonal presentation of goods, services, or ideas by an identified sponsor. The key aspects of this definition are: (1) that it is paid, which distinguishes advertising from publicity; and (2) that it is nonpersonal, which separates advertising from personal selling.

Concerns have long been raised regarding health care advertising. As seen in Table 12-1, consumers have mixed feelings toward this aspect of marketing. In two separate studies, Andaleeb assessed consumers' attitudes toward hospital advertising on a range of issues. The higher the value the stronger the agreement with the statement in Table 12-1. Thus, while consumers see advertising as increasing costs, they do see it as somewhat useful in choosing a hospital. Consumers also recognize that hospitals are really not different from other products, which may suggest some receptivity toward this marketing practice. Consumers, however, also express some distrust of hospitals that

Table 12-1	Attitude Toward Advertising	
Statement		Mean
Hospitals should not engage in advertising		3.09
Ads help win clients		2.92
Hospital ads increase costs		4.13
Hospitals with good reputations don't need to advertise		4.02
I don't trust hospitals that advertise		2.40
Hospital ads are no different than other products		3.52
To stay in business, hospitals need to advertise		2.27
Ads are useful in choosing hospitals		3.40
Hospital ads are often misleading		3.15
Hospital ads often exploit people's anxieties		3.18
Hospital ads make people aware of health-related issues		2.41

Scale was "1" very strongly disagree to "5" very strongly agree

Source: Adapted from Syed Sad Andaleeb, "How Consumers View Hospital Advertising," *Journal of Hospital Marketing,* Vol. 8, No. 2, 1994, pp. 73–85. Used by permission.

do advertise and question why those with good reputations need to engage in this practice. Thus, as with so much of society, advertising is a part of marketing that raises concerns. This chapter will discuss the value, the strategy, and tactics that make advertising a legitimate part of the marketing mix.

■ Common Classifications of Advertising

There are many forms of advertising with the two common classifications being *product* and *institutional*. Product advertisements focus on a particular product or service, while institutional advertisements build up or enhance an organization's image rather than a particular product. There are several variations within each form of advertising.

Product Advertising

Product advertising can assume one of several forms: informational, competitive, or reminder. Informational advertisements are used in the early stage of a new product or service introduction. These advertisements help to explain the service, how it can be accessed, or its objectives.

Competitive product advertisements are persuasive—they try to generate selective demand for the organization's service over that of competitors.[2] In traditional industries, this form of advertising makes specific comparisons of competing products. Few competitive advertisements have been seen in health care, where comparison are made to other provider organizations.

A final version of product advertising is purely reminder. For example, some hospitals have implemented nurse information lines so consumers can talk to a nurse regarding a medical question. When necessary, these nurses will provide callers with the names of health care providers to call for further examination or consultation. The University Health Care System of Augusta, Georgia, offers their "Ask-A-Nurse" health service center, a 24-hour, seven-day-a-week help line staffed by registered nurses with at least five years' experience. These nurses can assess symptoms, direct a caller to emergency services, prompt care, or physician referrals as necessary (www.universityhealth.org).

Institutional Advertising

Institutional advertising is frequently used in health care. These advertisements are used to build good will and to enhance the public's image of a particular organization. There are several variations of institutional advertising; some introduce or announce the opening of a new company or facility, some compare programs, and some advocate public policy positions.

The advertisement shown in EXHIBIT 12-1 is by Cooley Dickinson Hospital in Northampton, Massachusetts. In 2004, the federal government was strongly encouraging that health care workers be inoculated for smallpox. The physicians on the staff at the hospital analyzed this recommendation and felt it was not in the public's best interest. As a result, they took a stance against the government's position (a position that was ultimately followed by many other health care providers). The hospital ran a series of institutional advertisements as shown in this exhibit stating their reasoning in support of the public good.

Institutional advertisements occasionally can be competitive. These advertisements compare two or more organizational forms, showing one to be more effective than the others. In health care, this variation often appears with advertisements touting prepaid health care plans versus more traditional indemnity insurance programs.

As in product advertising, institutional advertising occasionally serves as a reminder to reinforce previous impressions in the target audience.

Another common form of institutional advertising is referred to as *advocacy*, in which an organization publicizes its position regarding a particular issue. For example, EXHBIBIT 12-2 shows an advertisement paid for by the American Chiropractic Association, which asked consumers to contact their congressional representatives about including chiropractic care when President Clinton proposed a major reform of health care during his administration.

Exhibit 12-1 Cooley Dickinson Hospital Institutional Advertisement

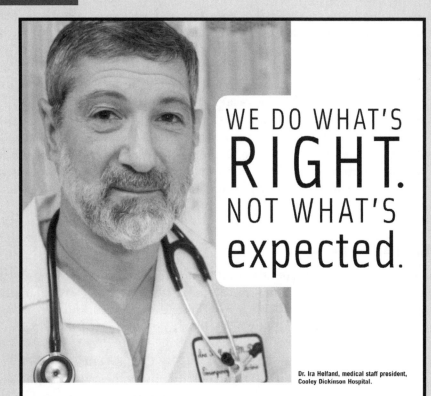

WE DO WHAT'S
RIGHT.
NOT WHAT'S
expected.

Dr. Ira Helfand, medical staff president,
Cooley Dickinson Hospital.

At Cooley Dickinson Hospital, we don't just act, we think about what we're doing and why. That's what we on the medical staff did when word went out that the state and federal governments were pushing to vaccinate health care workers against smallpox. The government is afraid that smallpox, a deadly virus that was eradicated in nature two decades ago, will be used as a weapon by terrorists. We don't question their concern. But we did question whether smallpox is an immediate danger in our community and, more important, whether the dangers of vaccination are greater than those posed by the hypothetical threat of bioterrorism using smallpox. The vaccine for smallpox can have adverse, potentially lethal, effects both on those who receive it and those they come in contact with. That concerned us. And, given that the vaccine is effective up to four days after someone is exposed to smallpox, we decided the risks of vaccination at this time outweigh the potential benefits. We opted out, because that's what we think is best for our community. The decision we made has put us in the news, because Cooley is the first hospital in the state to make such a choice. We believe others will join us, but we weren't about to wait for someone else to make the first move. That's not how things are done in our community. We follow our convictions rather than following the crowd.

COOLEY DICKINSON HOSPITAL
DARTMOUTH-HITCHCOCK ALLIANCE

30 Locust Street • Northampton, Massachusetts
413-582-2421
www.cooley-dickinson.org

Source: Institutional advertisement courtesy of Cooley Dickinson Hospital, Hampton, MA.

Exhibit 12-2   Sample Advocacy Advertisement

Find Out If Anyone Here Has A Backbone.

The health care reform bills are getting ready to come through Congress. And most don't include safe, cost-effective chiropractic care as a *guaranteed* benefit—something the big insurance companies couldn't take away.

For 20 million Americans who receive chiropractic care every year, that's more than bad policy. It's bad politics.

That's why we're asking everyone who believes chiropractic care ought to be a *guaranteed* benefit to give Congress a piece of their mind.

Send copies of the coupon on the right to your Senators and Representatives and let them know you want chiropractic care included in whatever health care reform bill they ultimately pass.

Who knows. For once, maybe we'll see some backbone in this town.

Watch My Back!   I expect you to stand up for my rights and lower health care costs by voting to include chiropractic care as a *guaranteed* benefit in any health care reform bill approved by Congress.

Name_____
Address_____
City_____State_____Zip_____

Mail to: (Your Representative or Dan
(Your Senator or Patrick Moynihan)   Rostenkowski)
U.S. Senate   U.S. House of Representatives
Washington, DC 20510   Washington, DC 20515

Or call 202-224-3121

AMERICAN CHIROPRACTIC ASSOCIATION • 1701 CLARENDON BLVD. • ARLINGTON, VIRGINIA 22209 • 1-703-276-8800

Source: Courtesy of Foot Levelers, Inc., Roanoke, Virginia.

■ Developing the Advertising Campaign

The development of an advertising campaign begins with the preparation of a **media plan,** which outlines the analysis and execution of the advertising campaign.

Define the Target Audience

Essential to a successful media plan is the first step—a definition of the **target audience.** The target audience specifies the group or groups to whom the organization is trying to communicate. This step is an organizational decision, determined by earlier market research and based on prior market segmentation decisions. The more detailed this section of the media plan, the easier subsequent decisions will be regarding placement of advertisements and advertising copy design. As in the earlier discussion of market segmentation, a target audience description will include demographics and, possibly, attitudinal profiles and lifestyle descriptions. Upon defining the target audience, the media plan must then specify the advertising campaign's objectives, budget, message, communication program, and manner for evaluation. These steps are shown in FIGURE 12-1 and are described in detail in the following pages.

Determine the Advertising Objectives

Advertising objectives are critical to any successful campaign. In setting objectives, it is best to consider how advertising works. Consumers do not view an ad and then buy a product or use a service. Rather, advertising facilitates moving consumers along a sequence of steps that have been described as a **hierarchy of effects**—the stages a buyer moves through from first seeing an advertisement ultimately to buying the product or using the service.[3,4] These stages include: awareness, interest, evaluation, trial, and adoption.

Awareness

This level of the hierarchy is necessarily the first. The consumer must recognize the ad or be cognizant of the fact that it exists. Canonsburg General Hospital of Canonsburg, Pennsylvania, selected consumer awareness as the advertising objective for its newly remodeled mammography center. The hospital conducted a five-week advertising campaign in several newspapers. Advertisements were also reprinted as flyers distributed to new residents.[5] Awareness was also the advertising objective for Mission Hospital Regional Medical Center of Orange County, California. The hospital wanted to target residents new to the area. The hospital purchased a mailing list of new arrivals and directly mailed a marketing package to residents in 13 ZIP codes. It also sent newcomers two cards. After sending out 8980 brochures in 1992, the hospital received a 2.7% response rate requesting more information.[6]

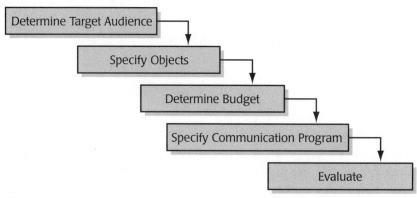

FIGURE 12-1 Developing the Advertising Campaign

Interest

After developing initial awareness, a consumer must have some inclination to seek additional information about the product. The organization's goal at this level of the hierarchy is to provide some information that will motivate further deliberation or action.

Evaluation

Before consumers will buy a product or seek out a service from a particular provider, they must compare that product or service with other available options. Organizational advertising must include dimensions that are important to the target market.

Trial

The initial use of a service is called trial. Advertising can only move a person to this level of the hierarchy. In order to have repeat purchases, a service must meet the customer's expectations. No amount of advertising can correct a bad experience with a hospital or medical group.

Adoption

This is the highest level of the hierarchy and the ultimate goal of advertising—the stage at which the customer becomes a regular user. If trial was satisfactory, reminder advertising plays an important role in this level of the hierarchy of effects.

Determine the Budget

Several methods are generally used to determine the appropriate amount to spend on advertising. Since there is no absolute formula, these methods tend to include one of the four following categories: percentage of sales, competitive parity, "all you can afford," and objective and task.

Percentage of Sales

This method involves determining a fixed percentage of sales or revenue to use as the basis for advertising allocations.[7,8] For example, a hospital might decide that one-half of one percent of last year's net revenue will be allocated to the current year's advertising. The advantage of this method is its simplicity. This method also provides some fiscal safeguard in tying advertising expenditures to organization resources. In spite of these advantages, however, this method has an inherent flaw that implies that sales or revenue causes advertising. Advertising should be seen as contributing to sales, not the other way around. Using this method, a company would reduce advertising expenditures when sales drop. In fact, this may be the period when additional monies must be spent to generate new sales. Hospitals that have large fixed-asset bases cannot afford to exist with large, idle capacity.[9]

Competitive Parity

This method is common in industries where there is a significant amount of trade data. The hospital sets the advertising budget based on industry norms or what it perceives the competitor is spending. Logic demands that an organization consider the competitor when determining any advertising budget.[10] Table 12-2 shows an example of such competitive comparison data collected in a recent study by Sutter Health of Sacramento, California, a health system consisting of hospitals, physicians, and a managed care plan. This study was conducted to determine norms regarding system advertising spending. Except for consideration of the competitor, the logic of this method is weak. It may well be that the competitor is trying to reach a different target market or has different goals. Moreover, this method assumes that the competitor knows what it is doing.

All You Can Afford

This approach is obvious by its name. Common to organizations that really don't believe in the value of advertising, it involves first allocating the budget to all important operations within the organization. If any money is left over, it might then be allocated to advertising.[11] While this method might address an organization's fiscal reality, it could lead to too much, as well as to too little, being spent on advertising. No consideration is given to the objectives of these methods.

Table 12-2	Competitive Parity Advertising Expenditures in Health Care		
	Advertising Expense Included		
Entity	Communications budget as a percent of system net patient revenues	Communications budget as a percent of system expenditures	Communications expenditures per system employee
Henry Ford Health System, Detroit	0.12%	0.13%	$138
Group Health Cooperative, Seattle	0.14	0.15	142
Sutter Health, Sacramento, CA	0.23	0.23	156
Baylor Health Care System, Dallas	0.25	0.27	184
Average	0.52	0.55	355
Health Midwest, Kansas City, Mo.	0.53	0.55	390
EHS Health Care, Oak Brook, IL	0.89	0.95	477
Alliant Health System, Louisville, KY	1.48	1.54	1000

Source: Adapted from Mary Chris Jaklevic, "Benchmarking Study Targets Communications Departments of Systems," *Modern Healthcare*, October 3, 1994, pp. 88–90.

Objective and Task

This fourth method is the most appropriate way to determine the advertising budget. The **objective and task** approach involves setting objectives along the hierarchy of effects and determining the tasks necessary to accomplish these objectives. The costs of these tasks ultimately determine the final budget needed.[12] EXHIBIT 12-3 offers examples of advertising objectives for each level of the hierarchy.

In using this method, for example, a marketing director must decide how to accomplish the first objective of getting referral physicians in the upper peninsula to be aware of helicopter service. In this instance, the director must determine the following tasks and costs:

One physician referral brochure (6,000 copies at $2 each)	$12,000
One full-page advertisement in *Michigan Medical Society* monthly magazine	1,500
One open house at medical center for area physicians	6,000
Total cost	$19,500

The total cost is the proposed budget. At this point, however, the marketing director determines how much can be afforded and adjusts the budget accordingly. Any further adjustment in the budget must be reflected in what can be accomplished regarding the objectives. The tasks will be redefined, and the budget subsequently adjusted.

In examining the objectives listed in Exhibit 12-3, it is important to note the ingredients for good, useful objectives. All of these objectives specify the target market. Each objective is time-based, whether it be 30 days or a quarter of a year. Finally, each objective is measurable. This last component is essential in order to prove the value of the campaign. In health care marketing, a common criticism of advertising relates to whether or not it achieved its objective. This concern is a result of not beginning with a measurable objective.

Exhibit 12-3   Advertising Objectives for the Hierarchy

Awareness: To have 10% of the elderly in the metropolitan area know of the existence of the meals-on-wheels program two months after opening.

Interest: To have our program director for industrial medicine be invited to make three new presentations a month to companies interested in our packed occupational/industrial medicine service.

Trial: In the next 30 days, to have 15% of the users at the new urgent care facility on the west side be first-time users.

Adoption: To have half the callers to the health information line define themselves as regular users of the program within one year of opening the service.

Develop the Message

The third step in designing the advertising program is the development of the message. Marketing research is essential at this stage to determine the attributes that are important to the consumer. In developing these messages, varying appeals are often used, including rational, emotional, and moral/social appeals.

Rational

These messages are directed at distinct functional attributes of the product. The purpose is to explain the value in using the particular service.

Emotional

An increasingly common advertising appeal is emotion, with fear and humor being used most often.[13] The use of fear in health care advertisements has some troubling ethical dilemmas, as noted in an earlier chapter. In fact, the Alliance for Health Care Strategy and Marketing, which was the major professional association for health care marketing professionals in the late 1980–1990s, developed a set of ethical guidelines for advertisers (reviewed later in this chapter). The group specifically noted that advertising should not use emotional appeals to take advantage of individuals who are vulnerable due to health care needs.[14] Within limits, however, fear appeals can be effective. One study used fear appeals in advertisements for acquired immune deficiency syndrome prevention to college-age students. Results of the study showed that an ad with a strong fear appeal generated tension, energy, and a more positive cognitive response than the milder version of the ad.[15]

Moral/Social Appeals

These messages focus upon causes or issues. Hospitals mount advertising campaigns to solicit funding for their medical foundation research. Likewise, the American Red Cross appeals to the community for participation in blood donation.

Pretesting

Any good advertising message should first be pretested. **Pretesting** involves assessing advertising copy options before their general use. Effective pretesting requires that it be conducted with the intended target audience.

In Chapter 5 on marketing research (Chapter 5), focus groups were discussed as one data-gathering methodology. Focus groups are used extensively in the early stages of advertising development and pretesting. Initially, focus groups can be used to identify the important dimension for the advertisements and alternative appeals that could be utilized. Other pretesting methods can be implemented, once a draft version of the advertisement is created. Pretests can be conducted to ensure that the target audience can interpret the advertisement, is interested in it, and prefers it over other versions. There are several ways to pretest an advertisement, including the use of portfolio tests, jury tests, and theater tests.

Portfolio Tests

This form of pretesting involves testing alternative copy. The test advertisement is placed in a grouping with other sample advertisements. Consumers are then asked to review all the samples. Upon completing the review, consumers are then asked to judge the advertisements on a series of dimensions such as interest, attention, likability, and informative value. When Fallon Health Plan in Worcester, Massachusetts initially embarked on its first health maintenance organization (HMO) advertising campaign, it pretested four different advertisements among consumers who belonged to traditional indemnity plans. In conducting the portfolio test, the Fallon HMO also showed variations of the advertisements to subscribers of a competing HMO.[16]

Jury Tests

In this version of a pretest, the advertisement or variations are shown to a panel of consumers. Similar to a portfolio test, researchers solicit consumer reactions on several dimensions in the advertisements.

Theater Tests

The most expensive and elaborate form of pretesting is the theater test. For example, consumers are invited to a special viewing of a new television show or movie. Inserted into the show are sample advertisements. When the viewing is over, consumers are asked to rate the show and provide reactions to the advertisements. In the most sophisticated theater tests, consumers can react immediately to the commercials and record their intensity of like or dislike by using a hand-held device while they view the advertisement.

Regardless of the degree of sophistication applied to the pretest, it is an essential step in advertising. In health care, pretesting often involves showing the advertisements to the physicians on staff or in the medical group to gain their approval. This step is important to ensure that any advertisement intended for the consumer be factually correct regarding any intervention or treatment discussed. Yet, unless the advertisement is directed to other physicians outside the organization, this kind of pretest would not be entirely valid. The advertisement also must be pretested with the target audience of intended consumers.

Specify the Communication Program

Once an advertisement's message is developed and pretested, the next step in the advertising campaign is to select the appropriate medium and vehicle for delivering the message to the target market. Related to this decision is determining the timing of the messages to be communicated. **Medium** refers to the form of communication selected, such as newspapers, radio, television, direct mail, or magazines. The **vehicle** is the advertising alternative chosen within each medium. For example, an advertiser might use magazines as the medium and *Modern Healthcare* magazine as the particular vehicle within that medium.

In selecting the appropriate medium, there are two objectives that often conflict within the constraints of any advertising budget. These are the goals of reach and frequency. **Reach** refers to the unduplicated audience that an advertising vehicle will deliver. The more people exposed to the message, the broader the reach. **Frequency** refers to the number of times the same person receives a message within a defined time period. The value of frequency was best shown by the advice to prospective advertisers from the 1800s shown in Chapter 4. Ideally, a company tries to maximize the reach and frequency of its advertising; however, based on definitions alone, it is easy to see that this would incur significant cost.

In addition to reach and frequency, advertisers must also consider the amount of waste, which refers to the people reached by a particular medium who do not belong to the intended target market. A magazine, for example, which counts family practitioners among its subscribers, as well as pediatricians, may have wasted coverage if the target is only pediatricians.

The price of most media advertising space is based upon the size and the purchasing power of the audience. The larger the audience of a radio station, the greater the charge to advertise on that particular station. Magazines such as *Architectural Digest* that target an upscale audience might charge more money for advertising than *Backpacker*.

Scheduling

After the organization determines the balance between reach and frequency, it must decide the timing for its messages. There are many variations by which an advertising campaign can deliver messages; the three most common are seasonal, steady, or flighting.

Seasonal

Some products and services have a seasonal pattern to their demand. For example, cold medicines have heavier demand in the winter months; a travel clinic might experience greater demand in the summer months. Advertising, therefore, is scheduled in heavier amounts at the onset of the peak demand period.

Steady

This schedule involves maintaining the same level of advertising exposure through the selected time period. Physician referral lines sponsored by hospitals often follow this scheduling pattern. On any given day, any number of people might need to avail themselves of this service. Maintaining a constant level of product or service awareness is necessary to reach each new consumer entering the adoption stage of the market.

Flighting

A common advertising schedule is called **flighting**, which involves a heavy amount of advertising for short time periods. FIGURE 12-2 shows three diagrams to represent flighting and two alternative scheduling patterns that are discussed below. The flighting

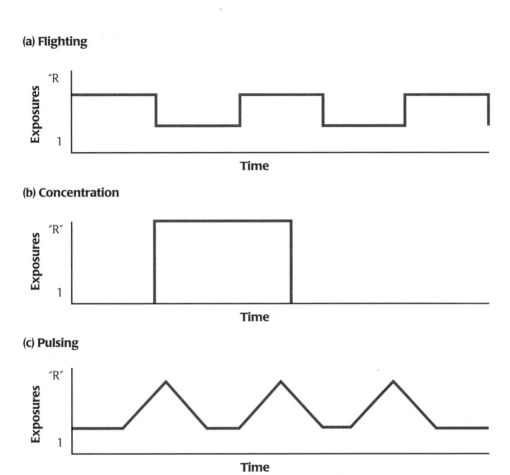

(a) Flighting

(b) Concentration

(c) Pulsing

FIGURE 12-2   Alternative Media Scheduling Patterns

approach has distinct periods when there are a large number of exposures. The logic of this approach is that advertising will have sufficient carryover effect to maintain awareness when there is little or no advertising. The risk of losing product awareness is represented by the gaps before the next burst in expenditures.

An alternative scheduling strategy is **concentration**, in which a company spends its advertising dollars and achieves exposure within a defined, relatively short time period. Or, an organization can follow a **pulsing** approach, in which advertising expenditures occur at a constant level with occasional, short, heavy expenditures.[17]

Selecting the Most Cost-Effective Approach

In choosing which medium to use, advertisers select the most cost-efficient vehicle possible. Every advertiser wants to minimize the amount of wasted coverage. In calculating the most cost-efficient advertising medium, advertisers can select one of several formulas based upon the particular medium being considered. These formulas vary as a function of the medium selected.

Cost-Per-Thousand

A common frame of comparing the cost of advertising media is the **cost-per-thousand,** or CPM formula. This measures the cost of a medium to deliver an audience. The formula is:

$$CPM = \frac{Cost\ of\ the\ Advertisement \times 1000}{Circulation}$$

Circulation is the number of people reached by the magazine or the newspaper. Using this formula, the advertiser can compare the cost of advertising in different magazines.

Cost-per-Point

In considering the cost of television advertising, advertisers use a different standard than the cost-per-thousand. The cost index in this medium is based on the audience that is delivered, or the rate. The rate is the program audience as a percent of the total television audience. In buying television advertising, however, advertisers schedule a package of advertisements across a number of different programs. The schedule is then determined in terms of its **gross rating points**, a measure of advertising reach calculated by multiplying the number of spots or ads times the rating.

Assume, for example, that *Monday Night Football* has a rating of 4.3 and the advertiser purchased 14 insertion spots during the season. The number of gross rating points would then be $14 \times 4.3 = 60.2$. The gross rating points are a measure of the reach times the frequency. The reach is reflected by the show's rating and the frequency by the number of insertions, or spots, purchased. This gross rating points system provides a common base that accounts for different-sized markets. The same gross rating points in two markets of very different sizes cannot be considered equivalent.

In buying advertising, advertisers often use the cost per rating point to make comparisons. Yet, the following example shows the caution that must be taken with that approach. One point appears to cost more in New York City than in Salt Lake City, yet, a point in New York has far greater reach than a point in Salt Lake City.

Consider the data below, which show two very different settings:

	Households with Televisions	Average Cost per Spot	Average Prime Time Rating
New York City	7,800,000	$3,200	19
Salt Lake City	925,000	$2,600	17

Assume the advertiser buys five spots:

$$\text{Cost-per-Point (CPP)} = \frac{\text{Cost of Schedule}}{\text{Gross Rating Points}}$$

$$\text{In Salt Lake City: CPP} = \frac{\$13,000}{85} = \$152.94$$

$$\text{In New York City: CPP} = \frac{\$16,000}{95} = \$168.42$$

Ultimately, in any comparison of rating points or costs, the advertiser must consider that the audience being delivered by any medium is the target audience that the organization wants to attract.

Picking the Right Medium

Advertisers have a variety of media from which to choose to place their message. Each of these media has distinct characteristics that must be assessed in the final advertising plan.

Television

Of all media available, television has the advantage of communicating sight, sound, and motion. These components afford the potential advertiser significant flexibility in the creation of the advertising copy. Today, almost 98% of all homes in the United States have television, providing the potential for enormous reach. Television's major disadvantage is its cost. Prime time spots can easily exceed $100,000. The production costs of television commercials also add significantly to the budget expense. Except for large national companies such as Cigna, Prucare, or Blue Cross Blue Shield, national advertising costs are not part of the average budget for most health care organizations.

In recent years, however, the advancement of local cable channels has made television advertising accessible and affordable for local advertisers such as hospitals or medical groups. The challenge of local market television advertising is in identifying the correct television station that will reach the desired target audience. As more households are wired for cable television, the number of station alternatives expands dramatically to 20, 40, or, in some markets, 80 channels, making vehicle selection all the more difficult for the local advertiser. Local television advertising is generally purchased by the time of the day rather than by a specific program. Because of this difference with national network advertising, local advertisers must again know the viewing habits of their target market at various times of day.

Another disadvantage of television advertising is the degree of clutter or competing messages that exists. It is difficult for one advertisement to stand out when so many commercials are packaged within a station break.

Radio

There are 10 times as many radio stations as there are television stations in the United States. Since the mid-1970s, the radio's major growth has been on the FM rather than the AM band. A wide array of formats and programs make radio a highly segmented medium for potential advertisers. Also, on a cost basis, radio compares very favorably to television. The average circulation cost-per-thousand for radio is $4. The cost of producing a radio commercial in local markets is often included in the rate charged to the advertiser.

The production of radio ads can usually be completed in a short time period, and St. Joseph's Hospital in Milwaukee has capitalized on this advantage. The hospital ran radio advertisements highlighting the birth of babies at its facility. The advertisements began with an announcer reporting the news of the day, followed by announcements of recent births at the hospital.[18] A final major advantage of this medium is that it reaches consumers out of their home. Peak listening times for radio are the morning and evening drive times.

Radio's major limitation is its lack of a visual means of communication. Also, because so many radio stations and varying formats are available, a potential advertiser has almost too many options. The advertiser must also accurately identify the radio station that attracts its particular target audience.

Newspaper

Of all media available, newspapers receive the most advertising dollars. In health care, this medium has been the most popular because the strength of newspapers is their coverage of local markets in which most health care organizations compete. Of all media, newspaper advertising is typically the best for generating immediate response. Coupons and special offers are common to newspapers. Newspapers are the medium of choice for physician referral lines or nurse information lines. Another advantage of newspapers is their cost. Newspaper rates are reasonable compared to other mass media like television, making it the medium of choice for local advertisers. Although in recent years, with the advent of cable television, the rate advantage of newspapers has been somewhat negated.

The segmentation possibilities in local newspapers are relatively limited. In recent years, however, most large metropolitan newspapers have developed zone editions that target specific geographic areas within their circulation. *The New York Times*, for example, has a regional edition as well as national edition sold in airport terminals throughout the United States. An additional advantage of newspapers is the short lead time required to place an advertisement. A hospital often will only need to wait a day or two before its advertisement can be run in the local newspaper.

Newspapers do have some disadvantages. Newspaper readership tends increasingly to be concentrated among older consumers. To overcome this problem, many local newspapers have followed the pattern of *USA TODAY*, using a glossy four-color approach and succinct writing to appeal to a younger, more visually oriented audience.

Magazines

Few media have grown as dramatically in recent years as magazines.[19] For the advertiser there is a vast array of specialized publications that allow an organization to target a specific market segment. Environmentally concerned consumers read *Garbage*, outdoor enthusiasts might peruse *Backpacker*, health-oriented consumers might subscribe to *Men's Health*, *Organic Gardening*, *Women's Health*, or a host of others. Within the magazine industry there is significant competition as varying publications compete for advertising dollars. And, like newspapers, many national publications have developed both zone and demographic editions targeted to particular subsets of their readership. All of these variations allow advertisers who know their target market to spend their advertising dollars efficiently.

Magazines have other advantages beyond the selectivity that they can deliver. Many publications have a long shelf life, meaning readers will keep them for weeks, months, or, in the case of the *National Geographic*, years. An advertisement in these publications may be read several times over the course of a publication's shelf life. An additional advantage of magazines is their excellent reproduction capabilities for advertisements. The quality of the printing and color separation in magazines far surpasses anything achieved to date by newspapers.

Like all other media, however, magazines have some disadvantages. The sheer number of magazines makes it more difficult to select the specific publication in which to advertise. Some publications also have a long lead time for the placement of an advertisement, often requiring delivery of ad copy four to six weeks prior to publication. Magazine advertisements thus must be used to support a longer running campaign rather than to generate an immediate response.

Outdoor Advertising

Outdoor media consist of a couple of variations, namely billboards or transit. Because of space and time exposure limitations for these media, outdoor advertising is typically viewed as a supplemental medium to support exposures in other media. Outdoor advertising is useful for its reminder appeal or in the introduction stage of a service to generate brand name or service recognition. This medium has also been useful in generating calls to referral lines or health information lines.[20] According to the Outdoor Advertising Association of America, the health care industry is the fastest growing segment of its business.[21]

The major advantage of outdoor advertising is the repetition it can provide through broad exposure of the message. Yet, its limitations are significant in terms of the degree of selectivity and the message that can be communicated. As a medium, outdoor advertising has an image problem. There are community concerns that billboards, in particular, are a form of visual pollution. Some communities have placed constraints on the presence and size of billboards. Four states (Alaska, Hawaii, Maine, and Vermont) have banned all outdoor billboards. Fewer constraints have been placed on transit advertising. These ads are common in larger communities that have public transportation.

Direct Marketing

Over the past 10 years there has been phenomenal growth in direct marketing as computers have allowed for more individually tailored messages and communication vehicles. This targeting ability is the major advantage of direct advertising. With increasing computer sophistication, many direct advertising pieces can make a highly personalized appeal to the recipient.

Critical to a successful direct mail approach is having a good list of prospects. There are two approaches most companies can use. The first is to develop their own refined lists of customers or prospects. Increasingly, companies are paying attention to what is referred to as database marketing, the process of developing and updating information about prospective customers. In effective database marketing, companies develop detailed profiles of their target market and can refine the list or access names based on qualifying variables such as income, age, or prior purchasing of particular products. A second approach is to purchase a list from a commercial list broker who can provide a customer database based on several classifications. This second approach can work, as was shown by Northwest Health in Springdale, Arkansas, in working with a commercial firm. In one campaign, the goal was to introduce a new pediatrician in an existing practice and improve market share by increasing the volume of appointments in the target market. The organization created a direct mail piece to offer a free outlet protector to parents who contacted the physician referral service of the hospital. Ten months after the campaign, a tracking system showed a 13.4% increase in the volume of patient visits and a correlating gain from charges resulting from those visits. A significant percentage of visits were patients who had never been to the health care organization.[22]

In a recent hospital survey, the prevalence of direct marketing efforts was clear. Almost 90% of hospitals surveyed indicated that their direct marketing budgets had increased. In citing their reasons for using this medium, hospitals reported four common objectives:

1. To increase hospital awareness
2. To generate leads for current programs
3. To promote special events
4. To enhance a facility's image[23]

Direct mail's limitations are its image and cost. Many consumers regard direct mail as junk mail. As consumers are increasingly deluged with large amounts of such material on a daily basis, getting one piece to stand out from the competition is difficult. Direct mail's cost must also be considered as its level of sophistication increases. Historically, the major cost of direct mail was postage. While this factor continues to be a concern as rates increase, production costs must also be factored into the cost equation. To attract attention, direct mail marketers have significantly increased the use of color, paper quality, and repetition to gain attention, all of which add greatly to total cost.

Internet Advertising

The Web is increasingly giving advertisers new and exciting ways to advertise. Online advertising is providing many advantages to potential advertisers. It allows sites to track users and how many times a site was clicked on as well as how deeply a site was looked at by a visitor. Did the person look at the first page of the medical group's site? Or, did the visitor also look at the page of the orthopedic department and the spine center services? There are many variations to Internet advertising. These are:

Banners—Rectangular graphics at the top or bottom of a Web page. They receive less than a 1% click-through rate.

Buttons—Small banner type advertisements placed anywhere on a page.

Pop-up ads—These advertisements appear on a screen while a page is being loaded or after the Web page has appeared. Recent technology has now blocked many of these pop-ups, which limits their effectiveness.

E-mail—Unsolicited email has been referred to as spamming. Many states are passing laws against spamming. While it is an easy way to communicate with perspective customers, it can be considered intrusive.

Evaluate the Response

Testing of advertising effectiveness occurs at two stages. As discussed earlier, the first form of evaluation, known as pretesting, ensures that the target audience receives the message in the way it is intended. Pretesting also determines preference and attention-getting value.

After selecting the media and placing advertisements, most organizations also conduct testing to determine the effects of their campaign. Testing formats vary, depending on the media used for advertising.

Companies often assess whether the advertising campaign has resulted in a change in attitudes toward the product or service being promoted through the use of surveys and posttest attitude tests.[24]

Broadcast

A common form of posttesting for television or radio is day-after recall. Typically, after a commercial is aired on television or radio, the advertiser conducts telephone surveys to determine whether people remember the advertisement. Recall can be either aided or unaided. In unaided recall, the telephone interviewer might ask, "Have you seen any advertisements on television for a women's health program?" The recall of the particular hospital's program could then be assessed. In aided recall, the interviewer would ask, "Have you seen any ads lately for St. Mary's Women's Health Center?"

Print

In the magazine industry, posttest scores are often collected through a syndicated data service referred to as Starch. Roper Starch Worldwide conducts personal reader interviews to determine the number of people who read a particular issue and whether they read the advertisement, the signature, or whether they read most of the ad. Starch provides companies with scores for the advertisements for the issues in which they were placed.

Direct Marketing

The advantage of direct marketing advertising is that customer response can be directly measured through follow-up inquiries or purchase orders. This direct form of measurement has led to the medium's growing appeal.

Internet

The advantage of the Internet is that it can be easily tracked with click-through, to measure how deeply someone is looking at the Web page, or by counting how often someone lands on the page. However, it is difficult to measure the retention of the information.

■ Working with Advertising Agencies

Many hospitals and health care organizations do not have the in-house resources needed to develop their own advertising materials. Those that do not can hire the services of an advertising agency. Advertising agencies vary in size and in the scope of the functions that they perform. A health care organization must identify the types of services needed to select the appropriate agency.

Alternative Advertising Agencies

The most comprehensive advertising agency, the **full service agency**, provides all the elements necessary to assume the total advertising function. These organizations typically offer sales promotion, public relations, direct marketing, consulting on design and identification, and even television programming.

The full service agency typically has several departments organized around creative services, account services, marketing, and administrative services. The creative department is responsible for producing all the advertising design and copy. Account services deals with the client—the health care organization. This professional has to understand the health care business and how to translate the client's goals and objectives to the creative department. The purchasing of media space and time is the responsibility of the marketing services department. Full service agencies often have marketing research functions residing within this area. The administrative and financial department handles billing and agency management.

Opposite of the full service agencies are the boutique, or specialized, firms. A **boutique agency** may offer a limited range of services, such as creative services or media buying services, or will act as a contractor to put together the range of services needed by the organization.

Agency Compensation

Advertising agencies are compensated in one of two ways: fees and commissions. Agencies paid by commission are, in effect, being paid by the media. In commission compensation, the agency places $200,000 of advertising in selected publications and in television. The agency keeps 15% of this billed amount as standard compensation. The media then provides $200,000 worth of advertising space. Although the client is paying the agency, the media is, in effect, subsidizing the commission by providing the full amount of media space or time.

A major buyers' concern about the commission system is that it provides agencies with an incentive to recommend more advertising than is necessary. Agencies have also felt that the commission-based compensation system may not be providing them with a fair return for the work they provide to a client. As a result, in recent years commissions have declined and some agencies have moved to a fee-based structure.[25] The fee is agreed upon by the agency and the client and is based upon the amount, type, and scope of work being provided.

■ Ethics in Advertising

Few aspects of marketing were of greater concern to health care professionals than the onset of advertising. Because of the sensitive nature of health care and the often precarious position of the health care buyer, there is heightened sensitivity to the use of this tool. The Alliance for Health Care Strategy and Marketing developed a set of voluntary guidelines regarding the concerns and issues that should be considered in health care advertising, shown in EXHIBIT 12-4.

Although advertising has become more common in health care, it is still a tactic that generates concern and criticism. In the March 28, 2005, issue of the *Annals of Internal Medicine,* a study was published that condemned the trend among respected academic

Exhibit 12-4 Health Care Advertising Guidelines

- Advertising should state and imply only documentable, normally expected outcomes.
- Advertising related to clinical outcomes should use the actual words and images of actual patients who have experienced the procedure or treatment being promoted.
- Advertising should place the good of the patient above other interests—especially a provider's economic interest, prestige, or image building.
- Advertising of health care services, including physician referral services, should acknowledge criteria used in identifying the list of service providers.

Source: "Ethical Guidelines for Healthcare Advertising," position paper, Alliance for Health Care Marketing and Strategy, 1993.

medical centers for using advertising strategies to promote services such as Botox and Lasik and fertility treatments. The study analyzed newspaper ads for 17 of the country's best known academic medical centers and concluded that the promotion placed profits before patient interests. The study underscored to a large degree that the information aspect of advertising is still not fully appreciated but also highlights that in health care great sensitivity must be made to the promotional claims made in any advertisement.[26]

The issue of ethics has extended to the Web. The Swiss-based Health on the Net (HON) Foundation has an eight-point code of ethics. If a health information provider abides by HON's code of ethics, it receives approval from the nonprofit to display the HON logo. In 2003 more than 3000 Web sites received such approval (including the Mayo Clinic) and displayed that they are in compliance with HON's ethical guidelines.[27]

Nonprofit Concerns

One final aspect of health care advertising warranting attention is the matter of an organization's nonprofit designation. Federal, state, and local government agencies have examined whether advertising by these organizations is excessive. Twenty of Pennsylvania's 224 nonprofit hospitals were required to provide services in place of property taxes to various taxing agencies after being judged as acting more like for-profit organizations in light of their advertising expenditures.[28]

■ Conclusions

Advertising is an important ingredient of any health care organization's promotional strategy. Developing an effective media plan begins with a specification of its objectives. From this foundation, a budget and appropriate tactics for media selection and scheduling can be determined. Any effective advertising requires that there be a mechanism both to pretest and posttest the campaign. Because of the serious nature of health care and the vulnerabilities of consumers engaged in the selection of health care services, significant attention is due to the ethical dimensions of the advertising strategy ultimately implemented.

■ Key Terms

Media Plan	Frequency
Target Audience	Flighting
Hierarchy of Effects	Concentration
Objective and Task	Pulsing
Pretesting	Cost-per-Thousand
Medium	Gross Rating Points
Vehicle	Full Service Agency
Reach	Boutique Agency

■ Chapter Summary

1. Advertising can take one of several forms; it can be product-based or institution-based.
2. The basis for an advertising campaign is the media plan, which is built on the definition of the target audience.
3. Advertising objectives are based on the hierarchy of effects model. A well-written objective is measurable, time-bound, and targeted to a well-specified audience.
4. Advertising budgets are often derived on a percentage of sales, competitive parity, or "all-that-can-be-afforded" basis. The most effective basis for determining the budget is an objective and task method.
5. The creation of effective advertising copy requires pretesting of the message with a sample similar to the target audience.
6. In selecting the media for use in an advertising campaign, an organization often must make trade-offs between reach and frequency.
7. There are several patterns by which advertising exposures can be scheduled: steady, seasonal, or flighting.
8. Advertising media must be selected to minimize wasted coverage. Media choices can be compared on a cost-per-thousand or cost-per-point basis.
9. Cable television has greatly reduced the cost of television advertising, while technological advances have affected both print and direct mail. Environmental constraints limit outdoor advertising.
10. Advertising agencies differ in the structure, fee, and range of services provided. In recent years, there has been a trend away from commission payment to a fee payment system.

■ Chapter Problems

1. Outline the advertising copy an HMO would use in advertisements that are: (a) competitive, product-based, (b) pioneering institutional, and (c) reminder institutional.
2. Write an awareness objective for a newly formed adolescent chemical dependency program whose target market consists of judges and social workers who refer to the facility. How would this objective change for the trial level of the hierarchy of effects?
3. As the newly hired hospital marketing director, you have your first meeting with the administrator. "Okay," he says, "we need to advertise our physical rehabilitation program. I'll give you a couple of days to tell me how much you'd like to spend. Is $5000 enough? I think we can afford a little more if you need it. And, based on what I've seen in the newspapers, St. Mary's seems to be spending a little less than that. Give me your thoughts in two days." Two days are up.

4. Recently, the physician marketing task force at State University Medical Center developed a physician referral directory and advertisement. The target was primary care physicians in the region who could refer patients to State University for tertiary care. A cardiologist who was an undergraduate English major chaired the committee and drafted the materials. Three months after distribution of the advertisement and directory, responses were disappointing. Explain how this process could have been improved to increase likely response.

5. The director of a cardiac rehabilitation program was recently approached by a sales representative from the community newspaper selling advertising space. The sales representative underscored the fact that the paper had the largest circulation of any of the three papers serving the area, and it had the lowest cost-per-thousand. Before deciding to use this medium, what other factors should the program director consider?

6. Robbinsdale Hospital is one of two hospitals among the six facilities in the city to have an intensive care (Level III) nursery. This facility is tailored to treat infants suffering from severe medical complications upon delivery. The program director is deciding whether to use an emotional or rational appeal in advertising copy. What are the considerations in this decision?

■ Notes

1. Tricia Bishop, "Health-care Advertising Gearing More towards Consumers," *The Baltimore Sun* (March 20, 2005), www.baltimoresun.com.

2. W. L. Wilkie and P. W. Farris, "Comparison Advertising: Problems and Potentials," *Journal of Marketing* 39, no. 4 (1975): 7–15.

3. R. J. Lavidge and G. A. Steiner, "A Model of Predictive Measurements of Advertising Effectiveness," *Journal of Marketing* 25, no. 2 (1961): 59–62.

4. C. L. Bovee and W. F. Arens, *Contemporary Advertising*, 3rd ed. (Homewood, IL: Richard D. Irwin, Inc., 1989), 228–233.

5. "Attention to Detail Pays Off," *Profiles in Healthcare Marketing*, no. 60 (1994): 50–51, 54.

6. "Finding New Families on the Block," *Profiles in Healthcare Marketing*, no. 52 (1993): 8–10.

7. C. H. Patti and V. Blanko, "Budgeting Practices of Big Advertisers," *Journal of Advertising Research* 21, no. 6 (1981): 23–30.

8. John Philip Jones, "Ad Spending: Maintaining Market Share," *Harvard Business Review* (January–February 1990), pp. 38–42.

9. E. J. McCarthy, "How Much Should Hospitals Spend on Advertising?," *Health Care Management Review* 12, no. 1 (1987): 47–54.

10. J. A. Schroer, "Ad Spending: Growing Market Share," *Harvard Business Review* 68, no. 1 (January–February 1990): 44–48.

11. D. Seligman, "How Much for Advertising?," *Fortune* 54, no. 12 (1956): 123–126.

12. J. E. Lynch and G. J. Hooley, "Increasing Sophistication in Advertising Budget Setting," *Journal of Advertising Research* 30, no. 1 (1990): 67–75.

13. K. Deveny, "Marketers Exploit People's Fears of Everything," *The Wall Street Journal* (November 15, 1993): B1, B6.

14. "Ethical Guidelines for Healthcare Advertising," Position paper, Academy for Health Services Marketing, Chicago, IL (February 23, 1993), 6.

15. M. S. LaTour and R. E. Pitts, "Using Fear Appeals for AIDS Prevention in the College Age Population," *Journal of Healthcare Marketing* 9, no. 3 (1989): 5–14.

16. B. Edelman-Lewis and G. W. Thomas, "The Development and Evaluation of a Multimedia Advertising Campaign," in *Marketing Is Everybody's Business*, ed. P. Sanchez (Chicago, IL: Alliance for Health Care Strategy and Marketing, 1988), 89–97.

17. P. Kotler, *Marketing Management*, 8th ed. (Englewood Cliffs, NJ: Prentice-Hall, 1994), 646.

18. K. Haley, "The Birth of Fast Ads in Milwaukee," *Healthcare Marketing Report* 12, no. 9 (1994): 10–11.

19. S. Pomper, "The Big Shake Out Begins," *TIME* 136, no. 1 (1990): 50.

20. L. Gintz Jasper and E. Lueders Terwilliger, "Advertising's Impact on Calls to a Women's Hotline," *Journal of Healthcare Marketing* 9, no. 3 (1989): 62–66.

21. "Madison Avenue and Managed Care," *Managed Healthcare* 14, no. 9 (1994): 37.

22. Robin Blair, "CRM Builds Market Share," *Health Management Technology* (February 2003) (www.healthmgttech.com/archives/h0203crm.htm).

23. J. W. Peltier, A. K. Kleimenhagen, and G. M. Naidu, "Taking the Direct Route," *Journal of Health Care Marketing* 14, no. 3 (Fall 1994): 22–27.

24. D. A. Aaker and D. M. Stayman, "Measuring Audience Perceptions of Commercials and Relating Them to Ad Impact," *Journal of Advertising Research* 30, no. 4 (1990): 7–17.

25. Kotler, *Marketing Management*, 628.

26. Michael Romano, "Pushing Procedures," *Modern Healthcare* 35, no. 14 (April 4, 2005): 8–9.

27. Scott D. Olson, "Success Is in the Details," *Marketing Health Services* 23, no. 2 (Summer 2003): 20–25.

28. J. Burns, "Hospitals Made To Justify Marketing's Worth," *Modern Healthcare* 23, no. 44 (1993): 52.

Sales and Sales Management

Learning Objectives

After reading this chapter you should be able to:

- Understand the range of alternative sales positions

- Know the sequence of the personal sales process

- Differentiate between alternative sales processes

- Recognize the elements in the management of a sales force

An integral part of the promotional mix is personal selling. Historically, personal selling involved direct, face-to-face communication between the buyer and the seller. In our age of advancing technology, personal selling now occurs via telephone, video conferencing, and computer networks.

In the health care industry, personal sales often had a somewhat negative connotation. The image of the salesperson was either that of the loud huckster on television or the medical detail representative rarely recognized for providing real value to the product. While few would dispute that the first image is less than desirable, the medical detail representative is an integral part of effective marketing strategy at a pharmaceutical company. This type of sales position represents just one of many variations of the sales functions that exist.

Personal sales representatives perform more than just the selling role. Personal sales jobs are multifaceted. An effective sales representative will be engaged not only in selling, but will also conduct important relationship-building activities with customers. Salespeople also serve as a source of ongoing market research information as they call upon their accounts. It is often the salesperson who first learns from physicians that a new preferred provider organization plan is being developed or that a competing hospital is establishing a physician–hospital organization. Health care organizations are wise to embrace this broader view of the sales function when developing a marketing program to maximize this component of the promotional mix.

■ Types of Sales Jobs

There are many variations to the sales job, several of which have particular relevance in health care settings.[1]

New Business Selling

When most individuals think of sales, they consider only this type of situation. This sales job requires a salesperson to go out and make calls to seek new business. The salesperson's primary responsibility is to identify, contact, and sell new accounts. New account selling is the most difficult aspect of sales, yet is becoming increasingly important in health care as the industry shifts to a managed care environment. University MED-NET, one of Ohio's largest multispecialty groups in Cleveland, has a sales force to handle contracting with employers and with third-party payers.[2]

On a more global scale of new business selling, the Cleveland Clinic and the Mayo Clinic maintain internationally based sales representatives and field offices.[3] These sales representatives develop new business for these respective clinics and compete for well paying patients who may seek sophisticated medical services anywhere across the world.

Trade Selling

A second variation of the sales job is trade selling, which focuses sales efforts on the intermediaries in the channel of distribution. Trade selling's goal is to gain intermediaries' support for the company's products. This sales function is common to many consumer food product companies whose sales forces make regular calls on their wholesalers and retailers. In health care, this aspect of sales has often been found in tertiary hospitals and academic medical centers. Sales representatives call on referral physicians to attract more business and to reinforce the existing referral base.

Missionary Selling

A major aspect of many sales jobs is the missionary task, in which the primary goal is to maintain business from existing customers. This has been identified as one of the least risky ways to achieve the greatest return on investment from a sales force. The sales person periodically calls the physician's office to thank the staff for referrals as well as to uncover any possible problems that may exist in terms of making referrals into the hospital or into the specialty practice.[4]

Technical Selling

Another type of sales job is the technical representative. This person generates volume by providing technical expertise and support to potential customers. A sales representative for an occupational medicine program often conducts this type of sales activity. This representative might analyze a company's worker compensation claims and develop a package of occupational medicine services to help reduce these claims.

These descriptions underscore the point that sales involves more than just selling to a prospect. Maintaining relationships, servicing customers, reinforcing experiences, monitoring service performance, and selling are all part of most sales jobs. The medical detail representative provides clients with information and often asks questions as an early part of the market research process. Most medical detail representatives do little actual selling. However, this type of sales detailing and information dissemination is not inexpensive. It has been estimated to be between $150 and $200 per visit.[5] Rather, the bulk of their efforts focus on the missionary aspects of their jobs. Because of the high cost of technical selling and detailing, in recent years more companies are beginning to experiment with E-detailing as a way to disseminate information about their products. In a national survey of 10,000 physicians, only 17% indicated that e-detailing was less informative than a live sales call.[6] The historical attitude that personal selling is wrong for health care reflects a naivety about the scope of sales functions that exist.

■ The Personal Sales Process

Personal selling involves several steps beyond just getting the customer to agree to the sale. FIGURE 13-1 shows the six steps in the sales process. Each step in this figure shows the sales process as it pertains to a managed care organization (MCO) sales representative selling this plan to a company.

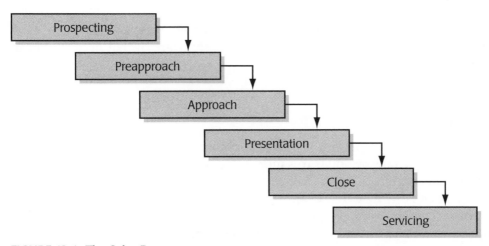

FIGURE 13-1 The Sales Process

Prospecting

Prospecting is the step in which the salesperson targets likely buyers, or **leads,** for sales calls. This is a difficult part of the sales process because it usually involves making **cold calls** by telephone or in person.[7,8] Cold calls are contacts with prospective buyers who did not initiate the process. For example, MCO salespeople make calls on large companies located in the MCO's business area. Doctors' Hospital in Columbus, Ohio, uses a nonclinician to generate the vast majority of the leads for its occupational health program.[9] As expected, cold calls can yield many rejections before turning up an interested party.

In this stage, the salesperson identifies **qualified prospects,** individuals who have a need for the product or service or are likely to buy. Physicians on the medical staff of a hospital are often the most qualified prospects. A goal of prospecting may well be to increase their level of utilization (a real sales target). This strategy has been effective for Columbus Regional Hospital in southeastern Indiana. Facing major competition from Indianapolis, Cincinnati, and even Louisville hospitals, the organization developed a sales force to call on physicians. The end result was a $2 million increase in internal medicine referrals alone in less than two years.[10] In generating leads of qualified buyers, companies use several sources, one of the most effective of which is personal references. For example, one physician might recommend that a salesperson call another physician who also might be interested in new diagnostic equipment. A reference from a knowledgeable source regarding another prospect reduces the salesperson's need to qualify the prospect. Advertising is often another source used to generate leads. For example, a hospital might advertise its industrial medicine program, and include in the ad copy a toll-free phone number for consumers to call for further information. A salesperson would receive the names of all callers and target these individuals as prospects.

At the prospecting stage, the salesperson tries to answer three key questions in qualifying the prospect:

1. Does the prospect have a need for my product or service?
2. Can I make the people responsible for buying so aware of that need that I can make the sale?
3. Will the sale be profitable to my company?[11]

Preapproach

The second step in the sales process is the preapproach. This is an information-gathering step in which the salesperson learns more about the customer and the customer's requirements. The more decision makers involved in buying the product, the longer and more complicated will be the preapproach stage. A corporation picking a health care plan for its employees might use a committee including the chief financial officer, the human resources director, and an employee representative to make this decision. Each committee member might have very different concerns regarding the selection of the health care plan. The salesperson's goal in the preapproach stage is to identify the issues for the buyer or buyers and to learn about their needs. Effective salespeople try to acquire as much information at this stage from secondary sources. The more knowledgeable the salesperson is about the prospect, the greater credibility he or she will have when trying to make the sale.

Approach

The **approach** stage of the sales process involves the initial meeting with the buyer. At this point, the MCO's sales representative tries to generate interest in the plan's offering and address the buyer's concerns and questions. This stage involves establishing trust and credibility with the buyer.

Presentation

The **presentation** stage is when the salesperson makes the pitch for the product or service. This step is where the actual selling effort occurs. The presentation is more difficult in service businesses than in product businesses. Usually, the best way to make a presentation is to demonstrate the product; however, this is difficult to do for a health care program.

In the presentation stage, the salesperson must become adept at handling buyer objections. Objections often take one of several forms. Timing objections are when the buyer delays the decision to purchase. The salesperson needs to identify the reasons for the delay and highlight the benefits the buyer could realize by immediate use of the MCO plan. A second common objection involves price. At this point, the salesperson must underscore the program's values and benefits relative to the price. Competitive objections are a third common form, when the buyer expresses satisfaction or loyalty to the health care provider presently under contract. It is essential for the salesperson to be familiar with competitive plans to focus the sales presentation on the differential advantages of the particular service being presented.

Another type of objection is called the logical objection, which is when buyers perceive a difference between their needs and the solution offered by the salesperson. These objections are usually focused on price, service characteristics, the salesperson's organization, or the firm's past experience. In most cases, such objections are negative. The salesperson must reestablish a positive set of objectives by getting the prospect to clarify the objection. A last set of objections is psychological and have no real logical basis. These objections often are based on the prospect's desire not to change existing habits or on the prospect's dislike of the sales process. The salesperson needs to minimize the degree of change. Citing testimonials from other new customers often can help reinforce the satisfaction others have felt since buying the service.

Within the presentation stage, a salesperson must learn how to counter any and all such objections. Several basic methods have been proposed for handling buyer objections.[12] These are:

1. Agree and counter—The salesperson agrees with the customer's concerns and then offers support for his or her own position.
2. List advantages and disadvantages—The sales representative specifically counters each negative with a positive perspective.
3. Positive conversion—The customer's objection is turned into the reason why the customer should buy the product. For example, the customer says, "We can't afford to change health care plans now." The salesperson responds, "Because of the real savings you are going to achieve, you cannot afford to stay with your existing plan."

The essential component of each method is that a well-trained salesperson must be able to diagnose the source of the objection. The sales representative must be adept at using one or more methods to counter the objection and move the prospect to the next stage of the sales process.

Close

The **close** is the stage of the sales process that involves asking the buyer for a commitment to purchase. All other steps of the sales process are irrelevant if the salesperson does not proceed to the close. Occasionally, a salesperson will use a *trial close* in which the salesperson asks the buyer for an opinion regarding the proposal. In this way, the salesperson can assess the buyer's readiness to decide without moving too quickly. An alternative approach to closing is known as the *assumptive close,* which involves asking the buyer to choose payment terms, delivery location, or the like, before there has been an actual agreement to purchase.

Servicing

The last step in the sales process—servicing—is often ignored by salespeople. This involves providing the buyer with post-sales follow-up and support. Table 13-1 shows the differing views of what a sale means to a buyer and a seller. From the buyer's perspec-

Table 13-1	The Differing Views of a Sales Interaction
The Seller's View	The Buyer's View
Culmination of a long sales negotiation	Initiation of a new relationship
Closure opens the way to culminating new potential clients	Concern about the support a new vendor will provide
Shift account from sales team to production team	How much attention and help will be received after the purchase decision
	Desire to continue to interact with the sales team

Source: From *Aftermarketing* by T. G. Vaura, Business One Irwin, 1992. Reprinted by permission of the McGraw-Hill Companies.

tive, closing the sale is not the end of the process, but the beginning of a relationship. In order to maintain repeat business, post-sales service and follow-up are essential.

■ Sales Approaches

There are several different approaches that are actually used in selling. Four common methods are the stimulus-response approach, the selling formula, the need satisfaction method, and consultative selling.

Stimulus-Response Sales Approach

The **stimulus-response sales approach** to sales presentations is based on psychological research conducted by Pavlov. As most introductory psychology students can recall, these experiments demonstrated that dogs that were given a stimulus (food) would yield a response (salivation). If the food was offered at the same time a bell was rung, the dog would begin to associate the bell with the food. And, if the bell alone was provided, the response of salivation would still occur even in the absence of food.[13] In effect, then, the bell became a substitute stimulus.

These experiments form the foundation of a sales approach in which the salesperson usually follows a canned presentation. A *canned presentation* is a set script through which the salesperson leads the prospect.[14] Following the stimulus-response method, then, the salesperson inserts questions within the presentation to encourage a particular response from the client.

For example, an MCO representative may follow a script such as the following:

Salesperson: Health care coverage is important to you and your family isn't it?

Prospect: Yes.

Salesperson: You wouldn't want your family not to have comprehensive coverage, would you?

Prospect: No.

Salesperson: Don't you think you should sign up for ABC MCO?

Prospect: Yes, you're right.

In reading this abbreviated version of a canned presentation, it is easy to discern that the salesperson dominates most of the discussion. The advantage of this approach is that it ensures that the salesperson will convey the intended corporate message. Sales training is relatively simple following a canned sales presentation. With practice, a canned sales presentation can be delivered relatively smoothly. The problems of this approach, however, are evident even in the abbreviated presentation. It does not require or encourage significant prospect involvement. It is not oriented to the prospect's concerns or specific issues. It also assumes that each prospect will react in the same way to a particular set of stimuli or questions. As a result, this type of presentation is best suited for low-priced products where the decision issues are relatively simple and similar. Selling products door-to-door, such as magazine subscriptions, is an example of a commonly used version of the stimulus-response approach.

The Selling Formula

The selling formula approach assumes that before customers agree to buy a product, they go through a series of steps. FIGURE 13-2 shows the formula for these steps, often referred to as "AIDA," which stands for attention, interest, desire, and action. The last step—action—is when the prospect agrees to buy. A trained sales professional recognizes the preconditions represented by these other steps and develops the potential customer's attention, interest, and desire in the service.

The AIDA approach's advantage is that the customer plays a more active part in the sales process. To gain customer interest and desire, the salesperson must engage the customer in conversation to assess how the product might match the customer's needs. Unlike the canned presentation, the salesperson has greater flexibility to direct more effort to the buyer's stage in the sales process. The challenge of this approach is that it does require a highly skilled salesperson. Buyers do not necessarily move through each stage in a distinct or timely fashion.

Need Satisfaction Method

This third sales method may well be the most marketing oriented. This approach focuses on identifying the customer's needs.[15] There are three stages of this sales method: need development, need awareness, and need fulfillment. In the first stage, the salesperson tries to identify the problems the customer is trying to solve. A hospital sales representative might ask a corporate health benefits officer questions such as:

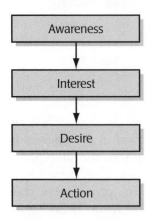

FIGURE 13-2 A-I-D-A

1. What are the most common reasons why workers' compensation claims are filed at your company?
2. Is there one division of the company where employees suffer more on-the-job injuries than they do in others?
3. Are there particular aspects of your company's business that workers have had physical difficulties accomplishing?

At the second stage of need awareness, the salesperson must ensure that the customer recognizes the same needs as the salesperson. For example, after assessing a company's needs, the salesperson might say something, such as:

It appears that most employee injuries are back-related, but these injuries don't occur on the loading dock. It seems from the data I've gathered and from the supervisors with whom I've met, that workers on the production line are suffering the greatest number of back injuries. These problems may not be due to lifting but rather to the ergonomics of their workstations.

At this stage, the salesperson will begin to highlight solutions available for resolving the customer's problems.

The last stage of this sales approach is need fulfillment. The salesperson now demonstrates how his company can meet the customer's needs. The presentation is customized to the buyer's needs rather than to what the selling organization wants to highlight. If ergonomic solutions are needed, talking about the industrial medicine toxicology components will not be helpful and may confuse the presentation.

Of the three sales approaches discussed so far, the needs satisfaction approach is the most customer-oriented and flexible. It requires a well-trained, sophisticated sales professional. The customer is an active participant in the sales process, but the salesperson must know how to engage the customer in the process and acquire the information necessary to ensure a match between the service being sold and the customer's needs.

Consultative Selling

This fourth sales approach focuses on problem identification. In this type of a sales strategy, the salesperson serves more as a consultant with a defined area of expertise.[16] A computer systems representative, for example, develops a proposal describing how a company can network its offices and explaining the potential values of such a network. Within the proposal, the sales representative provides a detailed specification list of the hardware requirements, as well as the necessary support services. Consultative selling will likely be used with greater frequency in health care as more organizations establish integrated delivery systems. For these organizations, a sales representative or consultant can analyze a business's specific health needs and tailor a package of services to meet the unique requirements of each customer.

■ Managing the Sales Function

A health care institution just establishing a sales force must address many dimensions and concerns inherent in sales management, including sales force organization, sales force size, recruitment and selection, training, compensation, and sales force evaluation and control.

Sales Force Organization

There are several ways a sales force can be structured. These variations include geographic, product, or customer organization.

Geographic Organization

This structure is the simplest way to organize a sales force. National companies can divide their sales forces by region, state, or even areas within states. The major advantage of this method is that it reduces the travel time and cost of sales personnel. And, only one company sales representative calls on customers within each sales territory.

The major disadvantage of this sales force organization is that salespeople must have a broad knowledge about all of the company's products and services. No sales specialization can be offered in this type of a structure. Sales representatives must also develop an ability to deal with a wide range of customers within their sales territory. Previously, this method had little applicability in health care. Most health care providers competed in relatively constrained geographical markets. Now, however, as more regional health care provider networks are being formed, geographic sales force structures might become more common.

Product Organization

FIGURE 13-3 shows a product organization structure for an integrated delivery system. In this design, there is a separate sales force for the Visiting Nurse Association (VNA) and separate sales forces for several clinical programs. Compared to the previous method, the primary benefit is that of product specialization. Since many of the clinical services require detailed technical or clinical knowledge, this structure allows the salesperson to develop the needed expertise in a particular field.

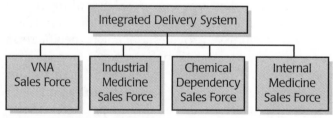

FIGURE 13-3 Product Organization Sales Structure

The disadvantages of this design can be readily appreciated. One customer could receive multiple calls by sales representatives from the same organization. This result can lead to potential ill will among customers, result in duplication of sales efforts, and increase sales costs.

Customer Organization

The third method of sales force structure is customer organization. As shown in FIGURE 13-4, this health care system has organized its sales force around its major customers: referral physicians, third-party payers, employers, and long-term care facilities. The major advantage of this structure is that the sales force can develop an expertise regarding customer requirements and concerns. Also, only one sales representative from the organization is assigned to call on a particular customer.

The major disadvantage to this sales force organization is that it requires each member of the sales force to have a broad understanding of the product and service mix of the health system. A company can compensate for this by having a sales team make a presentation to a customer when specific technical knowledge is required. This sales structure seems to be the most appropriate way for health care organizations to serve their diverse customer bases.

Sales Force Size

The most common method for determining the appropriate size of the sales force is called the **workload method**.[17] To use this method, management needs to estimate the work effort required to service the market. It does this by calculating the number of accounts to be called upon, the frequency with which each account is to be called, and the length of each sales call. To implement the workload method typically requires six steps.

The first step in the process requires that the organization classify its customers into sales volume categories. For example, a tertiary hospital might target the referral physician market and classify referrers as follows:

Class A physicians—heavy referrers: 550 physicians
Class B physicians—medium referrers: 700 physicians
Class C physicians—light/nonreferrers: 850 physicians

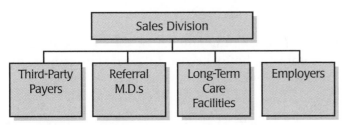

FIGURE 13-4 Customer Sales Force Organization

The second step requires a company to establish a call frequency for each class of account and the amount of time for each sales call. A hospital might decide that the heavy referral physician offices should be called upon six times per year. Class B physicians should receive four calls per year. Physicians who are categorized as Class C will receive two calls per year. For the Class A accounts, the sales calls might involve significant missionary work with the office and nursing staff, so these calls require 30 minutes. Classes B and C typically will require 15 minutes per call. With these call frequencies and call requirements established, each account class will require the following effort per year:

Class A—6 calls/year × 30 minutes per call = 3 hours
Class B—4 calls/year × 15 minutes per call = 1 hour
Class C—2 calls/year × 15 minutes per call = ½ hour

The third step involves determining the work required to cover the entire market.

Class A—550 accounts × 3 hours/account   = 1650 hours
Class B—700 accounts × 1 hour/account   =   700 hours
Class C—850 accounts × ½ hour/account   =   425 hours
                                               2775 hours

The fourth step is to determine the time available for each salesperson. A company must estimate the number of hours per week and the number of weeks per year that the salesperson works. Assume that the typical salesperson, working a 40-hour week, has 36 hours of effective selling time, which accounts for lunches and breaks. The salesperson might work a 48-week year:

36 hours × 48 weeks = 1728 hours

The fifth step is to determine the amount of time the salesperson spends in selling. As noted earlier, not all of a sales representative's time involves productive selling or account contact time. Some portion of the day is spent traveling or is involved in nonselling activities such as report completion, telephoning, and following up on problems.

Selling/account contact: 60% = 1036 hr/yr
Traveling: 20% = 346 hr/yr
Nonsales activities: 20% = 346 hr/yr
                                       1728 hr/yr

The sixth and final step involves calculating the number of salespeople needed. This is determined by dividing the number of hours needed to cover the accounts by the number of hours that is available for selling or account contact.

$$\frac{2775 \text{ hours}}{1036 \text{ hr/yr}} = 2.7 \text{ salespersons}$$

This number indicates that approximately three salespeople would be needed to cover the accounts for this medical center.

The workload method is one of the most common ways to determine sales force size. Its advantage is the relative ease at which estimates of size can be made. The disadvantage is that it does not account for differences in response by accounts if given varying levels of sales effort. Nor does it recognize that certain accounts within classes may still require higher levels of contact in order to maintain the existing relationships. The method also assumes that the cost of treating each account is identical, and that all salespeople use their time with the same level of efficiency. There are other methods for sales force size determination that go beyond the scope of this text. Suffice it to say that all of these methods require a sophisticated level of knowledge about customer response and the costs of accounts.

Recruitment and Selection

The effectiveness of any sales force ultimately is related to the quality of the individual recruited for a sales position. It is essential that the right person be matched with the position's job requirements.

The first step in identifying the type of individual to be recruited is an analysis of the sales job. This analysis must review the activities and tasks to be performed and their relative importance. From this perspective, a company can determine what traits are helpful in choosing the type of candidate to be recruited. Often it is valuable to analyze the characteristics of the existing sales force and those persons who either left their positions or were terminated for unsatisfactory performance. Studies have been unable to demonstrate that specific personality traits are useful predictors of successful salespeople, although there is some evidence that the following indicators have been found frequently among salespeople who fail. These are:

1. instability of residence
2. failure in business within the last two years
3. unexplained gaps in the person's employment record
4. excessive personal indebtedness.[18]

Recruitment

After a firm analyzes the types of sales skills needed for its sales positions, the next step involves recruiting qualified personnel. There are a variety of sources for finding qualified candidates, including educational institutions, other companies in the industry, professional associations, other departments within the company, and staff recommendations. Most universities, for example, have extensive placement services, and professional associations such as the Medical Group Management Association or the American Hospital Association have newsletters that frequently list job placement opportunities at various health care organizations. Depending on the level of the position being staffed, professional recruiting firms and employment agencies can be hired to match qualified applicants with the position.

Selection

Once a reasonable number of applicants is generated, an organization must have a strategy in place to select the best job candidate. Typically, selection involves several steps as shown in FIGURE 13-5. These include preliminary screening, personal history form, in-depth personal interview, testing, and background investigation.

The preliminary screening interview serves as a way to eliminate the most unqualified applicants. These interviews normally are conducted by a member of the human resources staff. The second step in the process is the personal history form. This form typically is more detailed than the initial application. Information collected on this form should relate only to the performance of the position being sought. Questions regarding race, sex, religion, age, and national origin are considered illegal discriminatory acts under federal equal opportunity guidelines.

A third step is the in-depth personal interview. This interview usually is conducted by the individual who will supervise the salesperson. In addition to obtaining insight into the candidate's background, the interview allows for judgments to be made about the candidate's communication style, personality, and mental abilities. Firms tend to use one of three interview methods. One method is the **structured interview**, which follows a set list of questions. The advantage of this approach is that it allows all candidates to be compared on the same dimensions. Its weakness is that the manager often cannot deviate from the list without compromising the interview process. As a result, many organizations have switched to **unstructured interviews**. In this interview format, the applicant is encouraged to talk freely on a range of subjects. The interviewer acts almost like a focus group moderator (as discussed in Chapter 5), asking a few probing questions; unstructured interviews require a well-trained interviewer. The third variation of the interview process is a **stress interview**. The interviewer places

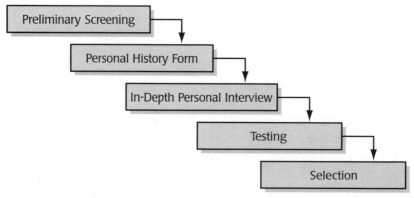

FIGURE 13-5 Sales Personnel Selection Process

the applicant under stress using role playing exercises such as handling multiple customer objections or a rude customer. The goal is to assess how the candidate will behave under actual on-the-job conditions.

Candidates who succeed in the screening and interview stages often may be required to take tests. Tests can include any of three forms: intelligence, aptitude, or personality tests. Because of concerns regarding discrimination, the Federal Equal Employment Opportunity Commission requires that tests used for selection be validated by focusing strictly on the job requirements and on tasks related to successful performance of the position.

Intelligence tests measure an individual's mental abilities to reason or to learn. Aptitude tests are designed to test a person's ability to learn to perform certain tasks or job requirements. One well-known aptitude test is the Strong Vocational Interest test, which asks candidates the type of setting they are most comfortable working in. The third type of test—personality—measures traits such as assertiveness, sociability, independence, and empathy. While all these tests provide some insight, companies must correlate test results with the successful performance by sales personnel. To avoid major issues regarding testing discrimination, it is suggested that tests be only one part of the selection process.

A final step in the selection process is the background investigation. This typically involves reference checks, credit information, and in some instances, lie detector tests. In the pharmaceutical industry, for example, background checks are an important part of the selection process. Since medical detail representatives have access to samples of prescription drugs, the applicant's integrity is an issue of paramount concern.

Training

Sales training is an ongoing activity for companies that want to maintain an effective sales force. Training begins when the candidate is first hired and often continues with on-the-job training.

Training the New Recruit

Most companies have a formal training program for new recruits. Large companies, such as consumer food product companies or life insurance firms, maintain a centralized sales training staff with a prescribed program for ongoing selection and recruitment of sales personnel. In smaller companies or in organizations that have smaller sales requirements, training activities are less formal and often are conducted within the marketing department.

The scope of the sales training typically involves issues such as the sales process. Salespeople receive information about the company and the industry, as well as about the organization's policies and procedures. Sales training for new recruits must focus on time and territory management and on customer requirements and product knowledge. Many organizations will also have a new salesperson shadow a more experienced representative in the field prior to the completion of the sales training. After this mentoring experience, sales training can focus on what was observed in real on-the-job settings.

Ongoing Training

Ongoing training of experienced personnel varies little from that of the new recruit. Companies typically provide annual updating of new services or changes within existing programs. This training helps to improve morale and refine existing sales techniques.

Compensation

A major issue in the management of any sales force is determining the compensation system. In developing an effective compensation plan, there are specific requirements important to the salesperson and valuable to the company.

Salespeople need to be assured that the compensation plan is equitable for the entire sales force. A well-designed plan should provide salespeople with a stable income, yet offer the motivation or incentive to perform. Finally, a sound compensation plan should be understandable, meaning the sales staff should understand the dimensions on which they are to be rewarded and what the organization values.

The design of the compensation plan should allow the company to attract and retain good salespeople. A well-designed plan should also provide to the company the ability to encourage or focus the sales force's efforts on specific tasks. A good plan allows for recognition of the differences between good and bad performers and provides the necessary balance between costs and results. While a good plan ultimately should be easy to administer, it must be constructed in such a way to ensure long-term customer relationships. Three basic types of compensation plans are used: the straight salary, the commission plan, and the combination plan.

Straight Salary

The **straight salary** compensation plan provides salespeople with a fixed salary. This plan's advantage is that it allows the salesperson to focus upon the nonsales aspects of the job. For the organization, another benefit is that the sales costs are easily determined and budgeted. The plan is also appropriate when it is hard to determine the effect of the salesperson's efforts on resulting volume. For example, a sales position that is primarily missionary in its focus might receive straight salary compensation.

One of the plan's disadvantages is its direct effects on motivation. Financial reward is not tied to any particular aspect of sales performance. As a result, the rationale for salary increases may not be easy to communicate. Also, the fixed-cost nature of the straight salary plan, while cited as an advantage, is also its limitation. When sales are rising and volume is high, compensation costs become a smaller percentage of total revenue. With declining sales volume, however, the fixed salary costs become a significant overhead expense.

Commission Plan

An alternative to a straight salary program is one that pays on **commission,** in which the salesperson is paid based on sales performance in terms of volume, net revenue, or margin. The advantage of this plan is that the salesperson is clearly focused upon the sales task. It also has the advantage of equity in that good performers are rewarded more highly than those who are less proficient. Unlike straight salary plans, commission compensation plans vary directly with the organization's revenue, allowing the firm a built-in cost advantage.

Commission plans have some major limitations, however, one being that the salesperson focuses too heavily on the sales tasks alone. Nonsales activities and missionary functions may not receive warranted attention in the short term as the salesperson tries to maximize income. Salespeople also have concerns about the security of a commission plan. These types of programs can lead to a high degree of variability in income from one pay period to the next.

Combination Plans

A **combination plan** for a sales force consists of a base salary plus commissions and bonuses. The base salary gives the salesperson some financial security as well as the motivation to perform the nonsales aspects of the job. The salesperson also receives a bonus, or commission, based on achieving particular sales quotas or other previously specified levels of performance. A **bonus** is a payment made for achieving a particular level of performance.

In developing a combination compensation plan, companies must consider the size of the incentive portion of compensation relative to that which is fixed. The incentive portion must be large enough to motivate the sales staff. The more important actual selling skills are to the salesperson's role, the higher the incentive proportion of the compensation plan should be. A second issue in any combination plan is whether it should set limits on incentive earnings. Limitations are often imposed so that the high performer's income is not so great as to affect the morale of those with lower performance ratings. Another concern is that a new service might be so positively received when first introduced in the market that the sales staff will be rewarded, even though their efforts contributed little to actual sales. Whenever a company implements a compensation plan with an incentive component, it is always useful to pretest the plan with past performance data. The company should assess what the relative compensation levels of the sales force would have been if the incentive plan was in place. This pretest can determine whether the plan reflects the performance levels of the sales personnel.

Supplemental Incentives

A growing element in sales compensation is the use of supplemental programs, such as sales contests or nonfinancial incentives, as shown in FIGURE 13-6. Sales contests typically reward personnel for short-term, highly focused activities. For contests to succeed, salespeople must believe they have an opportunity to compete for the prize. The objectives

Nonfinancial Incentives
Percentage of All Companies Using

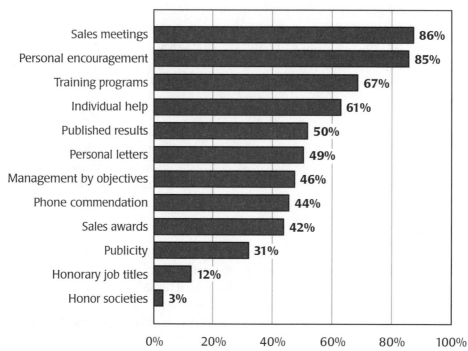

FIGURE 13-6 Nonfinancial Compensation Methods

Source: Ken Mack and Philip A. Newbold, *Health Care Sales* (San Francisco: Jossey-Bass Publishers, 1991), 61.

must be within the reach of each person. A contest that ties rewards to percentage improvement over last year's sales effort is one way to allow each person to compete. Programs should be simple and easy to communicate. Rewards should be attractive incentives, including cash, travel, or merchandise. With the use of nonfinancial incentives, the goal is to reward the salesperson through recognition—a personal letter, an award, or other publicity. The value of a nonfinancial incentive is to reinforce the salesperson's higher-order needs, such as self-esteem, as presented by Maslow (see Chapter 4).

Sales Force Evaluation and Control

The final step in the sales management process is the ongoing evaluation and control of the sales force. Evaluation of the sales force is based on both input and output measures. **Input measures** assess the effort expended by salespersons to perform their job. These measures might include number of calls per day, product knowledge, hours worked per day, or number of phone calls made. **Output measures** assess the results of the salesperson's efforts. These measures often include sales, gross revenue, number of referrals generated, number of new users, and expenses.[19] Organizations must decide whether to use single or multiple measures of performance. The advantage of a single measure is its administrative ease. In addition to being economical, single measure evaluation systems also are easy to communicate. Their chief limitation is that they often focus exclusively on sales. As discussed earlier in this chapter, selling is just one component of the salesperson's responsibilities.

There are many valuable sources of information that a company can use in the evaluation process. Company records are the primary source of evaluation data. Customers should also become part of the evaluation process, since it is the customer who might best be able to assess the salesperson's relationship-building methods and attitude. The limitation of this source is the validity of the information. Most consumer product companies have the sales manager accompany the salesperson on sales calls to assess on-the-job performance.

Regardless of the number of measures or sources used for evaluation, an organization needs to have an ongoing evaluation plan. The plan should be based on the requirements of the specific sales positions, and selling and nonselling tasks should be weighted according to their relative importance.

■ Conclusions

Use of personal selling in health care has been limited to a few areas in the past 10 to 15 years. While a common strategy for pharmaceutical companies and MCOs, personal selling has been a smaller component of the promotional mix among other segments of the industry. Now, as the health care environment shifts again from a capitated to a more competitive fee for service environment, competing for patients, referrals, and possibly direct contracts from employers will make the personal sales strategy assume greater importance.

To utilize a sales force effectively requires understanding the dimensions of all the sales functions. This way, effective recruiting programs can be implemented, sales force size determined, and compensation and evaluation systems put in place.

■ Key Terms

Leads
Cold Calls
Qualified Prospects
Approach
Presentation
Close
Stimulus-Response Sales Approach
Workload Method
Structured Interview

Unstructured Interview
Stress Interview
Straight Salary
Commission
Combination Plan
Bonus
Input measures
Output measures

■ Chapter Summary

1. Personal selling is an ingredient of the promotional mix. Sales positions involve a range of sales functions—from selling to customer relationship building.
2. There are six steps in the personal sales process: prospecting, preapproach, approach, presentation, close, and servicing.
3. In the stimulus-response approach to sales, a canned presentation is often used as a script to generate a customer response, while in the selling formula approach, the prospect is moved through a sequence from attention, interest, desire, to action.
4. The need satisfaction sales method is the most marketing-oriented because it focuses on the customer's problems. With the consultative selling method, the salesperson acts as a problem solver.
5. Sales forces can be organized geographically, by product, or by customer type.
6. A common method for determining the size of the sales force is the workload method, which estimates the work effort required to serve the market.
7. Prior to recruitment and selection of the salesperson, the company should conduct a job analysis. The selection process then follows several steps, including an interview that can be a structured, unstructured, or stress interview.
8. Sales force compensation can be either straight salary, commission, or a combination plan.
9. Sales staff evaluation should be based on input measures (a salesperson's efforts) and output measures (sales results).

■ Chapter Problems

1. What type of sales position would you recommend for: (a) a four-person gastroenterology practice that wants to maintain strong ties to its primary care referral physicians, (b) an MCO trying to penetrate a new market and have its plan offered as an option to employees within any local company, and (c) a health care data management firm that provides a program to hospitals for billing and quality assurance?
2. Develop a short sales presentation about a chemical dependency program that you would make to an employee assistance professional of a large company. Show how the presentation would change using: (a) the stimulus-response approach, (b) the selling formula, and (c) the need satisfaction method.
3. What method of sales force organization would be most appropriate for: (a) a national company that sells a computerized billing system for small physician practices, and (b) a manufacturer of adhesive bandages and sutures?

4. A major tertiary care medical center has decided to establish a sales force to call on physicians practicing in the medical center's three-state region. The marketing director has classified the physicians into the following categories:

Class A: loyal referrers—329 physicians
Class B: moderate referrers—480 physicians
Class C: potential referrers—620 physicians

She also estimates the following call pattern:

Class A: 4 calls per year @ 30 minutes per call
Class B: 3 calls per year @ 15 minutes per call
Class C: 2 calls per year @ 15 minutes per call

The average salesperson works 48 weeks a year, 40 hours a week and spends 80% of his time selling. Calculate the number of sales representatives needed to service this market.

5. A manufacturer of prosthetic devices has decided to review his company's sales compensation system. Historically, salespeople were paid on straight salary. While the company has grown in recent years, the president is convinced that the sales force could generate more sales volume. A major part of the sales job is missionary, yet with the increasing number of physician groups expanding into rehabilitation medicine, a new target market is possible. The manufacturer is also concerned that not all the products in the line have the same margin. What form of compensation would you recommend?

■ Notes

1. D. A. Newton, *Sales Force Performance and Turnover* (Cambridge, MA: Marketing Science Institute, 1973), 5.
2. W. S. Dempsey and S. H. Mandel, "It's No Longer Words and Music: Marketing in a Capitated Environment," *Group Practice Journal* 43, no. 3 (1994): 46–51.
3. "Taking U.S. Health Services Overseas," *Marketing Health Services* 22, no. 2 (Summer): 21–23.
4. Ken Mack, "Are You Ready to Invest in Business Development?," *Healthcare Financial Management* (October 2002): 70–74.
5. Terry Davidson and Eugene Savidas, "Details Drive Success," *Marketing Health Services* 24, no. 1 (Spring 2004): 20–25.
6. Davidson and Savidas, op. cit.
7. J. D. Lichenthal, S. Sikri, and K. Folk, "Teleprospecting: An Approach for Qualifying Accounts," *Industrial Marketing Management* 18, no. 1 (1989): 11–17.
8. M. A. Jolson, "Qualifying Sales Leads: The Tight and Loose Approaches," *Industrial Marketing Management* 17, no. 3 (1988): 189–196.

9. E. O. Wogensen, "Osteopathic Hospital Reaps Multiple Benefits through Occupational Health Program," *Strategic Health Care Marketing* 11, no. 7 (1994): 4–6.

10. Chris Taylor, "The Pioneers: In Some Industries, Having a Dedicated Sales Force Has Been Considered Taboo. But times have changed, and those same businesses are finding they need sales strategies like never before. Here's a look at trailblazers in three different sectors who are creating sales cultures from scratch." *Sales and Marketing Management* 157, no. 2 (February 25, 2005).

11. B. Shapiro, *Sales Force Management* (New York: McGraw-Hill, 1977), 160.

12. R. D. Balsey and E. P. Birsner, *Selling: Marketing Personified* (Hindsdale, IL: Dryden Press, 1987), 261–263.

13. I. P. Pavlov, *Conditioned Reflexes* (New York: Oxford University Press, 1927).

14. M. A. Jolson, "Canned Adaptiveness: A New Direction for Modern Salesmanship," *Business Horizons* 32, no. 1 (1989): 7–12.

15. M. Belch and R. W. Haas, "Using Buyer Needs To Improve Industrial Sales," *Business* 29, no. 5 (1979): 8–14.

16. R. Spiro and B. Weitz, "Adaptive Selling: Conceptualization, Measurement, and Nomological Validity," *Journal of Marketing Research* 27, no. 1 (1990): 61–69.

17. W. J. Talley, "How To Design Sales Territories," *Journal of Marketing* 25, no. 3 (1961): 7–13.

18. G. A. Churchill, Jr., et al., "The Determinants of Salesperson Performance: A Meta-Analysis," *Journal of Marketing Research* 22, no. 2 (1985): 103–118.

19. D. W. Jackson, Jr., J. E. Keith, and J. Schlacter, "Evaluation of Selling Performance: A Study of Current Practice," *Journal of Personal Selling and Sales Management* 31, no. 2 (1983): 43–51.

Controlling and Monitoring

Learning Objectives

After reading this chapter you should be able to:

- Explain the value of monitoring market share compared to using absolute measure of performance

- Recognize the value of sales, profitability, contribution, and variance analysis

- Understand the array of specific marketing mix control procedures to monitor mix-specific activities

- Describe the scope of an organization's marketing audit and elements of that audit

■ Controlling and Monitoring Marketing Performance

Essential to an effective marketing organization is the ongoing measurement and monitoring of outcomes. In health care, this aspect of marketing is particularly important. As noted in Chapter 1, for a long time the health care industry viewed marketing as an unnecessary expense and limited to advertising. Although there has been growing appreciation of marketing's role, concern still exists about whether the dollars spent on marketing are well invested. As health care organizations face more difficult resource allocation decisions, marketing managers will need to document their results. To accomplish this goal, marketing departments will need to have a system in place to monitor and measure results of marketing efforts continually.

To monitor marketing activities properly requires a multiple-step process, as shown in FIGURE 14-1. The initial requirement is to establish performance standards on an *a priori* basis. These standards, once specified, allow for the appropriate data requirements to be developed, and the internal system requirements to be established to collect data in a timely and accurate fashion. Data on the marketing activity can then be analyzed and corrective action taken or marketing strategy adjusted as needed.

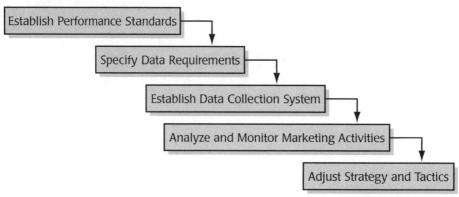

FIGURE 14-1 Monitoring the Marketing Process

Market Share Analysis

For some health care organizations, a major problem in developing an effective marketing strategy is complacency. Many health care providers believe they are doing well in the market simply by monitoring measures such as patient scheduling patterns for the physicians in the group. Many group medical practices often use measures of performance such as gross revenue, expense control, or net revenue that result in end-of-year payouts to the physicians. These measures are, in fact, all important indicators of performance. But, in a competitive market, these measures alone suffer from a major limitation—they are all absolute rather than relative indicators of performance. A group practice may believe it is performing well without fully understanding the dynamics of the marketplace or whether the revenue and patient increase it experiences is a result of its strategy or of a marketplace expansion.

Any organization in a competitive market must monitor its respective share of the market. Market share has the advantage of signaling when an organization needs to make changes. Market share is a measure of relative performance rather than an absolute indicator of performance. To understand the value of monitoring market share, consider the graph shown in FIGURE 14-2. In this graph, "Hypothetical" a hypothetical health maintenance organization (HMO) began its operation in 1975. This HMO was the first such plan to offer a prepaid version of health care in this small, southeastern metropolitan community. After several years of slow growth (the introductory stage of the life cycle for managed care in this market), the number of subscribers began to increase as more consumers recognized this option as a viable way to pay for health care coverage. In 1982, this HMO saw its first organized competition from a large national HMO. As can be seen, the number of subscribers increased dramatically as both health care plans began to advertise. The second HMO served to legitimize this form of health care in the marketplace.

The graph shows that the hypothetical HMO was not concerned about the competition, since the number of subscribers was increasing. Little evidence existed for

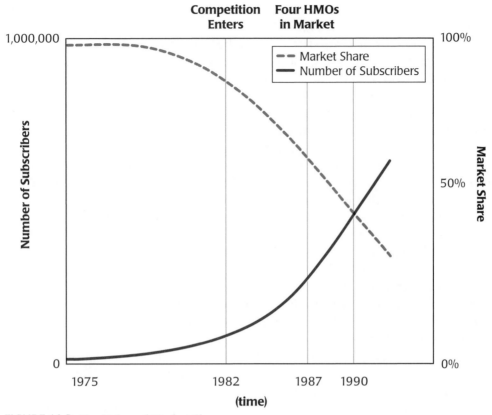

FIGURE 14-2 The Value of Market Share

revising the organization's strategy. By 1987, four HMOs were operating in the market, yet the hypothetical HMO still saw its number of subscribers rise. Its monitoring of an absolute performance measure indicated little cause for concern. An examination of market share, however, indicated the time for a possible strategic change. In 1975, the original HMO had a market share of 100%. As seen in the graph, its market share did not change significantly by the time a competitor entered the market in 1982. By 1990, however, this original HMO is no longer a market leader in terms of market share. Monitoring absolute measures (sales, number of subscribers) never suggested the need for this HMO to revisit its marketing strategy since the number of subscribers on an absolute basis increases. Yet, if market share had been monitored, the hypothetical HMO could have detected that, while its number of subscribers was growing, it may have had less to do with its strategy, and more to do with the fact that the entire market was expanding. If the company had been monitoring market share, it would have detected a fairly rapid erosion of its market position and recognized the need to reconsider its marketing mix. It could have opened a satellite office on the other side of the metropolitan area and changed its distribution mix. Or, the group could have offered an expanded benefit package including eye care (a product mix alteration), or changed the price of its premium.

Market share monitoring is an issue today in the health care marketplace. For many years, Kaiser Permanente Medical Group of Chula Vista, California, experienced significant continuing growth in the number of its subscribers. No doubt this was due to the quality of the medical plan and the fact that Kaiser was an early entrant into managed care in California. Yet, in the past few years, Kaiser has met considerable competition from other organized managed care plans in the state. Monitoring market share earlier might have indicated the need for a substantial revision in its service mix. In 1994, Kaiser experienced its first major decline in the number of enrollees in the state of California. That same year, Kaiser began to offer a point-of-service (POS) plan as a way to boost share growth and compete against other POS plans that already existed in the market. With its POS plan, Kaiser was a late entrant into the market.

When measuring performance based on market share, it is important to recognize that there are three types of market share measures to use:

1. **Overall market share:** This measure represents the company's sales as a percentage of total industry sales. For a national HMO like Cigna, market share would be calculated as the percentage of Cigna HMO enrollees to the total number of HMO enrollees in the United States.

2. **Served market share:** This indicator is a measure of the organization's sales as a percentage of the total sales of the served market. The served market represents all the buyers who are able and willing to buy or use the service. For most medical organizations, the market share basis is really on the served market. For example, a hospital will calculate its served market share of coronary bypass procedures, which is its total number of bypass procedures performed as a percentage of the total number of bypass procedures done in its service area. An organization's served market share is always larger than its total market share.

3. **Relative market share:** This indicator of market share is a calculation of the percentage of the organization's sales compared to that of the largest competitor, or often the combined sales of the three largest competitors. When calculating market share to that of the largest competitor, a relative market share greater than 100% would indicate a market leader.[1]

There is no one correct market share indicator to use. It is important, however, for a company to determine a market share indicator and then track data using that same indicator. It is also essential to determine initially which market share indicator to use so that the appropriate data can be obtained. In health care, market data can often be obtained from state or local health regulatory agencies or federal statistics. There are also private, commercial organizations that provide data to health care organizations for market share measurement.

Sales Analysis

A common method for monitoring marketing performance is **sales analysis**, which compares the actual sales generated with the goals that were established. In conducting a sales analysis, it is useful to examine sales at a level below that of gross sales, such as by analyzing results on one or more criteria, such as: (1) product line analysis, (2) customer size, (3) geographic region, or (4) discount level.

An innovative approach to sales analysis was conducted by Inova Health System for its Inova Fairfax Hospital. The hospital developed a two-step marketing campaign for its cardiology services. Using a sophisticated segmentation scheme, the hospital sent a direct mail letter to consumers inviting them to take a health risk assessment. Thirty-two versions of a follow-up postcard were sent based on the demographic and psychographic profiles of the individuals who received the invitations. The interesting aspect of the monitoring process of this campaign was that to accurately gauge the results of the "Don't Wait" campaign, Inova held out a control group that did not receive campaign materials against which it could compare the service utilization of individuals who received the campaign mailings. The control group had the same characteristics of those in the targeted group. Using its CRM database, Inova tracked both cardiology services utilization and noncardiology services utilization. Adjusting for the control group, approximately 1% of individuals had cardiology services for a net return on investment (ROI) of $225,008, while approximately 9% of individuals received noncardiology services for a net ROI of $578,605.[2]

Profitability Analysis

In Chapter 6, on market segmentation, the principle of heavy half segmentation was reviewed. As was noted, a large percentage of a product's sales are purchased by a small percentage of the customers. A useful method for monitoring marketing performance that incorporates this factor is **profitability analysis**, which examines the profitability of sales by customers, regions, products, or salespeople. For example, this type of analysis might reveal that there are some distinct differences among salespeople, as shown in Table 14-1. As seen in this analysis, salesperson A has the highest level of total sales. A more detailed examination of salesperson A's performance shows that, compared to salesperson C, A's level of sales resulted from selling possibly easier, less profitable

Table 14-1	Looking at Product Profitability		
Salesperson	A	B	C
Sales	$2,156,890	$1,768,925	$2,146,859
Direct Selling Expenses	$46,007	$57,809	$41,487
Gross Margin of Products Sold	$1,113,873	$876,931	$1,246,701
Average Gross Margin (Percent)	51.64%	49.57%	58.07%

products. This type of profitability analysis can help to refocus sales training efforts to encourage salespeople to sell more profitable items in the line. Profitability analysis can also indicate whether a company needs to redesign or change its sales compensation system to directly reward selling the more profitable products in the line.

In conducting an appropriate profitability analysis, a company needs to decide how to calculate costs. There are two options. One approach, referred to as **direct costing,** assigns only those costs to a product or service line that are directly associated with it. In **full costing,** both direct and indirect costs are assigned to the service unit and considered in the calculation of profitability.

Allocation of Costs

To conduct a full-costing analysis, a health care organization must assign both direct and indirect costs. Direct costs, as noted, pertain to costs directly associated with the program under analysis. Direct costs include any labor, technology, or supplies pertaining to the clinical program. There may also be direct marketing costs, if in fact specific advertisements were run for the program. Or, if a program manager made sales calls on possible accounts such as in an occupational medicine program, that person's salary would be a direct cost. **Indirect costs** are fixed costs that cannot be related to just one product line or service program. Indirect costs also include administrative management salaries unrelated to any specific program.

When using a full-costing method, a health care organization must decide to allocate costs to a particular program. While it is not incorrect to allocate costs, there are some concerns about what to use as the basis for the allocation. Is the allocation based on space utilized in the ambulatory building for a particular program? Or, is the basis for allocation the percentage of total hospital revenue generated by the program?[3] Ideally, the basis of allocation should be fair and consistent. Since there often are no exact determinations for the appropriate allocations, however, management should not spend excessive amounts of time resolving issues of cost allocations. Marketing's major concern about cost allocations is that they often distort the real value or profitability of a particular product. The result is that a low-volume product can often be identified as more profitable than a high-volume product, purely as a function of the cost allocation.[4] Because of the difficulties in assigning indirect costs, many companies prefer direct costing, which considers the contribution margin of a particular service. While overhead, or fixed costs, must be covered at some time, the contribution margin approach provides a clearer view of what would be gained or lost by dropping a particular clinical program.

Contribution Analysis

Another method for organizations to assess the market performance of a service or multiple services is contribution analysis. **Contribution analysis** considers the contribution of profit to fixed cost or overhead. Table 14-2 shows an analysis of four clinical serv-

Table 14-2	Examining Contribution to Profit			
	Product Profitability			
	Occupational Medicine	Substance Abuse	Rehab. Services	Executive Fitness
Number of Customers	375	222	97	75
Average Price per Employee	$127	$85	$320	$425
Variable Cost per Employee	$37.20	$22.50	$112.00	$97.00
Variable Contribution Margin per Employee Covered (Avg. Price − Variable Cost per Employee)	$89.20	$62.50	$208.00	$328.00
PVCM	70.23%	73.53%	65.00%	77.17%

ices offered by a medical center and the **percentage variable contribution margin** (**PVCM**) per service. The PVCM shows the percentage of each additional sales dollar available to the organization to cover its fixed costs. The calculation of this ratio is:

$$PVCM = \frac{Average\ Unit\ Price - Unit\ Variable\ Cost}{Unit\ Price}$$

The variable contribution margin is the price per unit sales less the variable cost per unit.

Insights from Contribution Analysis

The differences between using a contribution or full-cost approach are significant. Contribution analysis allows a marketing manager to calculate the incremental value of directing additional resources to a particular service line or customer account. Since contribution analysis considers only direct program costs, a company could estimate how much more sales or revenue would be obtained if additional marketing efforts were committed. Table 14-3 shows the analysis of three departments using a full-cost method. As seen with the allocation of indirect costs (administrative expenses and overhead),

Table 14-3	The Full Cost Approach			
	Totals	Clinical Service #1	Clinical Service #2	Clinical Service #3
Sales	$1,000,000	$500,000	$300,000	$200,000
Direct Costs	$800,000	$450,000	$250,000	$100,000
Contribution Margin	$200,000	$50,000	$50,000	$100,000
Indirect Costs Allocated	$110,000	$55,000	$33,000	$22,000
Net Profit	$90,000	($5000)	$17,000	$78,000

Table 14-4	The Contribution Approach			
	Totals	Clinical Service #1	Clinical Service #2	Clinical Service #3
Sales	$1,000,000	$500,000	$300,000	$200,000
Direct Costs	$800,000	$450,000	$250,000	$100,000
Contribution Margin	$200,000	$50,000	$50,000	$100,000
Indirect Costs Allocated	$110,000			
Net Profit	$90,000			

clinical service # 1 is losing $5,000, while clinical service # 3 saw net profit of $78,000. Consider the difference, however, when the contribution method is applied, as shown in Table 14-4. Without the allocation of indirect costs, clinical service # 1 provides incremental value by contributing $50,000 to fixed costs, or overhead.

The Beckham Company, a health care consulting firm reviewed several community hospitals, and found an inverse relationship between total inpatient revenue and contribution to operating margin. Traditionally, high revenue-producing services such as cardiology, internal medicine, and pulmonary medicine were creating the greatest losses. Some of the lowest inpatient revenue services—family practice, rheumatology, and obstetrics—had the most positive contribution margins.[5]

Variance Analysis

An important method for evaluating marketing efforts is through the use of **variance analysis**, which compares actual results to preestablished performance targets. Table 14-5 shows the results of a yearlong effort to enroll subscribers in a managed care plan. As seen in this table, the number of covered lives actually enrolled was 10,000 more than originally targeted. Yet, because there was intense competition from other

Table 14-5	Variance Analysis		
	Variance Analysis		
	Planned	Actual	Difference
Covered Lives	100,000	110,000	10,000
Premium per Subscriber	$1,400	$1,200	($200)
Direct Costs per Subscriber	400	400	—
Subscriber Gross Marketing Contribution	$1,000	$800	($200)
Sales	$140,000,000	$132,000,000	($8,000,000)
Direct Costs	40,000,000	44,000,000	(4,000,000)
Gross Margin Contribution	$100,000,000	$ 88,000,000	($12,000,000)

managed care plans, the premium dollar received per subscriber was less than originally projected. Many competitors aggressively discounted to encourage new enrollment. As a result, the gross marketing contribution fell below the targeted level.

Examining these data, it's evident that the decreases in gross marketing contribution resulted from two factors: the increase in the number of subscribers and the decrease in the premium dollar received. Which factor contributed more to the decrease in gross marketing contribution? It is possible to get an answer by examining the data in EXHIBIT 14-1. In this exhibit, one can see that the company enrolled more subscribers than anticipated. Such a difference between expected and real unit sales is called a **volume variance**. Yet because there was heavy discounting in the market, the contribution to gross marketing costs decreased. This difference between expected and real contribution

Exhibit 14-1   Sources of Variance

Variance Source

Differences Due to Changes in Gross Marketing Contribution:

Actual Gross Marketing Contribution	= Actual Subscriber Level × Actual Subscriber Gross Marketing Contribution
	= 110,000 × \$800 = \$88,000,000
Planned Gross Marketing Contribution	= Actual Subscriber Level × Planned Subscriber Gross Marketing Contribution
	= 110,000 × \$1,000 = \$110,000,000
Variance Due to Failure to get Subscriber Gross Marketing Contribution	= (\$110,000,000 − \$88,000,000)
	= (\$22,000,000)

Differences Due to Changes in Volume:

Annual Gross Marketing Contribution	= Planned Subscriber Level × Planned Subscriber Gross Marketing Contribution
	= 100,000 × \$1,000 = \$100,000,000
Planned Gross Marketing Contribution	= Actual Subscriber Level × Planned Subscriber Gross Marketing Contribution
	= 110,000 × \$1,000 = \$110,000,000

Increase in Gross Marketing Contribution Due to Subscriber Enrollment Success = \$10,000,000 margin is referred to as a **contribution variance** (or a price variance). By examining the variances calculated in Exhibit 14-1, one can assess which factor has a greater impact on the lower gross marketing contribution shown in Table 14-5. The analysis reveals that it was the lack of maintaining prices that resulted in the decreased gross margin contribution observed by the managed care plan.

Hospitals and other medical organizations have a wide array of products and services that they market. They can also assess market performance, therefore, by using a **product mix variance**, which refers to the difference between actual and targeted performance levels due to the composition of products or services offered. Consider the example shown in EXHIBIT 14-2. In this case, a hospital had established a company to sell durable medical equipment to nursing homes and long-term care facilities. The actual sales generated were $750,000. The exhibit also shows what the planned discounts and cost of goods sold were, based on the projected composition of products that were to be purchased. EXHIBIT 14-3 shows the sales and actual cost of goods that were sold. As can be seen, a higher cost of goods sold resulted because a different composition of products was ultimately purchased by the customers. The results, then, can be assessed to determine the impact of the product mix on the gross marketing contribution, as seen in Exhibit 14-3.

This type of analysis could also be conducted to assess whether there is a **price variance**, which is the difference between the actual price received and the targeted level because of discounting. Consider the original data shown in Exhibit 14-2 (price variance #1). In this case, the hospital planned to offer a planned discount level of 5%, or $37,500. In actuality, a new supplier of durable medical equipment entered the market, and, to retain customers and stay competitive, the hospital's actual discounts and allowances totaled $50,000. Results of this discounting are shown in EXHIBIT 14-4.

Exhibit 14-2 Performance Targets for Durable Medical Equipment

Sales	$750,000	100%	Actual Sales Percent
Discounts	37,500	5%	Planned Discount Percent
Net Sales	$712,500		
Cost of Goods Sold	360,000	48%	Planned Cost of Goods Sold
Gross Marketing Contribution	$352,500	47%	Planned Gross Marketing Contribution Percent
Direct Marketing Cost	51,300	6.84%	Direct Marketing Cost Percent
Net Marketing Contribution	$301,200		

Exhibit 14-3 Product Mix Variance

Sales	$750,000	100%	Actual Sales Percent
Discounts	37,500	5%	Planned Discount Percent
Net Sales	$712,500	95%	Net Sales Percent
COGS	384,000	51.20%	Actual COGS
Gross Marketing Contribution	$328,500	43.80%	Actual Product Mix Gross Marketing Contribution Percent
Direct Marketing Costs	51,300	6.84%	Direct Marketing Cost Percent
Net Marketing Contribution	$277,200	36.96%	Actual Net Marketing Contribution Percent

Actual Sales	$750,000
Planned Discount @ 5%	37,500
Expected Sales	$712,500
Planned COGS if Original Product Mix Sold @ 48%	360,000
Gross Marketing Contribution with Original Product Mix	$352,500
Gross Marketing Contribution with Actual Product Mix	$328,500
Decrease in Gross Marketing Contribution Due to Product Mix	($24,000)

Exhibit 14-4 Price Variance

	Price Variance	
	Actual	Planned
Sales	$750,000	$750,000
Discounts	50,000	37,500
Net Sales	$700,000	$712,500
Actual Cost of Goods Sold	384,000	384,000
Gross Marketing Contribution	$316,000	$328,500
Direct Marketing Costs	51,300	51,300
Net Marketing Contribution	$264,700	$277,200

Price Variance:

Actual Sales = $700,000
Planned Sales = 712,500
Price Variance = ($12,500)

Return on Investment

Return on Investment (ROI) is an additional approach to monitoring the performance of marketing expenditures. This approach is particular useful as a way to choose between marketing projects. And, it has been suggested as a useful tool for explaining resource allocation decisions. Many organizations will use a threshold level of an ROI before allocating dollars to a particular project.[6]

The formula for the calculation of an ROI is relatively simple:

$$[(\text{Returns} - \text{Expense})/\text{Expense}]/100$$

■ Sales Force Control

Control and measurement of the sales force can take several forms. Sales force control is relatively more straightforward than other aspects of marketing, since the compensation system often is tied directly to the performance expected. This is particularly true when the organization uses a commission system or a salary with bonus incentives. Even with these compensation systems, however, sales performance can be monitored by considering the allocation of effort, the result of the effort, and the investment required to generate the output.

In monitoring sales staff performance, companies can use several objective measures based on input to the job, which includes aspects such as the number of customer calls, the number of calls on new accounts versus existing accounts, the number of presentations made, and where necessary, the individual's service record. This last component is important for sales positions that are primarily missionary in nature. Monitoring sales behavior often requires a formal solicitation of evaluation from the respective customer.

In evaluating salesperson performance, a common control mechanism is the **sales/expense ratio**. To a large degree this ratio indicates the efficiency of the salesperson in generating output. The sales/expense ratio considers the amount of input required (in the form of sales expenses) relative to the output achieved (sales). Sales expenses might include but not be limited to travel costs, entertainment expenses, trial samples of products to give away, or promotional costs.

Several subjective measures can be used to measure salesperson performance. These include items such as job knowledge, territory management, and personal characteristics. Job knowledge pertains to how well the person knows the service lines represented, the health care organization's policies and procedures, and possibly the details and complexities of contract requirements. Management of the territory includes aspects such as report accuracy and scope, customer complaint handling, and planning of calls and accounts. Personal characteristics relate to the individual's motivation, initiative, appearance, or personality. This last dimension, while often included on evaluation reports of salespeople, is difficult to assess. While several studies have ex-

Table 14-6	A Multidimensional Approach to Salesperson Evaluation		
	Salesperson		
	A	B	C
Number of Accounts	87	69	79
Sales Potential	$1,568,000	$2,098,000	$989,000
Number of Sales Calls	198	202	272
Average Gross Margin	37.80%	41.20%	40.02%
Sales	$839,000	$1,230,083	$424,084
Sales Expense	$41,092	$36,798	$27,908
Cost per Call	$207.54	$182.17	$102.60
Percent of Potential	53.50%	58.63%	42.88%

amined the effect of personal characteristics on salesperson performance, results were disappointing.[7] A reasonably comprehensive approach to evaluating salespeople is shown in the framework in Table 14-6. In this table, salespeople are evaluated in terms of sales potential, margin contribution, and expense. This analysis provides an overview that extends beyond just the gross sales achieved by the individual. By examining the sales relative to quota, one can examine sales potential. For health care organizations that do not have established quotas for their salespeople, it is possible to develop an index of territory sales potential. To estimate sales potential for a territory, one needs to aggregate accounts based on sales potential. This information requires a list of potential accounts in the territory and an estimate of potential sales for the product mix at each account. The sales staff can provide this information by obtaining estimates of the amount or volume of a particular item or service used by an account.[8]

■ Advertising Control

Compared to many aspects of the marketing mix, monitoring and review of advertising is easy. As noted in Chapter 12, however, it is essential to specify advertising objectives prior to the beginning of any promotional campaign. Specifying these objectives then provides a benchmark against which to measure performance.

For most health care organizations, promotion and advertising are ongoing activities. They can establish a system that allows the comparison and review of a series of advertising campaigns with the use of media/service effectiveness ratios, as shown in Table 14-7. The table shows data for a hospital's advertising campaign for two new suburban primary care sites that were established in two neighborhoods. A different ad campaign ran for three months in each service area. Initially, the campaign's objectives were to gain awareness for the site. Measure A is the total number of families in the

Table 14-7	Monitoring Advertising Campaigns		
		Media/Service Effectiveness Ratio	
Measure		Neighborhood A	Neighborhood B
A	Total Families in Target Population	100%	100%
B	Aware of Service	88%	76%
C	Tried Service	11%	15%
D	Use Service Regularly	4%	2.5%
E	Media Effectiveness Ratio (B/A)	88%	76%
F	Creative Effectiveness Ratio (C/B)	12.5%	19.7%
G	Service Effectiveness Ratio (D/C)	36.4%	16.7%

target population. For both sites, this included all consumers over the age of 21 who lived within five miles of each new urgent care site. The hospital ran advertisements in local community shopping circulars and placed two advertisements on billboards on the major streets in each neighborhood. After four weeks, a telephone survey revealed an awareness level of 88% in neighborhood A, and 76% in neighborhood B. After eight weeks, a second random telephone survey revealed that 11% of consumers in neighborhood A had tried the new facility; 15% in neighborhood B had tried the other. At the end of the campaign, 4% of the consumers in neighborhood A said they were regular users, and 2.5% were regular users in neighborhood B.

Measures E through G are ratios that can be used to compare this campaign with other hospital campaigns. Ratio E is termed the *media effectiveness ratio*. This measure is the awareness over the total target population. This ratio suggests how well the organization did in identifying which media to use to reach the target population. As seen in neighborhood A, the media selection was more effective than in neighborhood B. Yet the creative effectiveness ratio indicates that the copy strategy employed in the advertisements in neighborhood B were more effective in moving people from the awareness level to the point of trial than in neighborhood A. The final ratio pertains more to the service itself than to the advertising. Advertising and promotion can move people through the hierarchy of effects (discussed in Chapter 12), but advertising and promotion cannot create regular customers. This objective can only be accomplished if the service meets customer expectations. The service effectiveness ratio indicates that the primary care site in neighborhood A is developing more loyal customers than that in neighborhood B. Now the objective of the marketing effort in the two neighborhoods will differ. In neighborhood A, a revision of the copy strategy is warranted based on the lower creative effectiveness ratio compared to neighborhood B (and, if this process is ongoing, based on other historical campaigns). In neighborhood B, the service itself must be analyzed relative to the customer satisfaction measures that are being obtained from the users at that clinic site.

The West Virginia University Health Science Center in Morgantown, West Virginia, used a monitoring approach to track physician referrals. The hospital held tailgate parties in the fall in conjunction with university football games. Potential referral physicians were invited to attend along with alumni, donors, and faculty. In the six months after the last party, 11 physicians referred to the Health Science Center for the first time. These physicians sent $595,000 worth of insured patient business to the Center.[9]

■ Customer Satisfaction Control

A large number of health care organizations today conduct ongoing customer satisfaction surveys. This should be an essential ingredient of any successful marketing strategy, considering that the cost of a dissatisfied patient can be significant. The Technical Assistance Research Programs, Inc. of Arlington, Virginia, a research and consulting firm specializing in customer satisfaction, has estimated that the cost of dissatisfaction for a hospital with 5000 annual discharges can be over $750,000.[10] Yet one recent study reported that only 20% of health care organizations conducting patient satisfaction surveys used them to provide feedback to clinical and administrative departments.[11]

Chapter 4 on buyer behavior presented a framework that showed how management should focus attention in the post-purchase evaluation stage of consumer decision making. As organizations monitor customer satisfaction, they can analyze these data by loyal or heavy half usage segments and determine how to change strategies.

The tendency in health care organizations, when dealing with medical staffs, is to respond to the physician who is the loudest complainer. Looking at physician satisfaction reports broken down by admission level (or, in managed care organizations [MCOs], by utilization) might result in a different response to the customer dissatisfaction. Consider Table 14-8, which shows this provider satisfaction by utilization. One can

Table 14-8	Controlling Customer Satisfaction		
	Average Satisfaction Levels		
Utilization level	Scheduling Ease	Laboratory Service	Ease of Use
light user	3.4	4.5	1.9
medium user	2.5	3.6	2.8
heavy user	5.2	2.8	1.7
Scale: '1' very satisfied to '7' very dissatisfied			

see that scheduling is a major problem for the heavy utilizer. It might be incorrect for a managed care plan to respond directly to this dissatisfaction. The more appropriate strategy might be to review the utilization pattern of this group of physicians and determine whether there is a way for these providers to be more efficient. This approach might reduce physician dissatisfaction with scheduling as well as save the managed care plan capitated revenue.

■ The Marketing Audit

Organizations should review periodically all aspects of their marketing operations. This process, called a **marketing audit,** is a systematic, critical review and appraisal of the total marketing operation. The audit reviews basic policies and assumptions, as well as procedures, personnel, and organization employed to implement marketing activities.[12] Because of the dynamic nature of the health care environment, health care organizations must periodically audit their total marketing activity and organization to ensure that it is responsive to market needs and preferences. A marketing audit has five major purposes:

1. It appraises the total marketing operation.
2. It centers on the evaluation of objectives and policies and the assumptions that underlie them.
3. It aims for prognosis as well as diagnosis.
4. It searches for opportunities and means for exploiting them, as well as for weaknesses and means for elimination.
5. It practices preventive as well as curative marketing practices.[13]

The marketing audit process has been described as a series of circles expanding outward from the consumer, as shown in FIGURE 14-3.[14] Beginning with the consumer market, a company examines how it is structured, how it can be divided, and how it is changing. To this information, a company can also add a review of its actions, policies, and plans. Internal constraints, organizational structure, and marketing programs can be reviewed. Within this context, the organization must conduct a detailed analysis of strengths and weaknesses. Finally, the audit must consider competitors and their respective programs, strengths, weaknesses, and trends.

As seen in this figure, the marketing mix variables—the controllable elements—cut across each aspect of this review. At each stage of the audit, the four marketing mix

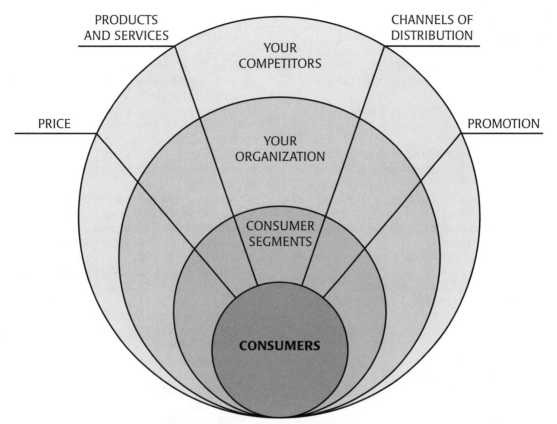

FIGURE 14-3 The Scope of the Marketing Audit

Source: From Berkowitz, E. N. and Flexner, W., "The Marketing Audit: A Tool for Health Service Organizations," from *Health Care Management Review*, Vol. 3, No. 4, p. 54, 1978. Used with permission of Lippincott Williams & Wilkins.

elements must be specifically considered: How are distribution channels changing for the market? Are new entities emerging that are gaining market share? How can functional shifting change the flow of patient volume?

The scope of issues reviewed in conducting the audit are far reaching. EXHIBIT 14-5 portrays a list of guiding questions that can be considered in a comprehensive audit of a health care organization.

Exhibit 14-5   Guiding Questions for the Market Audit

THE MARKET AND MARKET SEGMENTS

- How large is the territory covered by your market?
  How have you determined this?
- How is your market grouped?
  - Is it scattered?
  - How many important segments are there?
  - How are these segments determined (demographics, service usage, attitudinally)?
- Is the market entirely urban, or is a fair proportion of it rural?
- What percentage of your market uses third party payment?
  - What are the attitudes and operations of third parties?
  - Are they all equally profitable?
- What are the effects of the following factors on your market?
  - Age
  - Income
  - Occupation
  - Increasing population
  - Decreasing birthrate

  } demographic shifting
- What proportion of potential customers are familiar with your organization, services, programs?
  - What is your image in the marketplace?
  - What are the important components of your image?

THE ORGANIZATION

- Short history of your organization:
  - When and how was it organized?
  - What has been the nature of its growth?
  - How fast and far have its markets expanded?
  - Where do your patients come from geographically?
  - What is the basic policy of the organization? Is it on "health care," "profit"?
  - What has been the financial history of the organization?

- How has it been capitalized?
- Have there been any account receivable problems?
  - What is inventory investment?
  - What has been the organization's success with the various services promoted?
- How does your organization compare with the industry?
  - Is the total volume (gross revenue, utilization) increasing, decreasing?
  - Have there been any fluctuations in revenue,? If so, what were they due to?
- What are the objectives and goals of the organization? How can they be expressed beyond the provision of "good health care"?
- What are the organization's present strengths and weaknesses in:
  - Medical facilities
  - Management capabilities
  - Medical staff
  - Technical facilities
  - Reputation
  - Financial capabilities
  - Image
- What is the labor environment for your organization?
  - For medical staff (nurses, physicians, etc.)?
  - For support personnel?
- How dependent is your organization upon conditions of other industries (third party payers)?
- Are weaknesses being compensated for and strengths being used? How?
- How are the following areas of your marketing function organized?
  - Structure
  - Manpower
  - Reporting relationships
  - Decision-making power

Exhibit 14-5 Continued

- What kinds of external controls affect your organization?
  - Local?
  - State?
  - Federal?
  - Self-regulatory?
- What are the trends in recent regulatory rulings?

COMPETITORS

- How many competitors are in your industry?
  - How do you define your competitors?
  - Has this number increased or decreased in the last four years?
- Is competition on a price or nonprice basis?
- What are the choices afforded patients?
  - In services?
  - In payment?
- What is your position in the market—size and strength—relative to competitors?

PRODUCTS AND SERVICES

- Complete a list of your organization's products and services, both present and proposed.
- What are the general outstanding characteristics of each product or service?
- What superiority or distinctiveness of products or services do you have, as compared with competing organizations?
- What is the total cost per service (in-use)? Is service over/underutilized?
- What services are most heavily used? Why?
  - What is the profile of patients/ physicians who use the services?
  - Are there distinct groups of users?
- What are your organization's policies regarding:
  - Number and types of services to offer?
  - Assessing needs for service addition/deletion?

- History of products and services (complete for major products and services):
  - How many did the organization originally have?
  - How many have been added or dropped?
  - What important changes have taken place in services during the last ten years?
  - Has demand for the services increased or decreased?
  - What are the most common complaints against the service?
  - What services could be added to your organization that would make it more attractive to patients, medical staff, nonmedical personnel?
  - What are the strongest points of your services to patients, medical staff, nonmedical personnel?
  - Have you any other features that individualize your service or give you an advantage over competitors?

PRICE

- What is the pricing strategy of the organization?
  - Cost-plus
  - Return on investment
  - Stabilization
- How are prices for services determined?
  - How often are prices reviewed?
  - What factors contribute to price increase/decrease?
- What have been the price trends for the past five years?
- How are your pricing policies viewed by:
  - Patients
  - Physicians
  - Third party payers
  - Competitors
  - Regulators

continues

Exhibit 14-5 Continued

PROMOTION
- What is the purpose of the organization's present promotional activities (including advertising)?
  - Protective
  - Educational
  - Search out new markets
  - Develop all markets
  - Establish a new service
- Has this purpose undergone any change in recent years?
- To whom has advertising appeal been largely directed?
  - Donors
  - Patients
    - Former or current
    - Prospective
  - Physicians
    - On staff
    - Potential
- What media have been used?
- Are the media still effective in reaching the intended audience?
- What copy appeals have been notable in terms of response?
- What methods have been used for measuring advertising effectiveness?
- What is the role of public relations?
  - Is it a separate function/department?
  - What is the scope of responsibilities?

CHANNELS OF DISTRIBUTIION
- What are the trends in distribution in the industry?
  - What services are being performed on an outpatient basis?
  - What services are being provided on an at-home basis?
  - Are satellite facilities being used?
- What factors are considered in location decisions? When did you last evaluate present location?
- What distributors do you deal with? (e.g., medical supply houses, etc.)
- How large an inventory must you carry?

Source: Berkowitz, E. N. and Flexner, W., "The Marketing Audit: A Tool for Health Service Organizations," from *Health Care Management Review*, Vol. 3, No. 4, pp. 55–56. Used with permission of Lippincott Williams & Wilkins.

■ Conclusions

Health care organizations are facing a more competitive marketplace. Marketing strategies must be revised and changed continually to respond to the marketplace demands. To develop an effective marketing strategy, close monitoring and review of all marketing mix elements are necessary. Several control procedures and reports can be used to identify strategies or tactics that need to be refined. Periodically, the organization must conduct a systemwide review of all marketplace and organizational marketing efforts to ensure that strategy is directed appropriately to respond to the changing dynamics of the health care environment.

■ Key Terms

Overall Market Share
Served Market Share
Relative Market Share
Sales Analysis
Profitability Analysis
Direct Costing
Full Costing
Indirect Costs
Contribution Analysis
Percentage Variable Contribution Margin (PVCM)

Variance Analysis
Volume Variance
Contribution Variance
Product Mix Variance
Price Variance
Return on Investment
Sales/Expense Ratio
Marketing Audit

■ Chapter Summary

1. Market share provides a relative rather than absolute measure of performance. Market share can be either overall market share, served market share, or relative market share.
2. Sales analysis monitors sales performance relative to targets. It can be conducted on multiple bases for comparison.
3. Profitability analysis examines profitability by customers, regions, or products. The underlying premise is to monitor for a heavy half phenomenon.
4. A key issue in profitability analysis is the assignment of cost. It can be either a direct-cost or full-cost approach.
5. Contribution analysis considers performance of a service based on its contribution to profit or overhead.
6. Variance analysis compares actual results to targets. In conducting variance analysis it is possible to identify the source of the variance.
7. Variance can be due to volume, contribution, product mix, or price.
8. Return-on-Investment is a useful way to choose between projects. Many organizations set a threshold ROI.
9. Multiple measures of input and output are used in the monitoring of salespeople. A common efficiency indicator is the sales/expense ratio.
10. To monitor ongoing advertising efforts, an organization can establish media effectiveness, creative effectiveness, and service effectiveness ratios.
11. Customer satisfaction control is at the foundation of any effective marketing program. Dissatisfied customers have been found to represent a real dollar cost to the organization.
12. Periodically, every health care entity should conduct a marketing audit, which is a systematic review of all policies, procedures, and structures used to implement marketing activities.

■ Chapter Problems

1. At a recent strategic planning retreat of a 40-person multispecialty group, the administrator made a presentation that focused on the coming year's plans to establish the organization's first two primary care satellites, which would be located in the two growing suburbs of the community. These new additions would require the hiring of four family practitioners and other support staff. When the administrator finished her presentation, one of the most senior physicians stood up and said, "This is a foolish expenditure. We're so busy now in this group, we can't even see another patient. Our revenue was up 14% according to the previous financial presentation we heard. There is no reason to change what we're doing." How might you respond to this physician?

2. The administrator of a small, acute-care hospital is faced with his first managed care contract. He meets with representatives from the prepaid plan to discuss the amount to be paid to the hospital. The administrator is concerned because the managed care business does not look profitable—the hospital will be reimbursed below its current reimbursement levels. In what ways might the administrator evaluate this new managed care business in terms of its economic value to his institution?

3. A large national MCO recently entered a major southwestern metropolitan market. The managed care plan anticipated that, with an intensive advertising campaign and sales effort, it would have 75,000 subscribers after two years. They planned to charge a premium of $1800 per subscriber. Marketing and personnel costs directly related to this effort were anticipated to be $250 per subscriber. Prior to the MCO's entry into the market, two of the large tertiary facilities in the region began to offer their own managed care plans in a physician–hospital organization arrangement with their medical staffs. The result was aggressive discounting of the managed care premiums. The national MCO chain dropped its premium to $1400 per subscriber. Direct costs remained the same, yet because of the competition, the national MCO was able to enroll only 45,000 subscribers.
   a. What was the variance because of the failure to get the gross marketing contribution?
   b. What was the variance due to the lack of enrollment success?

4. The director of a large regional reference laboratory was reviewing the service's performance over the past year. The laboratory had gross revenues of $3,500,000. Some of the business was to managed care plans and to large-volume users that resulted in a discount of $350,000, which was $25,000 more than anticipated due to intense competition. The cost of providing the lab testing was $1,400,500, which was $250,000 higher than expected. Direct costs for salaries was $870,000. What was the product mix variance experienced by the laboratory service? What was the price variance?

5. A medical group recently conducted an advertising campaign for its new pediatric orthopedics department. After four weeks, a telephone survey found that 42% of the families with children under the age of 18 years were aware of the service. Six months later, it found that 12% had actually used the service, and 3% said they were regular users of the facility for their children's orthopedic needs. Compare this organization's advertising performance to that of the hospital discussed in Table 14-7. How does this organization compare in terms of its media, creative, and service effectiveness ratios? Where might the medical group need to make adjustments?

■ Notes

1. P. Kotler, *Marketing Management*, 8th ed. (Englewood Cliffs, NJ: Prentice Hall, 1994), 742–766.
2. "Inova Cardiology Program Achieves 10 Percent Response Rate, $803,613 ROI with CPM Program," *Business Wire Inc.* (September 1, 2004).
3. A procedure for allocating indirect costs has been proposed by Y. Goldschmidt and A. Gafai, "A Managerial Approach To Allocating Indirect Fixed Costs," *Health Care Management Review* 15, no. 2 (Spring 1990): 43–52.
4. R. Cooper and R. Kaplan, "How Cost Accounting Systematically Distorts Product Costs," in *Accounting and Management: Field Study Perspectives*, eds. W. J. Burns, Jr. and R. S. Kaplan (Cambridge, MA: Harvard University Press, 1987), 204–228.
5. D. Beckham, "Go Beyond Simple Revenues To Identify Best Specialties for Development," *Marketing To Doctors* (1990): 1–2.
6. Ann Klein and Tracy Swartzendruber, "A User's Guide to Marketing ROI," *Marketing Health Services* 23, no. 3 (Fall 2003): 33–36.
7. See for example, L. M. Lamont and W. J. Lundstrom, "Identifying Successful Industrial Salesmen by Personality and Personal Characteristics," *Journal of Marketing Research* 14, no. 4 (1977): 517–529.
8. C. D. Fogg and J. W. Rokus, "A Quantitative Method for Structuring a Profitable Sales Force," *Journal of Marketing* 37, no. 3 (1973): 8–17.
9. V. Hunt, "Tracking Physician Referrals through DocBase," *MPR Exchange* 19, no. 2 (1993): 2–3.
10. R. F. Ganey and M. P. Malone, "Satisfied Patients Can Spell Financial Well-Being," *Healthcare Financial Management* 45, no. 2 (1991): 34–42.
11. V. T. Dull, "Evaluating a Patient Satisfaction Survey for Maximum Benefit," *The Joint Commission Journal on Quality Improvement* 2, no. 8 (1994): 444–452.
12. A. Suchman, "The Marketing Audit: Its Nature, Purposes, and Problems," in *Analyzing and Improving Marketing Performance*, eds. A. Oxenfeldt and R.D. Crisp (New York: American Management Association, 1950) no. 32, 16–17.
13. Ibid.
14. E. N. Berkowitz and W. A. Flexner, "The Marketing Audit: A Tool for Health Service Organizations," *Health Care Management Review* 3, no. 4 (Fall 1978): 51–57.

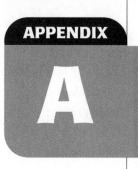

Glossary

Administered Vertical Marketing System: A system in which there is coordination between members of the *channel of distribution* but not common ownership.

Advertising: Any directly paid form of nonpersonal presentation of goods, services, and ideas.

Alternative Evaluation: Comparison by the consumer of the various choices that may best meet the individual's need.

Antimerger Act (1950): Regulation that strengthened the *Clayton Act* by broadening the federal government's power to prevent intercorporate acquisitions that would substantially reduce competition.

Approach: The stage in the sales process involving the initial meeting with the buyer.

Aspirational Reference Group: The reference group to which one aspires to belong.

Assumptive Close: Asking the buyer to choose payment terms, delivery location, or the like, before there has been an actual agreement to purchase.

Attitudes: A consumer's enduring cognitive evaluations, feelings, or action tendencies toward some person, object, or idea.

Autonomous Decisions: Decisions of lesser importance that individuals make independently.

BCG Matrix: A model based on *market growth rate* and *relative market share* for focusing company strategies in firms with multiple product lines.

Baby Boomers: The segment of the population born between 1946 and 1964.

Backward Integration: A strategy of incorporating new products and services that makes the firm its own supplier.

Barriers to Entry: Technological, regulatory, financial, strategic, or other conditions that a company must overcome in order to pursue a business opportunity.

Barriers to Exit: The costs of leaving a particular business or product line.

Benefit Segmentation: The grouping of people based on the benefits sought from the product.

Blended Family: The joining together of two households through remarriage.

Bonus: A payment that is made for reaching a certain level of performance.

Boutique Agency: An advertising agency that acts as a contractor to put together services needed by an organization, or one that offers a limited range of services.

Brand: Any name, term, colors, or symbol that distinguish one seller's product from another.

Brand Equity: The added value that a name *brand* gives to a product through associations made by the consumer.

Brand Loyalty: A situation in which the consumer regularly chooses the same product or service to fill a recognized need.

Breadth: The number of different product lines in a *product mix*.

Break-even Analysis: A mathematical determination of the level of sales required to cover *total cost* at a given price.

Bundled Pricing: A strategy that involves selling several items or services together for one total price.

Buying Center: The group of people involved in the decision to purchase a product or service.

Canned Presentation: A set script through which a salesperson leads a prospect.

Cannibalization: The situation when a company's own product steals share from other products within the company's line.

Census: A collection of data from an entire target population.

Channel: The means used to deliver a marketing message.

Channel Commander: The member of the *channel of distribution* who can dictate or control the activities of the other members.

Channel Intensity: The intensity with which a product is distributed that determines how available the product is to the ultimate consumer.

Channel of Distribution: The path a product takes as it goes from the manufacturer to the consumer.

Clayton Act (1914): Regulation forbidding certain actions likely to lessen competition, even if no actual damages occurred.

Close: The stage of the sales process that involves asking the buyer for a commitment to purchase.

Cluster Sampling: A sample in which the *sampling units* are selected in groups.

Co-branding: One organization markets its brand name alongside another organization's brand.

Cognitive Dissonance: A mental state of anxiety brought on because the consumer is unsure of the chosen alternative.

Cohort Segmentation: One of the newest ways to segment the market with the greatest strategic implication for health care organizations.

Cohort Segments: An approach to examining the market in which people are bound together by defining events that shape their attitudes and values. These events occur in their formative years (17-22) and these attitude/value shaping events affect their behaviors for the remainder of their lives.

Cohort: A group of consumers bound together in history by a set of events. These events shape their attitudes and values.

Cold Calls: Contacts with prospective buyers who did not initiate the process.

Combination Plan: A compensation plan for the sales force that consists of a base salary plus a *commission* or *bonus*.

Commission: Compensation to salespeople based on performance, in terms of volume, net revenue, or margin.

Competitor Orientation: Recognizing competitors' (and potential competitors') strengths, weaknesses, and strategies.

Complementary Products: Products or services for which the purchase of one will affect the purchase of another in that line.

Complex Decision Making: A decision-making situation requiring high involvement and extended search.

Concentration: An advertising schedule in which advertising dollars are spent and exposure achieved within a relatively short time period.

Concentration Strategy: (See *market concentration strategy*.)

Consolidation: A strategy of focusing a firm's business on a smaller set of markets, products, or services.

Consumer Decision-Making Process: A six-stage model of the decision-making process that includes *problem recognition*, *internal search*, *external search*, *alternative evaluation*, *purchase*, and *post-purchase evaluation*.

Consumer Goods: Products purchased by the ultimate consumer.

Consumer Price Index: A measure of monthly and yearly price changes for a broad range of consumer goods and services.

Contribution Analysis: An assessment of profitability of a product or service that considers the contribution of profit to fixed cost or overhead.

Contribution Variance: The difference between expected and real contribution margin.

Convenience Goods: Products that the consumer purchases frequently that require little deliberation or search prior to purchase.

Cooperatives: Agreements between members of the distribution channel who function on the same level.

Corporate Vertical Marketing System: A system that combines both the production and distribution of a product or service under one corporate ownership.

Corrective Advertising: Means of communications required by the Federal Trade Commission, by which a company must correct misimpressions formed in the marketplace.

Cost-per-Thousand (CPM): A common frame of comparing the cost of advertising media.

Culture: The values, customs, and conforming rules passed from one generation to the next.

Customer Contact Audit: A flow chart of the points of interaction between the customer and the service offering.

Customer Loyalty Pyramid: A progression of psychological commitment a consumer moves through that has seven stages from awareness to loyalty.

Customer Orientation: Having a sufficient understanding of the target buyers to be able to create superior value for them continuously.

Database Marketing: An automated system to identify people—both customers and prospects—by name, and to use quantifiable information about these individuals to define the best possible purchasers and prospects for a given offer at a given time.

Decoding: Translating the meaning of a message from words and symbols.

Demand-Minus Pricing: A pricing approach that involves determining what price the market is willing to pay and working backwards to compute costs.

Demand Schedule: A summary of the amounts of a product that are desired at each price level.

Demographics: Statistics to describe members of a population in terms of who they are, where they live, and the types of jobs they have.

Depth: The number of product items within each product line in a firm's product mix.

Derived Demand: The demand for one product or service that is derived from the demand for another product or service.

Differential Advantage: The incremental benefits of a product relative to competing products that are important to the buyer and perceived by the buyer.

Diffusion of Innovation: The rate at which a product is adopted by the market.

Direct Costing: An approach to costing in which only costs that are directly associated with the product or service are assigned to it.

Discretionary Income: The amount of money a consumer has left after paying for taxes and necessities.

Discrimination: The ability to determine differences between stimuli.

Disposable Income: The amount of money a consumer has left for food, clothing, and shelter after paying taxes.

Dissociative Reference Group: A reference group to which one does not wish to belong.

Diversification: A strategy of developing new products or services for new markets.

Divestment: The selling off of a business or product line.

Durable Good: A product that lasts over an extended period of time.

Encoding: Translating the meaning to be communicated into words or symbols.

Environment: The regulatory, social, technological, economic, and competitive factors to which the organization must be sensitive in developing strategy.

Evaluative Criteria: The criteria on which alternative products or services are judged, as determined by the consumer.

Exclusive Dealing: Condition under which a buyer is required to handle only the products of one manufacturer but not those of a competitor.

Experiment: A form of data collection where factors are manipulated to determine a causal relationship.

External (Information) Search: A consumer search for information from one or more sources after an internal search has failed.

Family Decision Making: Historical decision-making patterns within the traditional family life cycle.

Family Life Cycle: The stages the typical consumer passes through from childhood to the death of a spouse.

Federal Trade Commission Act of 1914: Legislation forbidding deceptive or misleading advertising and unfair business practices.

Feedback: Communication from the receiver to the sender.

Fixed Costs: Those costs that do not change based on the volume of product or service delivered.

Flexible Pricing Policy: A pricing approach in which a company charges different prices to different customers based on their ability to negotiate or on their respective buying power.

Flighting: Advertising heavily for short time periods.

Focus Groups: Interviews conducted with typically 8–10 people and a trained moderator following an interview guide for the purpose of examining and collecting data.

Forward Integration: A strategy of offering new products or services that are closer to the customer than existing products or services.

Forward Vertical Integration: The acquisition or development of operations that are closer to the final buyer in the *channel of distribution*.

Four Ps: Product, price, place, and promotion are the controllable variables that a firm uses to define its marketing strategy.

Franchising: A *vertical marketing system* in which a contract links elements of the manufacturing and distribution of a product or service.

Frequency: The number of times the same person receives a message within a defined time period.

Full Costing: An approach to costing in which both direct and indirect costs are assigned to the product or service unit and considered in the calculation of profitability.

Full Service Agency: An advertising agency that offers all the elements necessary to provide the total advertising function.

Functional Discounts: Discounts on price because the buyer agrees to perform or take over particular functions involved with the product or service.

Functional Shifting: The moving of different functions (credit, sorting, etc.) between the producer of a product or service and its intermediaries or the customer.

Gap Analysis: An approach to identify the gaps in effective service delivery.

GE Matrix: A multidimensional model for focusing company strategies in firms with multiple product lines based on dimensions of market attractiveness and business strength.

Generalizations: Extensions of past reinforced behavior to other stimuli.

Going-Rate Pricing: A pricing strategy that involves setting prices relative to the prevailing market price with less consideration for internal costs or margin requirements.

Gross Income: The total amount of money earned by a person or family in one year.

Gross Rating Points: A measure of advertising reach that is calculated by multiplying the number of spots or ads times the rating.

Growth Market Strategy: A strategy of gaining more sales from an existing business line or attempting to penetrate new markets.

HIPAA (Health Insurance Portability and Accountability Act of 1996): An act that requires national standards for the security and privacy of electronic health care transactions.

Harvesting: A consolidation strategy in which a firm gradually withdraws support for a product until there is little or no market demand.

Health Savings Account: A new insurance program in which consumers will be able to put pretax dollars into an account to pay for health care. It will allow them to directly pay for their health care and make economic trade-offs between consuming more services and the spending of their assets.

Heavy Half Consumer: A phenomenon observed within marketing in which a small group of consumers accounts for a disproportionate amount of a product's sales.

Hierarchy of Effects: The stages a buyer moves through from first seeing an advertisement ultimately to buying the product or using the service.

High Learning Product: A product that requires a significant introductory period because the immediate benefits might not be seen by the consumer.

Indirect Costs: Fixed costs that cannot be related to only one product line or service program.

Industrial Products: Products purchased for use in the production of other products.

Inflation: The decline in buying power when price levels rise faster than income.

Input Measures: Measures to assess the effort expended by salespersons to perform their jobs.

Integrated Delivery Systems: Health care systems in which care is coordinated and delivered at the level of intensity needed.

Interfunctional Coordination: Coordinating and deploying company resources in a manner that focuses on creating value for the customer.

Internal (Information) Search: Attempt by an individual to determine the solution to a recognized problem.

Invisible Value: The value that a producer or provider builds into a product or service.

Involvement: The level of the consumer's personal investment in the purchase decision.

Item Budget Theory: A theory suggesting that consumers set out with a predetermined price they are willing to pay for a particular item.

Joint Venture Business: A new corporate entity in which both partners have an equity position (often resulting from a strategic alliance).

Lanham Act: Legislation providing for the registration of a company's trademarks.

Leader Pricing: A strategy of attractively pricing an item in the product line and aggressively promoting it to encourage consumers to purchase it and other items in the line at the same time.

Leads: Likely buyers who are targeted for sales calls.

Learning: The changes in a person's behavior as a result of past experiences.

Lifestyle: The manner in which people live, as demonstrated by how they spend their time, what they think, and the interests they have.

Limited Decision Making: A decision-making situation involving extended search and low involvement.

Long-Term Focus: Adopting a perspective that includes a continuous search for ways to add value by making appropriate investments in the business.

Low Learning Product: A product for which the benefits are clearly seen by the consumer.

Majority Fallacy: The largest market segment is often not the most profitable due to its attractiveness to competitors.

Marginal Cost Pricing: A pricing approach based on the concept that the price per additional unit or service must equal or exceed the cost of the additional unit.

Markup Pricing: A pricing approach that involves calculating the per-unit cost of a product or service and determining the markup percentages needed to cover the cost of sales and profit.

Market Challenger: A firm that confronts the market leader.

Market Concentration Strategy: A marketing strategy in which only one segment of the market is targeted.

Market Development: A strategy of initiating sales of existing products and services in new markets.

Market Follower: A firm that competes in the market by following the market leader rather than by attacking it directly.

Market Growth Rate: The rate of sales growth in the market.

Market Leader: The firm that has the largest share and strives to dominate the competitors in the given market.

Market Modification: An attempt by a company to extend a product's life cycle by increasing use or creating new uses or users.

Market Niche: (See *niche strategy*.)

Market-Oriented Organization: An organization in which every distinct major market has its own marketing organization.

Market Penetration: A strategy to increase sales of existing products and services in present markets.

Market Segmentation: The process of grouping into clusters consumers who have similar wants or needs to which an organization can respond by tailoring one or more elements of the marketing mix.

Marketing: The process of planning and executing the conception, pricing, promotion, and distribution of ideas, goods, and services to create exchanges that satisfy individual and organizational objectives.

Marketing Audit: A systematic, critical review and appraisal of a firm's total marketing operation.

Marketing Information System: A structured, interacting complex of persons, machines, and procedures designed to generate an orderly flow of pertinent information collected from internal and external sources, for use as a basis for decision making.

Marketing Mix: The mix of controllable variables that the firm uses to pursue the desired level of sales. These variables are commonly classified as the *Four Ps*—product, price, place, and promotion.

Marketing Objectives: Quantitative measures of accomplishment by which the success of marketing strategies can be measured.

Marketing Orientation: The combination of *customer orientation*, *competitor orientation*, *interfunctional coordination*, *long-term focus*, and *profitability*.

Marketing Research: A process in which there is a systematic gathering of data from customers to identify their needs.

Mass Marketing: A strategy of treating the entire market as one target market and appealing to the broadest group.

Media Plan: The analysis and execution of an advertising campaign.

Medical Service Blueprints: The operational process mapping of a patient's or other external customer's interactions with a clinic or medical provider.

Medium: Form used for communication (television, radio, direct mail, magazines, newspapers).

Membership Reference Group: The reference group to which one belongs.

Message: The combination of symbols and words that the sender uses to transmit.

Modified Life Cycle: A modernized view of the family life cycle.

Monopolistic Competition: A situation where many companies have substitutable products.

Monopoly: A situation where there is only one company that sells a particular product.

Motivation: The goals or needs that propel a consumer to action.

Multibrand Strategy: A branding strategy in which the company places a different name on each product.

Multichotomous Questions: Questions that present the respondent with a fixed alternative.

Multiproduct Branding Strategy: A branding strategy in which the company places one brand name on all the products in its line.

Multisegment Marketing: A strategy of targeting multiple segments in the market in which a distinct marketing strategy might be developed for each group.

Multivariate Statistical Analysis: A quantitative analytical approach that considers the impact of multiple variables on a dependent variable.

Need: A condition in which there is a deficiency of something, or one requiring relief.

Niche: A very small specialized market segment with a highly defined set of needs.

Niche Strategy: A strategy of targeting a narrow segment or segments in the market with specialized products or services.

Noise: Anything that interferes with the effective communication of a message.

Nondurable Good: An item that can be consumed in some defined period of time.

Nonprobability Sample: A sample that was collected without the use of chance selection procedures.

Objective and Task: A promotional budgeting method that involves setting objectives along the hierarchy of effects and determining the tasks necessary to accomplish these objectives. The costs of the tasks determine the final budget needed.

Observational Research: Marketing research conducted by observing consumers either through a camera or by another individual.

Odd Pricing: A pricing approach in which items are priced just below whole dollar amounts.

Oligopoly: A situation where a few companies control a majority of the industry sales.

One-Price Policy: A pricing approach in which the company charges the same price to all customers who buy the product under the same set of conditions.

One-Stage Cluster Sample: A sampling method in which all the population elements in the selected subsets are included in the sample.

Opinion Leaders: People whose advice or experiences are often sought by others.

Organizational Mission: The organization's fundamental purpose for existing, as defined by its values and the customers it wishes to serve.

Organizational Objectives: The long-term performance targets that the company hopes to achieve.

Output Measures: Measures that assess the results of a salesperson's efforts.

Overall Market Share: A measure of a company's sales as a percent of total industry sales.

Penetration Price: A pricing strategy involving a low initial price relative to competing goods or services.

Perceived Risk: The concerns or anxieties a consumer anticipates regarding a product or service purchase.

Percentage Variable Contribution Margin (PVCM): A measure that shows the percentage of each additional sales dollar that is available to the organization to cover its fixed costs.

Perception: The psychological process by which individuals organize, select, and interpret information.

Personal Selling: Any paid personal presentation of goods, ideas, or services.

Place: The manner in which goods or services are distributed by a firm for use by consumers.

Population: The description of all people or elements of interest to researchers and from which a sample will be selected.

Post-Purchase Evaluation: A consumer's post-purchase assessment of a product that affects the possibility of repurchase or endorsement.

Presentation: The stage in the sales process involving the pitch for the product or service.

Prestige Pricing: A pricing strategy in which a high price is established relative to the competition or the true cost of production, in order to give the image of exclusivity or value.

Pretesting: Assessing advertising copy options before their general use.

Price: (1) The level of monetary reimbursement a firm demands for its goods or services, or (2) the economic value that the buyer provides to the producer in exchange for a product or service, or (3) the amount a customer is willing to pay for a product or service.

Price Elasticity: The change in demand for a product relative to a change in its price.

Price Lining: A pricing strategy in which products in a line are priced within a distinct price range that is significantly different from the prices of substitutes in the next range.

Price Variance: The difference between the actual price received and the targeted level due to discounting.

Primary Data: Information that is collected for a specific research question.

Primary Demand: Purchase interest in a class of product or service.

Problem Recognition: The first step in the consumer decision-making process in which the individual perceives a difference between the desired state and the actual state, and is motivated to close this gap.

Process Quality: A multidimensional construct that is one of four variables that comprise value to the customer.

Product: The goods, services, or ideas offered by a firm.

Product Development: A strategy of providing new products to existing markets.

Product Differentiation: A strategy of altering one or more elements of the marketing mix to respond differently to the various wants or needs of different groups in a multisegment strategy.

Product Life Cycle: The stages a product goes through as it exists in the market from its first introduction to its final withdrawal.

Product Lines: Groups of related products or services offered by a firm.

Product Mix: The entire range of products a firm offers.

Product Mix Variance: The difference between actual and targeted performance levels due to the composition of products or services offered.

Product Modification: Altering the product in some fashion by changing its quality, features, performance, or appearance.

Product-Oriented Organization: An organization in which each distinct product or related set of products has its own marketing organization.

Product Positioning: How a product is perceived in the minds of consumers relative to defined attributes and competing products.

Production Goods: Goods that are used to become part of the final product.

Profitability: Earning revenues sufficient to cover long-term expenses and to satisfy key constituencies.

Profitability Analysis: An approach to monitoring marketing performance that examines the profitability of sales by customers, regions, products, or salespeople.

Promotion: Any way of informing the market that the firm has developed a response to meet its needs.

Pruning: A consolidation strategy in which a firm reduces the number of products or services that it offers to the market.

Publicity: Any indirectly paid presentation of goods or services.

Pull: A strategy that involves bypassing or controlling the *channel of distribution* by appealing directly to the consumer and bypassing intermediaries.

Pulsing: An advertising schedule in which advertising expenditures occur at a constant level with occasional short, heavy expenditures.

Purchase: The act of selecting one brand over the others.

Pure Competition: A situation where every company has the same product.

Push: A strategy that involves controlling the *channel of distribution* by working through the channel.

Qualified Prospects: Individuals who have a need for the product or service or are likely to buy.

Quasi-Experimental Design: Research in which the data gathering is set up similar to a laboratory experiment, although lacking in control over all variables.

Reach: The unduplicated audience that an advertising vehicle will deliver.

Recovery System: An organized system that anticipates service delivery failures or problems and provides a defined script for service people to respond to the complaints that arise.

Reference Group: A group that influences an individual's thoughts or behaviors.

Regulation: The rules or restrictions placed on companies by federal or state governments.

Relationship Marketing: An organization's attempt to build long-term, cost-effective link with a customer.

Relative Market Share: The ratio of a product's share of business within the market compared to that of its largest competitor, or the combined share of the three largest competitors.

Requirement Contract: An agreement in which a buyer is required to purchase all or part of its needed products from one seller for a defined period of time.

Reseller Strategy: A branding strategy in which the company sells the product under the name of another company.

Retail Mix: The goods and services that an organization offers.

Retail Positioning Matrix: A model for retail positioning based on the breadth of the product line and the value added.

Retrenchment: A consolidation strategy in which a firm withdraws from certain markets.

Return on Investment: A useful way to assess alternative projects. The calculation is (Returns − Expense)/Expense/100.

Robinson-Patman Act (1935): Regulation against price discrimination between different buyers of the same product, where the effect may be to lessen competition and create a monopoly.

Routine Decision Making: A decision-making situation requiring repetitive purchasing.

SWOT Analysis: An examining of the strengths and weaknesses of the organization, and of the opportunities and threats relevant to the organization's future strategy.

Sales Analysis: An approach to monitoring marketing performance that examines the actual sales generated compared to the goals that were established.

Sales/Expense Ratio: A common control method for evaluating salesperson performance that indicates the efficiency of the salesperson in generating output.

Sales Promotion: Any short-term inducement or offer for a particular product or service.

Sample: A collection of data from only a portion of a target population.

Sampling Frame: The means of representing the sampling population.

Sampling Method: The way that sampling units are selected.

Sampling Unit: The elements of the population to be sampled.

Secondary Data: Information that was previously collected for a purpose other than that to which it is being applied.

Selective Comprehension: The way a consumer interprets information in a way that is consistent with past attitudes, beliefs, and knowledge.

Selective Demand: Interest in and preference for a company's products or services.

Selective Exposure: The way a consumer pays attention only to a particular set of advertisements.

Selective Retention: The way consumers retain only a fraction of the material to which they were exposed.

Served Market Share: A measure of the company's sales as a percentage of the total sales in the served market.

Services: Intangible activities or processes offered to customers to solve problems, for which the organization is often reimbursed.

Service Acquisition Cost: The effort the customer has to make to access the service value.

Sherman Antitrust Act (1890): Regulation forbidding contracts, combinations, or conspiracies in the restraint of trade.

Shopping Goods: Products in which the customer engages in some significant search to compare alternative brands on selected attributes.

Single Unit Sampling: A sample in which each sampling unit is selected individually.

Situational Assessment: An analysis of the organization's environment and of the organization itself.

Skimming Price: A pricing strategy involving a high initial price relative to competing products or substitutable services.

Social Class: Relatively stable and homogeneous divisions in society in which individuals, families, or groups share relatively similar interests, values, lifestyles, and behaviors.

Source Credibility: The target market's perception that the sender of a message can be believed.

Specialty Items: Products that the consumer specifically seeks out.

Spokesperson: The person who delivers the message in marketing communications.

Stakeholders: Any group with which the firm has, or wants to develop, a relationship.

Standard Industrial Classification (SIC) Code: A federal government classification system that groups organizations based on their major business activity or the major service or product they provide.

Stark II: Regulations published in 1993 by the Health Care Financing Administration that prohibited physician referrals to entities in which they held a financial interest; applies to both Medicare and Medicaid.

Stimulus-Response Sales Approach: An approach to selling that is founded in psychology.

Straight Salary: A compensation approach that provides a fixed salary.

Strategic Alliance: A formal arrangement with other companies to operate in a particular market.

Strategic Business Units: Businesses that operate as separate profit centers within a large organization.

Strategic Planning: A process that describes the direction an organization will pursue within its chosen environment and guides the allocation of resources and efforts.

Stress Interview: An interview in which the applicant is placed under stress to assess how he or she will act in similar situations.

Structured Interview: An interview that follows a set list of questions.

Substitutable Goods: Products that satisfy the same basic needs.

Support Goods: Items that are used to assist in the production of other products.

Survey Research: The collection of consumer data by telephone, personal interviews, focus groups, or mail.

Syncratic Decisions: Decisions in which the husband and wife participate jointly.

Syndicated Marketing Research: Commercial secondary data that regularly provide information on a particular question or problem area.

Target Audience: The group to whom an organization is trying to communicate.

Target Market: The group of customers whom the organization wishes to attract.

Target Pricing: A pricing approach that involves setting price to provide a targeted rate of return on investment for a standard level of production or service delivery.

Technology: Innovations or inventions from applied science and research.

Telemedicine: The delivery of health care through interactive audio, video, or data communications.

Total Cost: The total expense that the firm bears in delivering and marketing its product or service.

Trade Name: The commercial name under which a company does business.

Trademark: A *brand* or *trade name* given legal protection.

Trademark Law Revision Act (1988): Legislation granting a company *trademark* protection prior to actual use.

Trial Close: Asking the buyer for an opinion regarding a sales proposal.

Two-Stage Cluster Sample: A sampling method in which sample elements are collected from subsets of the population.

Tying Arrangement: Requirement by the seller of a product that the purchaser also buys another item.

Unstructured Interview: An interview in which the applicant is encouraged to talk freely on a range of subjects.

Utilities: Functions performed by intermediaries in the *channel of distribution*.

Variable Costs: Those costs that vary with the amount of the product or service delivered.

Variance Analysis: A method of evaluating marketing performance that compares actual results to preestablished targets of performance.

Vehicle: The advertising alternative chosen within each medium.

Vertical Integration: A strategy of incorporating products or services that are related to the firm's existing activities and that have usually been developed and offered by others to the marketplace.

Vertical Marketing Systems: Channels in which the intermediaries are integrated so that functions are performed at the most efficient place within the channel.

Visible Value: The value that can be seen by a consumer in a product or a service.

Volume Discounts: Discounts provided to buyers who purchase the product or service at some predetermined level.

Volume Variance: The difference between expected and real unit sales.

Want: A wish or desire for something.

Wheel of Retailing: A description of the process of how new retail forms enter the market and how they evolve over time.

Workload Method: A method for determining the appropriate size of the sales force based on work effort required to service the market.

Index